PHARMACOTHERAPEUTICS EXAM PREP:

CASE-BASED QUESTIONS

I0465542

By

Jim Carter, PhD

Table of Contents

SECTION I:QUESTIONS

SECTION II:ANSWERS

ACNE

1. Patient J is a 16-year-old male presenting with multiple comedones (blackheads and whiteheads) on his forehead and cheeks. He denies any pain or itching. What is the most likely diagnosis?

    a. Rosacea

    b. Acne vulgaris

    c. Folliculitis

    d. Seborrheic dermatitis

2. A 22-year-old female presents with large, painful nodules and cysts on her face and back. She reports these lesions have been increasing over the past few months despite over-the-counter treatments. What is the initial management strategy?

    a. Topical retinoid

    b. Oral antibiotics

    c. Isotretinoin (Accutane)

    d. Intralesional corticosteroids

3. A 30-year-old woman presents with acne predominantly on her lower face and jawline. She reports worsening of acne before menstruation and is otherwise healthy. What is the most appropriate initial treatment?

    a. Topical benzoyl peroxide

    b. Oral contraceptives

    c. Oral antibiotics

    d. Topical retinoid

4. A 25-year-old woman presents with multiple excoriated papules and pustules on her face. She admits to frequent picking and squeezing of acne lesions. What is the best approach to management?

    a. Topical antibiotics

    b. Oral isotretinoin

    c. Cognitive behavioral therapy

    d. Intralesional corticosteroids

5. A 35-year-old African American man presents with firm, keloid-like papules and plaques on the occipital scalp. He has a history of chronic shaving and reports itching and discomfort in the affected area. What is the likely diagnosis?

    a. Tinea capitis

    b. Acne rosacea

    c. Acne keloidalis nuchae

    d. Discoid lupus erythematosus

6. A 10-year-old boy presents with inflammatory papules and pustules on his cheeks and nose. He denies using any topical products or medications. What is the most appropriate management?

    a. Oral antibiotics

    b. Topical retinoid

    c. Topical benzoyl peroxide

    d. Observation without treatment

7. A 45-year-old woman presents with a sudden onset of acneiform eruptions on her face, chest, and back. She has recently started taking a new medication for hypertension. What is the most likely cause of her skin condition?

   a. Acne vulgaris

   b. Rosacea

   c. Drug-induced acneiform eruption

   d. Allergic contact dermatitis

8. A 55-year-old woman presents with persistent erythema, telangiectasias, and papulopustules on her central face. She denies a history of comedones or cysts. What is the most likely diagnosis?

   a. Acne vulgaris

   b. Acne rosacea

   c. Seborrheic dermatitis

   d. Perioral dermatitis

9. A 20-year-old Asian American woman presents with post-inflammatory hyperpigmentation following resolved acne lesions on her cheeks. What is the most appropriate treatment to address her concern?

   a. Topical retinoid

   b. Chemical peel

   c. Oral antibiotics

   d. Laser therapy

10. A 30-year-old man presents with severe nodulocystic acne associated with sinus tracts and hypertrophic scars on his back and shoulders. What is the most appropriate treatment?

    a. Topical retinoid

    b. Oral antibiotics

    c. Isotretinoin (Accutane)

    d. Intralesional corticosteroids

11. A 28-year-old pregnant woman presents with concerns about managing her acne. She has a history of moderate acne prior to pregnancy and is currently in her second trimester. What is the safest treatment option for her?

    a. Topical benzoyl peroxide

    b. Topical retinoid

    c. Oral antibiotics

    d. Azelaic acid

12. A 40-year-old man presents with atrophic scars and ice-pick scars on his cheeks and temples, which developed following severe acne during adolescence. What is the most appropriate treatment option?

    a. Topical retinoid

    b. Chemical peel

    c. Dermal fillers

    d. Oral antibiotics

13. A 25-year-old male athlete presents with acne primarily on his chest, back, and shoulders. He spends several hours daily in tight-fitting athletic gear. What is the most appropriate management strategy?

    a. Topical retinoid

    b. Oral antibiotics

    c. Topical benzoyl peroxide wash

    d. Isotretinoin (Accutane)

14. A 30-year-old woman presents with persistent acne despite multiple treatments including topical retinoids, oral antibiotics, and hormonal therapy. What is the next best step in management?

    a. Isotretinoin (Accutane)

    b. Dapsone gel

    c. Intralesional corticosteroids

    d. Photodynamic therapy

15. A 35-year-old man presents with painful, deep-seated nodules and abscesses in his axillae and groin, which discharge purulent material. He has no lesions on his face. What is the most likely diagnosis?

    a. Hidradenitis suppurativa

    b. Acne conglobata

    c. Folliculitis decalvans

    d. Pseudofolliculitis barbae

Allergic Rhinitis

1. Sarah, a 28-year-old female, presents with complaints of sneezing, watery eyes, and nasal congestion during the spring and fall seasons. Symptoms are worse outdoors and improve when she stays indoors. What is the most likely diagnosis?

    a. Viral rhinitis

    b. Allergic rhinitis

    c. Sinusitis

    d. Nasal polyps

2. A 10-year-old boy presents with symptoms of sneezing, itching of the eyes, and clear rhinorrhea. His symptoms worsen when he plays outside in the grassy fields and improve when he stays indoors. What is the first-line treatment for his condition?

    a. Oral antihistamines

    b. Intranasal corticosteroids

    c. Decongestants

    d. Mast cell stabilizers

3. Mark, a 35-year-old man, complains of nasal congestion, postnasal drip, and headache. His symptoms have persisted for several weeks, and he reports a history of similar episodes every spring. Which additional symptom would help differentiate allergic rhinitis from sinusitis in this case?

    a. Fever

    b. Halitosis

    c. Facial pain or pressure

    d. Decreased sense of smell

4. A 50-year-old woman with a history of seasonal allergies presents with complaints of chronic nasal congestion and occasional epistaxis. Physical examination reveals pale, boggy nasal mucosa. What is the likely diagnosis?

    a. Allergic rhinitis

    b. Chronic sinusitis

    c. Nasal polyps

    d. Deviated nasal septum

5. A 25-year-old man presents with complaints of sneezing, nasal congestion, and itchy, watery eyes. His symptoms have worsened since moving into a newly carpeted apartment. Which allergen is most likely responsible for his symptoms?

    a. Pollen

    b. Dust mites

    c. Pet dander

    d. Mold spores

6. A 30-year-old pregnant woman presents with complaints of nasal congestion, postnasal drip, and sneezing. She prefers non-pharmacological treatments. What is the most appropriate initial recommendation?

    a. Intranasal corticosteroids

    b. Oral antihistamines

    c. Saline nasal irrigation

    d. Decongestant nasal spray

7. A 45-year-old man with a history of asthma presents with complaints of nasal congestion, facial pain, and purulent nasal discharge. He reports a fever of 101°F (38.3°C). What is the likely diagnosis?

    a. Allergic rhinitis

    b. Acute viral rhinitis

    c. Sinusitis

    d. Nasal polyps

8. A 12-year-old boy presents with sneezing, nasal congestion, and itchy eyes. He has a history of allergic rhinitis and his symptoms are not controlled on oral antihistamines alone. What is the most appropriate next step in management?

    a. Increase the dose of oral antihistamines

    b. Add intranasal corticosteroids

    c. Switch to a different class of antihistamines

    d. Initiate allergen immunotherapy

9. A 60-year-old woman presents with complaints of chronic nasal congestion and decreased sense of smell. Physical examination reveals bilateral nasal polyps. What underlying condition is commonly associated with nasal polyps?

    a. Allergic rhinitis

    b. Chronic sinusitis

    c. Nasal septal deviation

    d. Olfactory nerve damage

10. A 40-year-old man presents with recurrent sneezing, nasal congestion, and itchy, watery eyes. His symptoms occur year-round and worsen in certain environments. What type of allergic rhinitis is he likely experiencing?

    a. Seasonal allergic rhinitis

    b. Perennial allergic rhinitis

    c. Occupational allergic rhinitis

    d. Mixed allergic rhinitis

11. A 55-year-old woman presents with complaints of sneezing, nasal congestion, and itchy eyes. She has a history of allergic rhinitis and asthma. Which class of medications should be avoided in her treatment regimen due to potential exacerbation of asthma?

    a. Oral antihistamines

    b. Intranasal corticosteroids

    c. Decongestants

    d. Leukotriene receptor antagonists

12. A 30-year-old man presents with complaints of recurrent sneezing, nasal congestion, and itchy, watery eyes. He works in a flower shop and his symptoms worsen during work hours. What type of allergic rhinitis is he likely experiencing?

    a. Seasonal allergic rhinitis

    b. Perennial allergic rhinitis

    c. Occupational allergic rhinitis

    d. Mixed allergic rhinitis

13. A 20-year-old woman presents with complaints of recurrent sneezing, nasal congestion, and itchy, watery eyes. Her symptoms occur during spring and fall seasons. What is the most appropriate initial step in managing her condition?

   a. Prescribe oral antihistamines

   b. Recommend allergen avoidance measures

   c. Initiate intranasal corticosteroids

   d. Perform allergy testing

14. A 40-year-old man presents with complaints of sneezing, nasal congestion, and itchy eyes. His symptoms occur only during the summer months. What type of allergic rhinitis is he likely experiencing?

   a. Seasonal allergic rhinitis

   b. Perennial allergic rhinitis

   c. Occupational allergic rhinitis

   d. Mixed allergic rhinitis

15. A 25-year-old woman presents with complaints of chronic nasal congestion and postnasal drip. She denies any seasonal variations in symptoms and reports persistent symptoms year-round. What type of allergic rhinitis is she likely experiencing?

   a. Seasonal allergic rhinitis

   b. Perennial allergic rhinitis

   c. Occupational allergic rhinitis

   d. Mixed allergic rhinitis

Alzheimer's Disease

1. A 72-year-old woman presents with progressive forgetfulness and difficulty managing finances. On examination, she shows mild cognitive impairment with impaired short-term memory. MRI shows medial temporal lobe atrophy. What is the most likely diagnosis?

    a. Vascular dementia

    b. Frontotemporal dementia

    c. Lewy body dementia

    d. Alzheimer's disease

2. A 65-year-old man with a history of hypertension and diabetes presents with recent memory loss and difficulty finding words. He becomes disoriented in familiar surroundings and has trouble managing his medications. What is the most likely initial management step?

    a. Start donepezil

    b. Perform a lumbar puncture

    c. Order an MRI of the brain

    d. Screen for depression

3. A 78-year-old woman presents with progressive decline in cognition over the past year. She is now unable to perform her usual activities independently. Neurological examination reveals apraxia and aphasia. Which subtype of Alzheimer's disease is most likely?

    a. Amnestic subtype

    b. Posterior cortical atrophy

    c. Logopenic variant

    d. Frontal variant

4. A 70-year-old man presents with fluctuating cognition, visual hallucinations, and sleep disturbances. His wife reports episodes of him acting out his dreams. What is the most likely diagnosis?

    a. Frontotemporal dementia

    b. Vascular dementia

    c. Parkinson's disease dementia

    d. Lewy body dementia

5. A 62-year-old woman presents with worsening memory loss and behavioral changes. She has difficulty with language and frequently repeats herself. MRI shows left posterior temporoparietal atrophy. What is the likely diagnosis?

    a. Semantic variant of primary progressive aphasia

    b. Alzheimer's disease

    c. Frontotemporal dementia

    d. Corticobasal degeneration

6. A 68-year-old man presents with progressive memory loss and difficulty with executive function. He has no significant medical history. On examination, he has a positive Romberg sign. What is the most likely diagnosis?

    a. Alzheimer's disease

    b. Normal pressure hydrocephalus

    c. Frontotemporal dementia

    d. Creutzfeldt-Jakob disease

7. An 80-year-old woman presents with recent memory loss and difficulty finding her way around familiar places. She becomes disoriented in new surroundings. Neurological examination reveals no focal deficits. What is the most appropriate initial step in management?

   a. Initiate treatment with memantine

   b. Order an MRI of the brain

   c. Perform genetic testing for familial Alzheimer's disease

   d. Screen for depression

8. A 75-year-old man presents with recent memory loss and confusion. His family reports episodes of him wandering and getting lost in familiar places. He is found to have elevated levels of tau protein in the cerebrospinal fluid. What is the most likely diagnosis?

   a. Alzheimer's disease

   b. Vascular dementia

   c. Creutzfeldt-Jakob disease

   d. Frontotemporal dementia

9. A 70-year-old woman presents with progressive memory loss and difficulty with language. She has preserved motor function and no other neurological deficits. MRI shows left perisylvian atrophy. What is the likely diagnosis?

   a. Alzheimer's disease

   b. Semantic variant of primary progressive aphasia

   c. Corticobasal degeneration

   d. Normal pressure hydrocephalus

10. A 60-year-old man presents with progressive memory loss and behavioral changes. His family notes he has become socially withdrawn and has developed repetitive behaviors. On examination, he shows early signs of parkinsonism. What is the likely diagnosis?

    a. Alzheimer's disease

    b. Frontotemporal dementia

    c. Vascular dementia

    d. Lewy body dementia

11. A 72-year-old woman presents with progressive memory loss and difficulty with complex tasks. She frequently misplaces items and struggles with basic arithmetic. Neurological examination is normal. What is the most likely diagnosis?

    a. Alzheimer's disease

    b. Frontotemporal dementia

    c. Normal pressure hydrocephalus

    d. Creutzfeldt-Jakob disease

12. A 68-year-old man presents with recent memory loss and difficulty with spatial orientation. He has trouble recognizing faces and has difficulty with calculations. MRI shows bilateral posterior parietal and occipital lobe atrophy. What is the most likely diagnosis?

    a. Alzheimer's disease

    b. Posterior cortical atrophy

    c. Frontotemporal dementia

    d. Vascular dementia

13. A 75-year-old man presents with progressive memory loss and difficulty with language. He has developed anxiety and depression. MRI shows asymmetric frontotemporal atrophy. What is the likely diagnosis?

    a. Alzheimer's disease

    b. Semantic variant of primary progressive aphasia

    c. Corticobasal degeneration

    d. Normal pressure hydrocephalus

14. A 70-year-old woman presents with progressive memory loss and difficulty with executive function. She frequently repeats herself and struggles with word-finding. Neurological examination shows no focal deficits. What is the most appropriate next step in management?

    a. Initiate treatment with donepezil

    b. Perform a lumbar puncture

    c. Order an MRI of the brain

    d. Screen for depression

15. A 72-year-old man presents with progressive memory loss and difficulty with language. He has developed behavioral changes and impulsivity. MRI shows left frontal lobe atrophy. What is the likely diagnosis?

    a. Alzheimer's disease

    b. Semantic variant of primary progressive aphasia

    c. Frontotemporal dementia

    d. Normal pressure hydrocephalus

Anemia

1. A 45-year-old woman presents with fatigue, pale skin, and shortness of breath on exertion. She reports heavy menstrual periods. Laboratory findings reveal a hemoglobin level of 9.5 g/dL. What is the most likely type of anemia?

   a. Iron deficiency anemia

   b. Vitamin B12 deficiency anemia

   c. Anemia of chronic disease

   d. Sickle cell anemia

2. A 30-year-old vegetarian presents with tingling sensations in the hands and feet, along with difficulty walking and a sore tongue. Laboratory tests reveal a low hemoglobin level and macrocytic red blood cells. What is the likely cause of this patient's anemia?

   a. Iron deficiency anemia

   b. Vitamin B12 deficiency anemia

   c. Thalassemia

   d. Sickle cell anemia

3. A 25-year-old African-American male presents with recurrent episodes of pain in the joints, especially in the fingers, toes, and hips. He has a history of similar episodes since childhood. Laboratory findings show low hemoglobin levels and sickle-shaped red blood cells on peripheral blood smear. What type of anemia does this patient most likely have?

   a. Iron deficiency anemia

   b. Vitamin B12 deficiency anemia

   c. Anemia of chronic disease

   d. Sickle cell anemia

4. A 60-year-old man presents with weakness, fatigue, and chest pain. He has a history of coronary artery disease and diabetes mellitus. Laboratory findings reveal a low hemoglobin level and normal MCV. What is the likely cause of anemia in this patient?

    a.   Iron deficiency anemia

    b.   Vitamin B12 deficiency anemia

    c.   Anemia of chronic disease

    d.   Hemolytic anemia

5. A 35-year-old pregnant woman presents with fatigue, pallor, and shortness of breath. Laboratory tests show a low hemoglobin level and low MCV. What is the most likely cause of anemia in pregnancy?

    a.   Iron deficiency anemia

    b.   Folate deficiency anemia

    c.   Hemolytic anemia

    d.   Sickle cell anemia

6. A 55-year-old man presents with fatigue, dizziness, and unintentional weight loss. He has a history of alcohol abuse. Laboratory tests show low hemoglobin levels and macrocytic red blood cells. What is the likely cause of his anemia?

    a.   Iron deficiency anemia

    b.   Vitamin B12 deficiency anemia

    c.   Anemia of chronic disease

    d.   Alcohol-induced anemia

7. A 20-year-old woman presents with a history of irregular menstrual periods and fatigue. Laboratory findings show a low hemoglobin level and normal MCV. What is the likely cause of her anemia?

    a. Iron deficiency anemia

    b. Thalassemia

    c. Anemia of chronic disease

    d. Sickle cell anemia

8. A 45-year-old man of Mediterranean descent presents with weakness, fatigue, and jaundice. Laboratory tests reveal low hemoglobin levels and microcytic, hypochromic red blood cells. What is the likely diagnosis?

    a. Iron deficiency anemia

    b. Vitamin B12 deficiency anemia

    c. Thalassemia

    d. Sickle cell anemia

9. A 65-year-old man presents with easy bruising, gum bleeding, and petechiae. He has a history of hypertension and has been taking aspirin regularly. Laboratory findings show low hemoglobin levels and normal MCV. What is the likely cause of his anemia?

    a. Iron deficiency anemia

    b. Vitamin B12 deficiency anemia

    c. Aplastic anemia

    d. Drug-induced thrombocytopenia

10. A 28-year-old woman presents with fatigue, palpitations, and dyspnea on exertion. She reports a recent history of recurrent infections. Laboratory tests show low hemoglobin levels and normal MCV. What is the likely cause of her anemia?

    a. Iron deficiency anemia

    b. Vitamin B12 deficiency anemia

    c. Autoimmune hemolytic anemia

    d. Chronic kidney disease

11. A 50-year-old man presents with severe abdominal pain and dark, tarry stools. He has a history of peptic ulcer disease and is taking NSAIDs regularly. Laboratory findings show low hemoglobin levels and normal MCV. What is the likely cause of his anemia?

    a. Iron deficiency anemia

    b. Vitamin B12 deficiency anemia

    c. Gastrointestinal bleeding

    d. Autoimmune hemolytic anemia

12. A 35-year-old man presents with a history of progressive fatigue, muscle weakness, and paresthesias in the hands and feet. He is a strict vegan and avoids all animal products. Laboratory tests show low hemoglobin levels and macrocytic red blood cells. What is the likely cause of his anemia?

    a. Iron deficiency anemia

    b. Vitamin B12 deficiency anemia

    c. Thalassemia

    d. Sickle cell anemia

13. A 25-year-old woman presents with jaundice, dark urine, and abdominal pain. She recently had a viral illness. Laboratory findings show low hemoglobin levels and elevated LDH. Peripheral blood smear reveals fragmented red blood cells. What is the likely cause of her anemia?

    a. Iron deficiency anemia

    b. Vitamin B12 deficiency anemia

    c. Thalassemia

    d. Hemolytic anemia

14. A 30-year-old pregnant woman presents with fatigue, pale skin, and shortness of breath. She has a history of a previous pregnancy with similar symptoms. Laboratory tests show low hemoglobin levels and low MCV. What is the likely cause of her anemia?

    a. Iron deficiency anemia

    b. Folate deficiency anemia

    c. Sickle cell anemia

    d. Thalassemia

15. A 40-year-old man presents with joint pain, fatigue, and dark urine. He has a family history of similar symptoms. Laboratory tests reveal low hemoglobin levels and elevated serum bilirubin. Peripheral blood smear shows spherocytes. What is the likely cause of his anemia?

    a. Iron deficiency anemia

    b. Vitamin B12 deficiency anemia

    c. Hereditary spherocytosis

    d. Autoimmune hemolytic anemia

Angina Pectoris

1. A 58-year-old male presents with chest pain that occurs upon exertion and is relieved by rest or nitroglycerin. He has a history of hypertension and hyperlipidemia. Which of the following is the most likely diagnosis?

    a. Myocardial infarction

    b. Stable angina

    c. Unstable angina

    d. Variant angina

2. Which of the following is a typical trigger for stable angina?

    a. Emotional stress

    b. Resting after a meal

    c. Exposure to cold weather

    d. Sudden loud noise

3. A patient presents with chest pain at rest that lasts for more than 20 minutes. ECG shows ST-segment depression. What is the most likely diagnosis?

    a. Stable angina

    b. Unstable angina

    c. Variant angina

    d. Silent ischemia

4. A 45-year-old smoker presents with severe chest pain at rest. ECG shows transient ST-segment elevation followed by normalization. Which of the following is the most likely diagnosis?

    a. Stable angina

    b. Unstable angina

    c. Variant angina

    d. Silent ischemia

5. Which of the following medications is commonly used for both the acute and chronic management of stable angina?

    a. Aspirin

    b. Nitroglycerin

    c. Clopidogrel

    d. Statins

6. A patient with stable angina is started on a beta-blocker. Which of the following is a potential adverse effect of beta-blockers in this patient?

    a. Hypotension

    b. Bradycardia

    c. Hypercholesterolemia

    d. Hyperkalemia

7. Which of the following is a typical finding in the history of a patient with stable angina?

    a. Chest pain that wakes the patient from sleep

    b. Chest pain relieved by exertion

    c. Chest pain that is sharp and stabbing

    d. Chest pain worsened by nitroglycerin

8. A 65-year-old patient with stable angina presents with increasing chest pain that now occurs at rest and is not relieved by nitroglycerin. What is the most appropriate next step in management?

    a. Immediate angiography

    b. Increase the dose of nitroglycerin

    c. Start aspirin therapy

    d. Initiate oxygen therapy

9. A patient with stable angina experiences chest pain while shoveling snow. Which of the following medications should be prescribed to this patient?

    a. Aspirin

    b. Ranolazine

    c. Nitroglycerin

    d. Clopidogrel

10. A 60-year-old male with stable angina has persistent symptoms despite maximum tolerated doses of beta-blockers and nitrates. Which of the following medications may be considered to improve his symptoms?

    a. Diltiazem

    b. Furosemide

    c. Allopurinol

    d. Warfarin

11. A 52-year-old woman with stable angina presents with chest pain that resolves spontaneously within a few minutes. ECG during pain shows ST-segment elevation. What is the most likely diagnosis?

    a. Stable angina

    b. Unstable angina

    c. Variant angina

    d. Silent ischemia

12. Which of the following factors is not a typical risk factor for the development of stable angina?

    a. Hypertension

    b. Diabetes mellitus

    c. Low HDL cholesterol

    d. Young age (20-30 years)

13. A 62-year-old man presents with chest pain at rest that started 2 days ago. His ECG shows ST-segment depression. Troponin levels are normal. What is the most likely diagnosis?

    a. Stable angina

    b. Unstable angina

    c. Variant angina

    d. Non-cardiac chest pain

14. A patient with stable angina has been compliant with nitroglycerin for relief of chest pain. However, recently he has noticed that the nitroglycerin spray is less effective in relieving his symptoms. What is the most appropriate next step?

    a. Increase the dose of nitroglycerin

    b. Add a calcium channel blocker

    c. Add ranolazine

    d. Evaluate for drug tolerance

15. Which of the following is a characteristic feature of stable angina as compared to unstable angina?

    a. Chest pain at rest

    b. ECG changes during pain

    c. Pain relieved by nitroglycerin

    d. Normal troponin levels

Anxiety Disorders

1. A 32-year-old female presents with excessive worry, restlessness, fatigue, difficulty concentrating, and muscle tension for the past 6 months. She reports difficulty falling asleep due to worrying about her job and relationships. Which of the following is the most likely diagnosis?

    a. Major Depressive Disorder

    b. Panic Disorder

    c. Generalized Anxiety Disorder (GAD)

    d. Social Anxiety Disorder

2. A 45-year-old male presents with recurrent episodes of sudden-onset palpitations, sweating, trembling, shortness of breath, and feelings of impending doom. He worries about having another attack and avoids situations where escape might be difficult. What is the most likely diagnosis?

    a. Generalized Anxiety Disorder (GAD)

    b. Panic Disorder

    c. Social Anxiety Disorder

    d. Specific Phobia

3. A 28-year-old female avoids public speaking and social gatherings due to intense fear of being embarrassed or humiliated. She experiences anticipatory anxiety before such events and endures them with intense distress. What is the most likely diagnosis?

    a. Panic Disorder

    b. Specific Phobia

    c. Social Anxiety Disorder

    d. Obsessive-Compulsive Disorder (OCD)

4. A 20-year-old male student experiences intrusive thoughts about germs and contamination. He engages in repetitive handwashing rituals and avoids touching objects in public places. What is the most likely diagnosis?

    a. Panic Disorder

    b. Generalized Anxiety Disorder (GAD)

    c. Social Anxiety Disorder

    d. Obsessive-Compulsive Disorder (OCD)

5. A 35-year-old female presents with recurrent episodes of intense fear and discomfort, accompanied by physical symptoms such as palpitations, sweating, trembling, and a feeling of choking. These episodes occur unexpectedly and she worries about having another attack. What is the most likely diagnosis?

    a. Generalized Anxiety Disorder (GAD)

    b. Panic Disorder

    c. Social Anxiety Disorder

    d. Specific Phobia

6. A 50-year-old male complains of chronic worry, difficulty concentrating, irritability, muscle tension, and sleep disturbances for the past 9 months. His symptoms are not related to any specific stressors and cause significant impairment in daily functioning. What is the most likely diagnosis?

    a. Major Depressive Disorder

    b. Panic Disorder

    c. Generalized Anxiety Disorder (GAD)

    d. Adjustment Disorder

7. A 25-year-old female has an intense fear of flying, which causes her to avoid air travel. She experiences marked distress when thinking about flying and recognizes her fear as excessive. What is the most likely diagnosis?

   a. Generalized Anxiety Disorder (GAD)

   b. Panic Disorder

   c. Social Anxiety Disorder

   d. Specific Phobia

8. A 30-year-old male is preoccupied with thoughts that his hands are contaminated with germs, despite regular handwashing. He spends hours each day washing his hands and avoids touching objects in public places. What is the most likely diagnosis?

   a. Generalized Anxiety Disorder (GAD)

   b. Panic Disorder

   c. Social Anxiety Disorder

   d. Obsessive-Compulsive Disorder (OCD)

9. A 40-year-old female experiences recurrent intrusive thoughts of harming her children. She knows these thoughts are irrational but cannot stop worrying about them. She avoids sharp objects and worries constantly about potential harm to her children. What is the most likely diagnosis?

   a. Panic Disorder

   b. Generalized Anxiety Disorder (GAD)

   c. Social Anxiety Disorder

   d. Obsessive-Compulsive Disorder (OCD)

10. A 22-year-old male experiences recurrent episodes of palpitations, sweating, trembling, and feelings of derealization. He fears that these episodes indicate a serious medical condition and frequently visits the emergency department. What is the most likely diagnosis?

    a. Panic Disorder

    b. Generalized Anxiety Disorder (GAD)

    c. Social Anxiety Disorder

    d. Adjustment Disorder

11. A 55-year-old female has an intense fear of driving over bridges. She avoids driving over bridges and experiences marked anxiety when she must do so. What is the most likely diagnosis?

    a. Panic Disorder

    b. Generalized Anxiety Disorder (GAD)

    c. Social Anxiety Disorder

    d. Specific Phobia

12. A 30-year-old male is preoccupied with thoughts of having a serious illness. Despite normal medical evaluations, he continues to worry excessively about his health and frequently seeks reassurance from healthcare providers. What is the most likely diagnosis?

    a. Hypochondriasis

    b. Generalized Anxiety Disorder (GAD)

    c. Panic Disorder

    d. Adjustment Disorder

13. A 25-year-old female reports sudden, intense fear and discomfort, accompanied by palpitations, sweating, and a sense of impending doom. These episodes occur in specific situations, such as public speaking or performing in front of others. What is the most likely diagnosis?

    a. Generalized Anxiety Disorder (GAD)

    b. Panic Disorder

    c. Social Anxiety Disorder

    d. Specific Phobia

14. A 35-year-old male presents with a persistent fear of snakes, leading to avoidance of parks and hiking trails. He experiences marked anxiety when confronted with pictures of snakes or actual encounters. What is the most likely diagnosis?

    a. Panic Disorder

    b. Generalized Anxiety Disorder (GAD)

    c. Social Anxiety Disorder

    d. Specific Phobia

15. A 28-year-old female worries excessively about her job performance, health, and relationships. She finds it difficult to control her worrying and experiences sleep disturbances and irritability. What is the most likely diagnosis?

    a. Major Depressive Disorder

    b. Panic Disorder

    c. Generalized Anxiety Disorder (GAD)

    d. Adjustment Disorder

Asthma

1. A 30-year-old female presents to the emergency room with sudden onset of dyspnea, cough, and wheezing. She has a history of seasonal allergies and occasional wheezing with colds. On physical exam, she has audible wheezing and decreased air movement on auscultation. Which of the following is the most likely diagnosis?

    a. Pneumonia

    b. Pulmonary embolism

    c. Asthma exacerbation

    d. Chronic obstructive pulmonary disease (COPD)

2. A 45-year-old male presents with a persistent dry cough, worse at night and early morning, and wheezing for the past 3 months. He denies any history of allergies or smoking. Physical exam reveals diffuse expiratory wheezing. What is the most likely diagnosis?

    a. Asthma

    b. Chronic bronchitis

    c. Bronchiectasis

    d. Pulmonary fibrosis

3. A 10-year-old boy presents with cough and wheezing that worsens during exercise or at night. He has a history of allergies and eczema. On physical exam, he has diffuse expiratory wheezing. What is the initial treatment of choice?

    a. Oral corticosteroids

    b. Short-acting beta agonist (SABA)

    c. Long-acting beta agonist (LABA)

    d. Inhaled corticosteroid (ICS)

4. A 60-year-old female presents with chronic cough and progressive dyspnea. She has a long history of smoking. On physical exam, there are scattered expiratory wheezes and decreased breath sounds at the lung bases. What diagnostic test would be most appropriate?

    a.   Chest X-ray

    b.   Pulmonary function tests (PFTs)

    c.   Bronchoscopy

    d.   High-resolution CT scan (HRCT)

5. A 25-year-old male presents with episodic shortness of breath and chest tightness that occurs after exercise and exposure to allergens. He has a history of hay fever. On physical exam, there are diffuse expiratory wheezes. What is the most likely diagnosis?

    a.   Chronic bronchitis

    b.   Asthma

    c.   Pulmonary embolism

    d.   Pneumonia

6. A 40-year-old female presents with a history of intermittent cough, wheezing, and dyspnea, worsened by exposure to dust and pets. She has a history of atopic dermatitis. On physical exam, there are diffuse expiratory wheezes. What is the most appropriate initial treatment?

    a.   Montelukast

    b.   Oral corticosteroids

    c.   Inhaled corticosteroids (ICS)

    d.   Long-acting muscarinic antagonist (LAMA)

7. A 50-year-old male presents with chronic cough and dyspnea on exertion. He has a history of smoking for the past 30 years. On physical exam, there are diffuse expiratory wheezes. Pulmonary function tests (PFTs) show airflow limitation that is not reversible with bronchodilators. What is the most likely diagnosis?

   a. Asthma

   b. Chronic bronchitis

   c. Bronchiectasis

   d. COPD

8. A 35-year-old female presents with a history of recurrent sinus infections and chronic cough with large amounts of purulent sputum production. She reports that her symptoms worsen during respiratory infections. On physical exam, there are diffuse crackles and coarse breath sounds. What is the most likely diagnosis?

   a. Asthma

   b. Chronic bronchitis

   c. Bronchiectasis

   d. Pneumonia

9. A 20-year-old male presents with acute dyspnea, tachypnea, and wheezing. He has a history of mild intermittent asthma treated with albuterol as needed. On physical exam, he is using accessory muscles for breathing and has diffuse expiratory wheezes. What is the initial treatment of choice?

   a. Inhaled corticosteroids (ICS)

   b. Long-acting beta agonist (LABA)

   c. Short-acting beta agonist (SABA)

   d. Oral corticosteroids

10. A 55-year-old female presents with a 3-month history of progressive dyspnea on exertion and a chronic non-productive cough. She has no history of allergies or smoking. On physical exam, there are fine bibasilar inspiratory crackles. What is the most likely diagnosis?

    a. Asthma

    b. Chronic bronchitis

    c. Pulmonary fibrosis

    d. Bronchiectasis

11. A 25-year-old female presents with episodic cough, wheezing, and dyspnea that occur after exposure to pet dander and dust. She has a history of atopic dermatitis. On physical exam, there are diffuse expiratory wheezes. Which of the following tests would be most appropriate for confirming the diagnosis?

    a. Chest X-ray

    b. High-resolution CT scan (HRCT)

    c. Pulmonary function tests (PFTs)

    d. Bronchoscopy

12. A 40-year-old male presents with chronic cough and dyspnea on exertion. He has a history of smoking for the past 20 years. On physical exam, there are scattered expiratory wheezes. Pulmonary function tests (PFTs) show airflow limitation that is partially reversible with bronchodilators. What is the most likely diagnosis?

    a. Asthma

    b. Chronic bronchitis

    c. Bronchiectasis

    d. COPD

13. A 30-year-old female presents with chronic cough, wheezing, and dyspnea on exertion. She has a history of allergic rhinitis and eczema since childhood. On physical exam, there are diffuse expiratory wheezes. What is the most appropriate initial treatment?

    a. Oral corticosteroids

    b. Short-acting beta agonist (SABA)

    c. Long-acting beta agonist (LABA)

    d. Inhaled corticosteroid (ICS)

14. A 50-year-old male presents with chronic cough and dyspnea on exertion. He has a history of smoking for the past 30 years. On physical exam, there are diffuse expiratory wheezes. Pulmonary function tests (PFTs) show airflow limitation that is not fully reversible with bronchodilators. What is the most likely diagnosis?

    a. Asthma

    b. Chronic bronchitis

    c. Bronchiectasis

    d. COPD

15. A 45-year-old female presents with a history of intermittent dyspnea and wheezing, worse at night and early morning. She denies any history of allergies or smoking. On physical exam, there are diffuse expiratory wheezes. What is the most likely diagnosis?

    a. Asthma

    b. Chronic bronchitis

    c. Pulmonary embolism

    d. Pneumonia

Atherosclerosis

1. Mr. Johnson, a 55-year-old smoker with a family history of heart disease, presents with intermittent claudication. Which of the following is the most likely underlying pathology?

    a. Coronary artery spasm

    b. Aortic dissection

    c. Atherosclerosis of peripheral arteries

    d. Thromboangiitis obliterans

2. A 60-year-old woman with poorly controlled diabetes mellitus and hypertension presents with acute onset chest pain. ECG shows ST-segment elevation in leads II, III, and aVF. Which of the following mechanisms is most likely responsible for her symptoms?

    a. Myocardial infarction due to plaque rupture and thrombosis

    b. Vasospasm of the coronary arteries

    c. Myocardial ischemia due to microvascular disease

    d. Pulmonary embolism

3. A 45-year-old man presents with sudden-onset right-sided weakness and slurred speech. CT scan shows a left middle cerebral artery infarct. What is the most likely underlying cause?

    a. Embolic stroke due to atrial fibrillation

    b. Atherosclerotic plaque rupture in the carotid artery

    c. Thrombotic stroke from atherosclerosis in the intracranial arteries

    d. Lacunar stroke from hypertension

4. A 50-year-old obese male with dyslipidemia presents with exertional chest pain that resolves with rest. Which of the following is the most appropriate initial step in management?

   a. Coronary angiography

   b. Cardiac stress test

   c. Lifestyle modification and pharmacotherapy

   d. Immediate coronary artery bypass graft surgery

5. A 65-year-old woman with a history of smoking and hypertension presents with sudden severe abdominal pain and hypotension. Imaging reveals an abdominal aortic aneurysm with signs of impending rupture. What is the most likely cause?

   a. Atherosclerosis of the abdominal aorta

   b. Trauma to the abdomen

   c. Syphilitic aortitis

   d. Connective tissue disorders

6. A 55-year-old man presents with erectile dysfunction. He has a history of diabetes mellitus and hypertension. What is the most likely underlying cause of his symptoms?

   a. Neurological damage

   b. Venous leakage

   c. Atherosclerosis of pelvic arteries

   d. Psychological factors

7. A 70-year-old man presents with exertional dyspnea and ankle edema. Echocardiography shows severe aortic stenosis. What is the most common cause of aortic stenosis in elderly patients?

   a. Rheumatic heart disease

   b. Bicuspid aortic valve

   c. Atherosclerosis of the aortic valve

   d. Idiopathic calcification

8. A 60-year-old woman with hyperlipidemia and a sedentary lifestyle presents with persistent leg pain at rest. Which of the following arteries is most likely affected?

   a. Carotid artery

   b. Coronary artery

   c. Popliteal artery

   d. Radial artery

9. A 45-year-old man presents with a history of transient ischemic attacks (TIAs). MRI reveals multiple small infarcts in the cerebral cortex. What is the most likely underlying etiology?

   a. Atrial fibrillation

   b. Atherosclerosis of intracranial arteries

   c. Migraine with aura

   d. Vasculitis

10. A 55-year-old woman with a history of smoking presents with progressive pain in her calves during exercise. Which of the following arteries is most likely affected?

    a. Internal carotid artery

    b. Coronary artery

    c. Femoral artery

    d. Pulmonary artery

11. A 65-year-old man with hypertension and diabetes presents with chronic non-healing ulcers on his feet. What is the most likely underlying cause?

    a. Peripheral neuropathy

    b. Venous insufficiency

    c. Atherosclerosis of peripheral arteries

    d. Osteomyelitis

12. A 70-year-old man presents with sudden-onset speech difficulty and right-sided weakness. CT scan shows a left middle cerebral artery infarct. What is the most likely cause?

    a. Atherosclerotic plaque rupture

    b. Hypertensive hemorrhage

    c. Embolic stroke

    d. Migraine with aura

13. A 50-year-old man presents with chest pain that occurs at rest and is relieved by nitroglycerin. ECG shows ST-segment depression. What is the most likely underlying cause?

    a. Coronary artery spasm

    b. Aortic dissection

    c. Atherosclerotic plaque rupture

    d. Pericarditis

14. A 60-year-old woman presents with sudden-onset severe abdominal pain radiating to the back. CT scan shows a ruptured abdominal aortic aneurysm. What is the most likely underlying cause?

    a. Atherosclerosis of the abdominal aorta

    b. Trauma to the abdomen

    c. Syphilitic aortitis

    d. Familial aortic aneurysm

15. A 55-year-old man with a history of smoking and hypertension presents with exertional dyspnea and chest discomfort. Echocardiography shows reduced left ventricular function with global hypokinesis. What is the most likely cause?

    a. Aortic dissection

    b. Myocardial infarction

    c. Chronic ischemic heart disease

    d. Pericarditis

Bipolar Disorder

1. John, a 32-year-old man, presents with a history of alternating episodes of euphoria, increased energy, decreased need for sleep, and racing thoughts followed by periods of profound sadness, hopelessness, and decreased energy. He reports these episodes have been occurring for the past 5 years. What is the most likely diagnosis?

    a. Major depressive disorder

    b. Bipolar disorder

    c. Schizophrenia

    d. Generalized anxiety disorder

2. Sarah, a 26-year-old woman, has been admitted to the hospital during a manic episode. She presents with grandiosity, decreased need for sleep, pressured speech, and excessive involvement in pleasurable activities that have a high potential for painful consequences. What is the initial treatment of choice?

    a. Lithium

    b. Olanzapine

    c. Fluoxetine

    d. Lorazepam

3. Mark, a 40-year-old man, has been stabilized on lithium for his bipolar disorder for several years. He presents with symptoms of diarrhea, tremor, and confusion. What is the most likely explanation for his symptoms?

    a. Lithium toxicity

    b. Bipolar depressive episode

    c. Olanzapine side effects

    d. Antidepressant discontinuation syndrome

4. Emily, a 30-year-old woman with bipolar disorder, is planning to become pregnant. Which of the following medications is generally considered safest during pregnancy?

    a. Lithium

    b. Valproate

    c. Carbamazepine

    d. Lamotrigine

5. David, a 35-year-old man with bipolar disorder, presents with a history of multiple episodes of depression and mania. He has tried several medications without sustained improvement. What is the next appropriate step in management?

    a. Augment current medication with a second mood stabilizer

    b. Switch to a different class of antidepressant

    c. Start electroconvulsive therapy (ECT)

    d. Consider referral for cognitive behavioral therapy (CBT)

6. Anna, a 25-year-old woman, presents with a history of recurring depressive episodes and has recently started experiencing periods of increased energy, racing thoughts, and decreased need for sleep. She denies any history of manic episodes. What is the most likely diagnosis?

    a. Bipolar II disorder

    b. Major depressive disorder

    c. Schizoaffective disorder

    d. Cyclothymic disorder

7. Michael, a 50-year-old man with bipolar disorder, has been stable on lithium for many years. He presents with complaints of excessive thirst, frequent urination, and weight gain. What is the most likely cause of his symptoms?

    a. Lithium-induced nephrogenic diabetes insipidus

    b. Lithium-induced hypothyroidism

    c. Lithium toxicity

    d. Lithium-induced hyperparathyroidism

8. Julia, a 28-year-old woman, presents with a history of multiple episodes of mania and depression. She has rapid cycling bipolar disorder. Which of the following treatments is often used to stabilize mood in rapid cycling bipolar disorder?

    a. Lithium

    b. Carbamazepine

    c. Lamotrigine

    d. Valproate

9. Matthew, a 45-year-old man with bipolar disorder, presents with complaints of weight gain, increased appetite, and daytime sleepiness. He is currently taking olanzapine. What is the likely cause of his symptoms?

    a. Olanzapine-induced metabolic syndrome

    b. Bipolar depressive episode

    c. Olanzapine-induced akathisia

    d. Hypothyroidism

10. Rachel, a 30-year-old woman with bipolar disorder, presents with recent onset of irritability, racing thoughts, and decreased need for sleep. She has never experienced manic episodes before. What is the most appropriate initial treatment?

    a. Antidepressants

    b. Lithium

    c. Olanzapine

    d. Psychotherapy

11. Eric, a 38-year-old man, has been diagnosed with bipolar disorder. He is currently experiencing a depressive episode and has not responded adequately to antidepressants alone. What is the recommended treatment approach?

    a. Add lithium or lamotrigine

    b. Increase the dose of the current antidepressant

    c. Switch to a different class of antidepressant

    d. Start cognitive behavioral therapy (CBT)

12. Sophia, a 24-year-old woman with bipolar disorder, has been prescribed lithium. What is the recommended monitoring schedule for lithium levels in a stable patient?

    a. Every month

    b. Every 3 months

    c. Every 6 months

    d. Every year

13. Daniel, a 55-year-old man with bipolar disorder, has been taking carbamazepine for several years. He presents with nausea, vomiting, and confusion. What is the likely cause of his symptoms?

    a. Carbamazepine toxicity

    b. Bipolar depressive episode

    c. Carbamazepine-induced hyponatremia

    d. Hypothyroidism

14. Olivia, a 30-year-old woman with bipolar disorder, presents with a recent history of rapid mood swings, irritability, and impulsivity. She reports feeling energetic but also easily angered. What is the most likely diagnosis?

    a. Borderline personality disorder

    b. Bipolar disorder, mixed episode

    c. Panic disorder

    d. Schizoaffective disorder

15. Thomas, a 42-year-old man with bipolar disorder, presents with severe agitation, psychosis, and insomnia. He has a history of non-adherence to medications. What is the initial treatment of choice?

    a. Intramuscular olanzapine

    b. Oral lithium

    c. Electroconvulsive therapy (ECT)

    d. Cognitive behavioral therapy (CBT)

Bronchitis

1. A 45-year-old male presents with a persistent cough productive of greenish-yellow sputum for the past 10 days. He reports a low-grade fever and mild chest discomfort exacerbated by coughing. On examination, there are coarse crackles heard on auscultation over both lung bases. What is the most likely diagnosis?

    a. Acute bronchitis

    b. Chronic bronchitis

    c. Pneumonia

    d. Asthma

2. A 55-year-old heavy smoker complains of a chronic cough with expectoration of copious amounts of purulent sputum most mornings for the past 3 months. He also experiences dyspnea on exertion and wheezing. What is the most likely diagnosis?

    a. Acute bronchitis

    b. Chronic bronchitis

    c. Bronchiectasis

    d. Asthma

3. A 30-year-old otherwise healthy individual presents with a 5-day history of non-productive cough, sore throat, rhinorrhea, and low-grade fever. There are no abnormal findings on chest examination. What is the most likely diagnosis?

    a. Acute bronchitis

    b. Chronic bronchitis

    c. Viral upper respiratory tract infection

    d. Atypical pneumonia

4. A 65-year-old female with a history of chronic obstructive pulmonary disease (COPD) presents with worsening dyspnea, increased sputum production, and generalized fatigue over the past week. On examination, she has prolonged expiratory phase, wheezing, and bilateral coarse crackles. What is the most likely cause of her exacerbation?

   a. Acute bronchitis

   b. Chronic bronchitis

   c. Pneumonia

   d. COPD exacerbation

5. A 50-year-old male presents with a persistent cough for 2 weeks, initially dry but now productive of mucoid sputum. He denies fever or significant shortness of breath. On examination, there are no abnormal lung sounds. What is the most appropriate management?

   a. Empirical antibiotics

   b. Antitussive therapy

   c. Bronchodilators

   d. Supportive care

6. A 60-year-old male smoker presents with a chronic cough productive of yellow-green sputum nearly every day for the past 2 years. He has had occasional exacerbations requiring antibiotics and oral corticosteroids. What is the most likely diagnosis?

   a. Acute bronchitis

   b. Chronic bronchitis

   c. Bronchiectasis

   d. Asthma

7. A 25-year-old female presents with a 3-week history of persistent cough, fever, and increasing dyspnea. She is a non-smoker and denies any significant medical history. On examination, there are coarse crackles heard over the right lower lung fields. What is the most likely diagnosis?

    a. Acute bronchitis

    b. Chronic bronchitis

    c. Pneumonia

    d. Tuberculosis

8. A 35-year-old otherwise healthy female presents with a persistent cough and wheezing for the past 2 weeks. She denies fever or sputum production. On examination, there are expiratory wheezes heard bilaterally. What is the most likely diagnosis?

    a. Acute bronchitis

    b. Chronic bronchitis

    c. Asthma

    d. Pneumonia

9. A 40-year-old male presents with a persistent productive cough for the past 6 months. He is a heavy smoker and reports increasing dyspnea on exertion. On examination, there are prolonged expiratory phase and scattered wheezes. What is the most likely diagnosis?

    a. Acute bronchitis

    b. Chronic bronchitis

    c. Emphysema

    d. Asthma

10. A 50-year-old male presents with recurrent episodes of cough with foul-smelling sputum, hemoptysis, and recurrent pulmonary infections despite appropriate antibiotic treatment. Chest X-ray shows cystic bronchiectatic changes. What is the most likely diagnosis?

    a. Acute bronchitis

    b. Chronic bronchitis

    c. Bronchiectasis

    d. Lung abscess

11. A 30-year-old non-smoker presents with a dry cough and mild chest discomfort for the past 5 days. There is no history of fever or significant respiratory symptoms. On examination, lung auscultation is clear. What is the most likely diagnosis?

    a. Acute bronchitis

    b. Chronic bronchitis

    c. Viral upper respiratory tract infection

    d. Early-stage asthma

12. A 60-year-old male with a history of recurrent bronchitis presents with increased sputum production and dyspnea over the past week. He is noted to have cyanosis, digital clubbing, and bilateral coarse crackles on lung auscultation. What is the most likely diagnosis?

    a. Acute bronchitis

    b. Chronic bronchitis

    c. Bronchiectasis

    d. Pneumonia

13. A 45-year-old male presents with a productive cough and mild fever for the past 7 days. He denies dyspnea or significant medical history. On examination, there are scattered rhonchi heard bilaterally. What is the most appropriate initial management?

    a. Empirical antibiotics

    b. Corticosteroids

    c. Bronchodilators

    d. Antitussive therapy

14. A 55-year-old male smoker presents with a chronic cough productive of copious amounts of sputum nearly every day for the past 6 months. He reports occasional wheezing and dyspnea on exertion. What is the most appropriate initial step in management?

    a. Empirical antibiotics

    b. Chest X-ray

    c. Pulmonary function tests

    d. Smoking cessation counseling

15. A 35-year-old female presents with recurrent episodes of wheezing, cough, and chest tightness, especially at night and early morning. She denies significant sputum production or fever. On examination, there are expiratory wheezes heard bilaterally. What is the most likely diagnosis?

    a. Acute bronchitis

    b. Chronic bronchitis

    c. Asthma

    d. Pneumonia

Cancer

1. A 55-year-old former smoker presents for routine health maintenance. He smoked a pack of cigarettes daily for 30 years and quit 5 years ago. What is the most appropriate screening test to recommend?

    a. Colonoscopy

    b. Mammography

    c. Low-dose CT scan of the chest

    d. PSA (Prostate-specific antigen) test

2. A 45-year-old woman presents with a painless lump in her left breast that she discovered during a self-examination. On examination, a firm, non-mobile mass is palpated in the upper outer quadrant. What is the next appropriate step?

    a. Order a mammogram and ultrasound

    b. Perform a core needle biopsy

    c. Refer to a breast surgeon for excisional biopsy

    d. Start empirical treatment with antibiotics

3. A 60-year-old man with no significant medical history presents for a routine check-up. He asks about prostate cancer screening. According to current guidelines, what should be recommended?

    a. Annual PSA (Prostate-specific antigen) test

    b. Digital rectal examination (DRE) every 2 years

    c. PSA test every 2 years

    d. Shared decision-making regarding PSA testing

4. A 55-year-old man presents with new-onset rectal bleeding and changes in bowel habits, including alternating diarrhea and constipation. He has no family history of colorectal cancer. What is the next appropriate step?

    a. Start empirical treatment for hemorrhoids

    b. Order a colonoscopy

    c. Refer to gastroenterology for sigmoidoscopy

    d. Perform a fecal occult blood test (FOBT)

5. A 40-year-old fair-skinned woman presents for her annual check-up. She reports a history of blistering sunburns during childhood and uses sunscreen regularly now. What is the most appropriate recommendation?

    a. Perform a full-body skin examination

    b. Refer to dermatology for a biopsy of suspicious lesions

    c. Order a PET-CT scan for surveillance

    d. Recommend genetic testing for melanoma

6. A 35-year-old woman presents for a routine gynecological examination. She has no significant medical history and is not vaccinated against HPV. What is the recommended screening test?

    a. Pap smear every 3 years

    b. HPV DNA testing every 5 years

    c. Pap smear and HPV testing annually

    d. Colposcopy with biopsy

7. A 50-year-old woman presents with persistent bloating, pelvic pain, and early satiety. She has no significant medical history. What is the most appropriate initial investigation?

    a. Transvaginal ultrasound

    b. CA-125 blood test

    c. CT scan of the abdomen and pelvis

    d. Colonoscopy

8. A 25-year-old man presents with a painless lump in his left testicle that he noticed during a self-examination. On examination, a firm, non-tender mass is palpated. What is the next appropriate step?

   a. Order a scrotal ultrasound

   b. Refer to urology for orchiectomy

   c. Perform a testicular biopsy

   d. Start empirical treatment with antibiotics

9. A 60-year-old man presents with new-onset jaundice, weight loss, and clay-colored stools. He has a history of heavy alcohol use. What is the most appropriate initial investigation?

   a. Abdominal ultrasound

   b. MRI of the abdomen

   c. CT scan of the abdomen and pelvis

   d. Endoscopic retrograde cholangiopancreatography (ERCP)

10. A 55-year-old man presents with progressive dysphagia to solids. He reports unintentional weight loss and occasional regurgitation of food. What is the most appropriate initial investigation?

    a. Upper endoscopy with biopsy

    b. Barium swallow

    c. CT scan of the chest and abdomen

    d. Esophageal manometry

11. A 40-year-old woman presents with a painless lump in her neck that she discovered while bathing. On examination, a firm, non-tender mass is palpated in the right lobe of the thyroid gland. What is the next appropriate step?

    a. Order a thyroid ultrasound

    b. Refer to otolaryngology for thyroidectomy

    c. Perform a fine-needle aspiration (FNA) biopsy

    d. Start empirical treatment with thyroid hormone replacement

12. A 65-year-old man presents with painless gross hematuria. He reports a history of smoking and occasional lower abdominal discomfort. What is the most appropriate initial investigation?

    a. Urine cytology

    b. Renal ultrasound

    c. CT urogram

    d. Cystoscopy with biopsy

13. A 70-year-old man presents with elevated PSA levels on routine screening. He has no lower urinary tract symptoms. Digital rectal examination reveals a firm nodule on the right side of the prostate gland. What is the next appropriate step?

    a. Repeat PSA test in 6 months

    b. Order a transrectal ultrasound (TRUS) and biopsy

    c. Refer to urology for prostatectomy

    d. Start empirical treatment with antibiotics

14. A 55-year-old woman presents with left-sided flank pain and hematuria. She reports unintentional weight loss and fatigue over the past few months. What is the most appropriate initial investigation?

    a. Renal ultrasound

    b. CT scan of the abdomen and pelvis

    c. Urine cytology

    d. MRI of the abdomen

15. A 25-year-old man presents with painless lymphadenopathy in the cervical and supraclavicular regions. He reports night sweats and unintentional weight loss over the past few months. What is the most appropriate initial investigation?

    a. Fine-needle aspiration (FNA) biopsy of a lymph node

    b. CT scan of the chest, abdomen, and pelvis

    c. PET-CT scan

    d. Complete blood count (CBC) with differential

Candidiasis

1. A 30-year-old woman presents with complaints of vaginal itching and thick, white vaginal discharge. She reports no history of similar symptoms before. On examination, the vaginal mucosa appears erythematous with a cottage cheese-like discharge. What is the most likely diagnosis?

    a. Bacterial vaginosis

    b. Trichomoniasis

    c. Candidiasis

    d. Gonorrhea

2. A 65-year-old diabetic man presents with complaints of oral discomfort and burning sensation. On examination, white plaques are noted on the buccal mucosa and tongue that can be scraped off, leaving a red, raw surface. What is the most likely diagnosis?

    a. Oral lichen planus

    b. Oral thrush

    c. Oral herpes simplex virus infection

    d. Oral leukoplakia

3. A 50-year-old woman presents with complaints of dysphagia and odynophagia. She has a history of recurrent episodes of esophagitis and is HIV-positive. Endoscopy reveals whitish plaques on the esophageal mucosa. What is the most likely diagnosis?

    a. Herpes esophagitis

    b. Candida esophagitis

    c. Eosinophilic esophagitis

    d. Barrett's esophagus

4. A 2-month-old infant presents with persistent diaper rash despite frequent diaper changes and use of barrier creams. On examination, there are well-defined erythematous plaques with satellite lesions in the diaper area. What is the most likely diagnosis?

    a. Irritant contact dermatitis

    b. Allergic contact dermatitis

    c. Candidal diaper dermatitis

    d. Atopic dermatitis

5. A 45-year-old man with poorly controlled diabetes mellitus presents with a complaint of groin itching and discomfort. On examination, there are erythematous plaques with satellite papules and pustules in the inguinal folds. What is the most likely diagnosis?

    a. Tinea cruris

    b. Candidal intertrigo

    c. Psoriasis

    d. Erythrasma

6. A 60-year-old woman presents with chronic paronychia and nail changes characterized by nail plate separation and yellow discoloration. There is no history of trauma or contact dermatitis. What is the most likely diagnosis?

    a. Onychomycosis

    b. Psoriasis

    c. Eczematous dermatitis

    d. Candidal nail infection

7. A 35-year-old woman presents with persistent redness and scaling between her toes. On examination, there are white, macerated areas with a slightly pungent odor. She reports no improvement with over-the-counter antifungal creams. What is the most likely diagnosis?

    a. Tinea pedis

    b. Candidal interdigital infection

    c. Erythrasma

    d. Psoriasis

8. A 25-year-old woman presents with recurrent episodes of pruritic, red, scaly patches in the skin folds of her axillae and inframammary areas. She reports worsening during hot and humid weather. What is the most likely diagnosis?

    a. Psoriasis

    b. Tinea versicolor

    c. Candidal intertrigo

    d. Erythrasma

9. A 30-year-old sexually active woman presents with vulvar itching and burning. On examination, there are erythematous plaques with satellite papules and pustules. She denies any recent antibiotic use. What is the most likely diagnosis?

    a. Bacterial vaginosis

    b. Trichomoniasis

    c. Vulvar dermatophytosis

    d. Candidal vulvovaginitis

10. A 50-year-old man presents with chronic mucocutaneous candidiasis, recurrent oral thrush, and nail infections. He has a history of autoimmune disease. What underlying condition is most likely contributing to his susceptibility to Candida infections?

    a. Diabetes mellitus

    b. HIV infection

    c. Chronic corticosteroid use

    d. Autoimmune polyendocrinopathy-candidiasis-ectodermal dystrophy (APECED)

11. A 70-year-old man presents with dysphagia and odynophagia. He has a history of esophageal cancer treated with chemotherapy and radiation therapy. Endoscopy reveals whitish plaques on the esophageal mucosa. What is the most likely diagnosis?

    a. Radiation-induced esophagitis

    b. Candida esophagitis

    c. Chemotherapy-induced mucositis

    d. Barrett's esophagus

12. A 35-year-old man presents with chronic diarrhea and abdominal pain. He has a history of HIV infection with a CD4 count of 120 cells/mm³. Stool studies are negative for pathogens. Colonoscopy reveals multiple yellowish plaques adherent to the colonic mucosa. What is the most likely diagnosis?

    a. Cytomegalovirus colitis

    b. Candida colitis

    c. Clostridioides difficile colitis

    d. Crohn's disease

13. A 55-year-old woman presents with chronic nasal congestion, facial pain, and headache. She has a history of allergic rhinitis and diabetes mellitus. Physical examination reveals unilateral erythematous nasal mucosa with purulent discharge. What is the most likely diagnosis?

    a. Allergic rhinitis

    b. Chronic sinusitis

    c. Nasal polyps

    d. Fungal sinusitis

14. A 45-year-old man presents with complaints of persistent itching and discomfort in the groin area. On examination, there are well-defined erythematous plaques with satellite papules and pustules. He reports no improvement with antifungal creams. What is the most likely diagnosis?

    a. Tinea cruris

    b. Candidal intertrigo

    c. Erythrasma

    d. Seborrheic dermatitis

15. A 60-year-old man with poorly controlled diabetes mellitus presents with complaints of a painful, swollen right big toe. On examination, the toe is erythematous, warm to touch, and there is purulent discharge from the nail bed. What is the most likely diagnosis?

    a. Gouty arthritis

    b. Septic arthritis

    c. Paronychia

    d. Candidal nail infection

Celiac Disease

1. A 30-year-old woman presents with chronic diarrhea, bloating, and weight loss over the past few months. She reports feeling fatigued and irritable. Laboratory tests show iron deficiency anemia and positive tissue transglutaminase antibodies (tTG-IgA). What is the most likely diagnosis?

    a. Irritable bowel syndrome

    b. Crohn's disease

    c. Celiac disease

    d. Ulcerative colitis

2. A 25-year-old man presents with chronic abdominal pain, steatorrhea, and muscle wasting. He has a history of type 1 diabetes mellitus. Laboratory tests reveal vitamin deficiencies (A, D, E, K) and malabsorption. What is the most likely cause of his symptoms?

    a. Pancreatic insufficiency

    b. Celiac disease

    c. Giardiasis

    d. Inflammatory bowel disease

3. A 45-year-old woman presents with chronic constipation, intermittent abdominal pain, and occasional episodes of diarrhea. She has a family history of autoimmune diseases. Physical examination is unremarkable. What initial investigation is most appropriate?

    a. Colonoscopy with biopsy

    b. Serum anti-tTG antibodies

    c. Upper endoscopy with duodenal biopsy

    d. Stool culture for pathogens

4. A 35-year-old man presents with recurrent canker sores (aphthous stomatitis), bloating after meals, and a history of infertility. He mentions his sibling was recently diagnosed with Celiac disease. What is the most appropriate initial step in management?

    a. Refer for genetic testing

    b. Initiate gluten-free diet

    c. Order serum anti-tTG antibodies

    d. Perform upper endoscopy

5. A 50-year-old woman with chronic diarrhea, fatigue, and joint pain presents for evaluation. She reports no improvement with over-the-counter medications. Laboratory tests show elevated liver enzymes and positive anti-endomysial antibodies (EMA). What is the most likely diagnosis?

    a. Non-celiac gluten sensitivity

    b. Autoimmune hepatitis

    c. Celiac disease

    d. Rheumatoid arthritis

6. A 55-year-old man presents with chronic anemia despite iron supplementation. He has a history of osteoporosis and recurrent oral ulcers. Laboratory tests show low serum iron, ferritin, and vitamin B12 levels. What investigation should be performed next?

    a. Stool occult blood test

    b. Serum anti-tTG antibodies

    c. Colonoscopy

    d. Bone density scan

7. A 40-year-old woman presents with chronic diarrhea, abdominal pain, and unintentional weight loss. She reports no relief with antispasmodics. On examination, she has signs of malnutrition. What is the next appropriate step in management?

    a. Refer for genetic testing

    b. Initiate gluten-free diet

    c. Order HLA typing

    d. Perform upper endoscopy with biopsy

8. A 30-year-old man presents with chronic bloating, abdominal pain, and intermittent diarrhea. He has a history of type 1 diabetes mellitus. Laboratory tests show vitamin deficiencies and positive serum anti-tTG antibodies. What is the most appropriate initial step in management?

    a. Initiate gluten-free diet

    b. Perform upper endoscopy with biopsy

    c. Check serum total IgA levels

    d. Screen for other autoimmune diseases

9. A 25-year-old woman presents with chronic diarrhea and abdominal distension. She reports frequent headaches and muscle pain. Laboratory tests show low serum calcium and vitamin D levels. What is the most likely diagnosis?

    a. Irritable bowel syndrome

    b. Celiac disease

    c. Inflammatory bowel disease

    d. Lactose intolerance

10. A 35-year-old man presents with chronic fatigue, anemia, and unexplained weight loss. He has a history of recurrent mouth ulcers and dermatitis herpetiformis. Laboratory tests show positive serum anti-tTG antibodies and HLA-DQ2 genotype. What is the likely diagnosis?

    a. Non-celiac gluten sensitivity

    b. Crohn's disease

    c. Dermatitis herpetiformis

    d. Celiac disease

11. A 40-year-old woman presents with chronic diarrhea, fatigue, and occasional joint pain. She reports feeling bloated after consuming bread or pasta. Laboratory tests show low serum iron and positive serum anti-tTG antibodies. What is the next step in management?

    a. Initiate gluten-free diet

    b. Perform upper endoscopy with biopsy

    c. Check serum total IgA levels

    d. Refer for genetic testing

12. A 50-year-old man presents with chronic diarrhea, bloating, and unintentional weight loss. He has a family history of autoimmune diseases. Laboratory tests show positive serum anti-endomysial antibodies (EMA) and vitamin deficiencies. What is the most likely diagnosis?

    a. Celiac disease

    b. Crohn's disease

    c. Ulcerative colitis

    d. Irritable bowel syndrome

13. A 30-year-old woman presents with chronic fatigue, joint pain, and frequent headaches. She reports having abdominal bloating and intermittent diarrhea. Laboratory tests show vitamin deficiencies and positive serum anti-tTG antibodies. What is the next appropriate step in management?

    a. Initiate gluten-free diet

    b. Perform upper endoscopy with biopsy

    c. Check serum total IgA levels

    d. Refer for genetic testing

14. A 35-year-old man presents with chronic diarrhea, abdominal pain, and unintended weight loss. He has a history of migraines and recurrent mouth ulcers. Laboratory tests show low serum iron and positive serum anti-tTG antibodies. What is the likely diagnosis?

    a. Irritable bowel syndrome

    b. Crohn's disease

    c. Celiac disease

    d. Ulcerative colitis

15. A 40-year-old woman presents with chronic bloating, abdominal pain, and intermittent diarrhea. She has a family history of autoimmune diseases. Laboratory tests show low serum calcium and vitamin D levels, and positive serum anti-tTG antibodies. What is the most appropriate next step in management?

    a. Initiate gluten-free diet

    b. Perform upper endoscopy with biopsy

    c. Check serum total IgA levels

    d. Refer for genetic testing

Chronic Kidney Disease

1. A 55-year-old man with a history of hypertension presents with fatigue, swelling in the ankles, and decreased urine output over the past month. Laboratory tests show elevated serum creatinine and decreased estimated glomerular filtration rate (eGFR). What stage of CKD is most likely present?

    a. Stage 1

    b. Stage 2

    c. Stage 3

    d. Stage 4

2. A 65-year-old woman with diabetes presents with nausea, vomiting, and confusion. Laboratory findings show severe metabolic acidosis and markedly elevated serum potassium levels. What complication of CKD is she likely experiencing?

    a. Hyperphosphatemia

    b. Hyperkalemia

    c. Hypocalcemia

    d. Hypomagnesemia

3. A 70-year-old man presents with pruritus (itching), bone pain, and pathologic fractures. Laboratory tests show elevated serum phosphorus and parathyroid hormone levels, along with low serum calcium. What complication of CKD is he likely experiencing?

    a. Metabolic acidosis

    b. Renal osteodystrophy

    c. Anemia

    d. Peripheral neuropathy

4. A 60-year-old woman presents with dyspnea, pedal edema, and hypertension. She has a history of CKD and is on dialysis. Physical exam reveals crackles at lung bases. What is the likely cause of her symptoms?

    a. Volume overload

    b. Hypertensive crisis

    c. Pulmonary embolism

    d. Cardiac tamponade

5. A 45-year-old man presents with weakness, paresthesias in the hands and feet, and muscle cramps. He has a history of CKD and is on multiple medications. Laboratory tests show decreased serum calcium and elevated serum phosphate levels. What is the likely cause of his symptoms?

    a. Hyperphosphatemia

    b. Hypocalcemia

    c. Hyperkalemia

    d. Metabolic acidosis

6. A 50-year-old woman presents with frequent urination, nocturia, and swelling in her legs. She has a history of diabetes and hypertension. Laboratory tests show albuminuria and elevated serum creatinine. What is the most likely cause of her symptoms?

    a. Acute kidney injury

    b. Chronic kidney disease

    c. Urinary tract infection

    d. Renal artery stenosis

7. A 55-year-old man presents with fatigue, nausea, and metallic taste in the mouth. He has a history of CKD and is on hemodialysis. Laboratory tests show a markedly elevated serum urea level. What is the likely cause of his symptoms?

   a. Uremia

   b. Metabolic acidosis

   c. Hyperkalemia

   d. Anemia

8. A 60-year-old man presents with severe lower back pain and oliguria. He has a history of CKD and is on peritoneal dialysis. Physical exam reveals tenderness over the lumbar spine. What complication of CKD should be suspected?

   a. Peritonitis

   b. Renal osteodystrophy

   c. Urinary tract infection

   d. Renal colic

9. A 70-year-old woman with CKD presents with confusion, restlessness, and seizures. Laboratory tests show severe metabolic acidosis with markedly elevated serum potassium levels. What complication of CKD is she likely experiencing?

   a. Hyperphosphatemia

   b. Hyperkalemia

   c. Hypocalcemia

   d. Hypomagnesemia

10. A 55-year-old man presents with shortness of breath and chest pain. He has a history of CKD and hypertension. ECG shows hyperkalemia. What cardiac complication of CKD should be suspected?

    a. Myocardial infarction

    b. Pericarditis

    c. Arrhythmia

    d. Heart failure

11. A 65-year-old man presents with generalized weakness, bone pain, and fractures. He has a history of CKD and has been on dialysis for the past 5 years. Laboratory tests show elevated serum phosphate levels and low serum calcium levels. What complication of CKD is he likely experiencing?

    a. Hyperphosphatemia

    b. Hypocalcemia

    c. Metabolic acidosis

    d. Renal osteodystrophy

12. A 50-year-old woman presents with severe pruritus (itching), especially in the evenings and at night. She has a history of CKD and diabetes. Laboratory tests show elevated serum phosphate levels. What complication of CKD is she likely experiencing?

    a. Hyperphosphatemia

    b. Hypocalcemia

    c. Hyperkalemia

    d. Metabolic acidosis

13. A 45-year-old man presents with weakness, fatigue, and shortness of breath. He has a history of CKD and diabetes. Laboratory tests show decreased hemoglobin levels and normal MCV. What is the likely cause of his anemia?

    a. Iron deficiency anemia

    b. Vitamin B12 deficiency anemia

    c. Anemia of chronic disease

    d. Renal anemia

14. A 60-year-old woman presents with fatigue, muscle weakness, and paresthesias in the hands and feet. She has a history of CKD and is on hemodialysis. Laboratory tests show decreased serum calcium levels and elevated serum phosphate levels. What is the likely cause of her symptoms?

    a. Hyperphosphatemia

    b. Hypocalcemia

    c. Hyperkalemia

    d. Metabolic acidosis

15. A 55-year-old man presents with confusion, peripheral edema, and decreased urine output. He has a history of CKD and hypertension. Laboratory tests show elevated serum creatinine and low urine output. What is the likely cause of his symptoms?

    a. Acute kidney injury

    b. Chronic kidney disease progression

    c. Urinary tract infection

    d. Renal artery stenosis

Chronic Obstructive Pulmonary Disease (COPD)

1. A 60-year-old male smoker presents with progressive dyspnea on exertion and chronic cough with sputum production for the past 3 years. Physical examination reveals decreased breath sounds and prolonged expiration. What is the initial diagnostic test?

    a. Chest X-ray

    b. Pulmonary function tests (PFTs)

    c. High-resolution CT scan

    d. Arterial blood gas (ABG) analysis

2. A 70-year-old man with known COPD presents to the emergency department with increased dyspnea, increased sputum production, and wheezing for 2 days. He is afebrile. What is the initial management?

    a. Oral corticosteroids and antibiotics

    b. Nebulized short-acting bronchodilators

    c. Non-invasive positive pressure ventilation (NIPPV)

    d. Chest X-ray and ABG analysis

3. A 50-year-old woman presents with episodic wheezing, dyspnea, and cough, worsened by exposure to allergens and cold air. She has a history of atopy. What diagnostic test would help differentiate between asthma and COPD?

    a. Chest X-ray

    b. PFTs before and after bronchodilator

    c. CT scan of the chest

    d. Methacholine challenge test

4. A 65-year-old man with severe COPD continues to smoke despite multiple exacerbations. He expresses interest in quitting. What is the most effective intervention for smoking cessation?

   a. Nicotine replacement therapy (NRT)

   b. Varenicline (Chantix)

   c. Bupropion (Zyban)

   d. Combination of NRT and behavioral counseling

5. A 72-year-old woman with severe COPD presents with worsening dyspnea and peripheral edema. Arterial blood gas analysis shows PaO2 of 55 mmHg. What is the appropriate therapy?

   a. Home oxygen therapy

   b. Nebulized bronchodilators

   c. Inhaled corticosteroids (ICS)

   d. Non-invasive positive pressure ventilation (NIPPV)

6. A 68-year-old man with moderate COPD presents with acute onset fever, productive cough, and pleuritic chest pain. Chest auscultation reveals crackles over the right lower lobe. What is the initial management?

   a. Start empirical antibiotics

   b. Perform chest X-ray

   c. Order sputum culture and sensitivity

   d. Administer nebulized bronchodilators

7. A 60-year-old woman with severe COPD experiences frequent exacerbations and dyspnea despite optimal medical therapy. What intervention would most likely improve her exercise capacity and quality of life?

   a. Long-term oxygen therapy (LTOT)

   b. Influenza vaccination

   c. Pulmonary rehabilitation

   d. Continuous positive airway pressure (CPAP)

8. A 55-year-old man with moderate COPD complains of persistent dyspnea despite using short-acting bronchodilators as needed. What is the most appropriate initial step-up therapy?

    a. Add inhaled corticosteroids (ICS)

    b. Switch to long-acting beta-agonist (LABA)

    c. Combine LABA and ICS

    d. Prescribe phosphodiesterase-4 (PDE-4) inhibitor

9. A 70-year-old man with severe COPD and hypertension presents with worsening dyspnea and lower extremity edema. ECG shows new-onset atrial fibrillation. What should be the next step in management?

    a. Initiate beta-blocker therapy

    b. Perform echocardiogram

    c. Increase diuretic therapy

    d. Refer for coronary angiography

10. A 65-year-old woman with moderate COPD presents with persistent sadness, loss of interest, and poor sleep. She denies suicidal ideation. What is the initial management approach?

    a. Start selective serotonin reuptake inhibitor (SSRI)

    b. Refer for cognitive behavioral therapy (CBT)

    c. Increase COPD medication regimen

    d. Monitor closely without intervention

11. A 70-year-old man with severe COPD experiences unintentional weight loss and decreased appetite. What intervention is most appropriate to address his nutritional needs?

    a. Oral nutritional supplements

    b. Enteral tube feeding

    c. Intravenous nutrition

    d. Encourage high-calorie diet

12. A 60-year-old woman with moderate COPD is concerned about indoor air quality. What intervention would be most effective in reducing exposure to indoor pollutants?

    a. Encourage use of air purifiers

    b. Advise on smoking cessation

    c. Recommend opening windows for ventilation

    d. Use of dust masks during cleaning

13. A 65-year-old man with severe COPD has frequent exacerbations despite optimal medical therapy. What additional intervention would most likely reduce exacerbation frequency?

    a. Long-term macrolide therapy

    b. High-dose oral corticosteroids

    c. Prophylactic antibiotics

    d. Inhaled anticholinergics

14. A 55-year-old man with moderate COPD asks about vaccinations. Which vaccination is recommended for all COPD patients annually?

    a. Pneumococcal polysaccharide vaccine (PPSV23)

    b. Influenza vaccine

    c. Hepatitis B vaccine

    d. Meningococcal vaccine

15. A 60-year-old woman with severe COPD presents with dyspnea on minimal exertion and frequent exacerbations. What benefit can she expect from pulmonary rehabilitation?

    a. Reduced use of bronchodilators

    b. Decreased need for supplemental oxygen

    c. Improved exercise tolerance and quality of life

    d. Slower progression of COPD

Congestive Heart Failure (CHF)

1. A 65-year-old man presents with progressive dyspnea on exertion, orthopnea, and paroxysmal nocturnal dyspnea. On examination, he has bilateral crackles on lung auscultation and elevated jugular venous pressure. What is the initial diagnostic test?

    a. Chest X-ray

    b. Echocardiogram

    c. Electrocardiogram (ECG)

    d. B-type natriuretic peptide (BNP) assay

2. A 70-year-old woman with known CHF presents with sudden onset dyspnea at rest, frothy pink sputum, and bilateral crackles on lung auscultation. She is tachycardic and has elevated blood pressure. What is the initial management?

    a. Intravenous diuretics

    b. Non-invasive positive pressure ventilation (NIPPV)

    c. Inotropes (dobutamine)

    d. Anticoagulation therapy

3. A 60-year-old man with history of myocardial infarction presents with worsening dyspnea and fatigue. His echocardiogram shows an ejection fraction of 25%. What medication is most beneficial for improving his prognosis?

    a. Loop diuretics

    b. Angiotensin-converting enzyme (ACE) inhibitors

    c. Beta-blockers

    d. Calcium channel blockers

4. A 65-year-old woman with hypertension presents with exertional dyspnea and fatigue. Her echocardiogram shows preserved ejection fraction (>50%). What medication is beneficial for symptom management?

   a. Loop diuretics

   b. Angiotensin receptor blockers (ARBs)

   c. Beta-blockers

   d. Mineralocorticoid receptor antagonists

5. A 68-year-old man with CHF presents with muscle weakness and fatigue. Laboratory tests show serum potassium of 2.9 mEq/L. What is the initial management?

   a. Oral potassium supplementation

   b. IV potassium supplementation

   c. Discontinue diuretics

   d. Check magnesium levels

6. A 70-year-old man with severe CHF on optimal medical therapy presents with persistent symptoms despite treatment. What intervention is indicated to improve his symptoms and reduce hospitalizations?

   a. Implantable cardioverter-defibrillator (ICD)

   b. Cardiac resynchronization therapy (CRT)

   c. Permanent pacemaker insertion

   d. Coronary artery bypass graft (CABG)

7. A 65-year-old woman with CHF presents with worsening peripheral edema and decreased urine output. Her serum creatinine is elevated. What is the initial management?

   a. Reduce diuretic dose

   b. Increase ACE inhibitor dose

   c. Start angiotensin receptor-neprilysin inhibitor (ARNI)

   d. Perform renal ultrasound

8. A 60-year-old man with history of rheumatic fever presents with exertional dyspnea and lower extremity edema. Cardiac auscultation reveals a diastolic murmur at the apex. What diagnostic test is most appropriate?

    a. Transthoracic echocardiogram

    b. Cardiac catheterization

    c. Exercise stress test

    d. Coronary angiography

9. A 70-year-old woman with CHF presents with recurrent hospitalizations for exacerbations despite medication therapy. What intervention is most appropriate?

    a. Increase medication doses

    b. Simplify medication regimen

    c. Switch to IV diuretics

    d. Perform coronary angiography

10. A 65-year-old man with CHF presents with new-onset atrial fibrillation. His CHA2DS2-VASc score is 4. What is the most appropriate management strategy?

    a. Start warfarin therapy

    b. Initiate direct oral anticoagulant (DOAC)

    c. Monitor without anticoagulation

    d. Perform electrical cardioversion

11. A 68-year-old woman with CHF presents with dyspnea and weight gain. On examination, jugular venous pressure is elevated, and she has crackles in both lung bases. What is the initial management?

    a. Increase loop diuretic dose

    b. Reduce salt intake

    c. Initiate intravenous fluids

    d. Order BNP assay

12. A 70-year-old man with CHF complains of exercise intolerance and fatigue despite optimal medical therapy. What intervention would most likely improve his exercise capacity?

    a. Coronary artery bypass graft (CABG)

    b. Cardiac rehabilitation program

    c. Inotropes (dobutamine)

    d. Heart transplant evaluation

13. A 65-year-old woman with CHF presents with worsening dyspnea and fatigue. Laboratory tests show hemoglobin of 9.5 g/dL. What intervention is appropriate?

    a. Start erythropoietin therapy

    b. Increase loop diuretic dose

    c. Refer for iron supplementation

    d. Perform blood transfusion

14. A 60-year-old man with CHF presents with excessive daytime sleepiness and morning headaches. Polysomnography shows severe obstructive sleep apnea. What intervention is indicated?

    a. Continuous positive airway pressure (CPAP)

    b. Increase loop diuretic dose

    c. Refer for bariatric surgery

    d. Initiate supplemental oxygen

15. A 68-year-old man with severe CHF and reduced ejection fraction despite optimal medical therapy is considered for advanced heart failure therapy. What intervention improves survival in similar patients?

    a. Implantable cardioverter-defibrillator (ICD)

    b. Left ventricular assist device (LVAD)

    c. Coronary artery bypass graft (CABG)

    d. Transcatheter aortic valve replacement (TAVR)

Crohn's Disease

1. A 25-year-old female presents with chronic abdominal pain, diarrhea, and weight loss over the past 6 months. She also complains of intermittent fever and fatigue. On physical exam, there are diffuse abdominal tenderness and palpable mass in the right lower quadrant. What is the most likely diagnosis?

    a. Irritable bowel syndrome (IBS)

    b. Crohn's disease

    c. Ulcerative colitis

    d. Diverticulitis

2. A 35-year-old male presents with recurrent episodes of abdominal pain and diarrhea over the past year. He has noticed blood in his stool occasionally. On physical exam, there are perianal fissures and mild tenderness on palpation of the lower abdomen. What is the most appropriate initial diagnostic test?

    a. Colonoscopy with biopsy

    b. Stool culture for pathogens

    c. Abdominal ultrasound

    d. CT scan of the abdomen and pelvis

3. A 30-year-old female presents with chronic diarrhea, abdominal pain, and fatigue. She has a history of oral ulcers and has noticed occasional perianal abscesses. On physical exam, there are aphthous ulcers in the mouth and perianal fistulas. What is the most likely diagnosis?

    a. Crohn's disease

    b. Ulcerative colitis

    c. Celiac disease

    d. Irritable bowel syndrome (IBS)

4. A 40-year-old male presents with recurrent episodes of abdominal pain and diarrhea, which are worse after meals. He also reports feeling bloated and has noticed weight loss over the past few months. On physical exam, there are diffuse abdominal tenderness and palpable abdominal mass. What is the most likely finding on imaging?

    a. Skip lesions in the small intestine

    b. Continuous colonic involvement

    c. Diffuse thickening of the rectum

    d. Sigmoid colon strictures

5. A 55-year-old female presents with chronic diarrhea, weight loss, and occasional rectal bleeding over the past year. She has a history of autoimmune thyroiditis. On physical exam, there is tenderness on palpation of the left lower quadrant. What is the most likely diagnosis?

    a. Crohn's disease

    b. Ulcerative colitis

    c. Diverticulitis

    d. Infectious colitis

6. A 45-year-old male presents with chronic abdominal pain, diarrhea, and occasional fever for the past 3 years. He has a history of smoking. On physical exam, there are signs of malnutrition with muscle wasting and dermatologic manifestations such as erythema nodosum. What is the most appropriate initial treatment?

    a. Mesalamine

    b. Corticosteroids

    c. Methotrexate

    d. Infliximab

7. A 50-year-old female presents with chronic diarrhea, abdominal pain, and weight loss. She has a history of anemia and osteoporosis. On physical exam, there are oral ulcers and signs of malnutrition. What is the most likely finding on colonoscopy?

    a. Continuous involvement of the colon

    b. Cobblestone appearance of the mucosa

    c. Pseudopolyps in the rectum

    d. Diffuse rectal strictures

8. A 35-year-old male presents with recurrent episodes of abdominal pain, diarrhea, and fever. He has a history of oral aphthous ulcers and occasional perianal abscesses. On physical exam, there are diffuse abdominal tenderness and palpable mass in the right lower quadrant. What is the most appropriate initial imaging test?

    a. Abdominal ultrasound

    b. CT scan of the abdomen and pelvis

    c. MRI of the small intestine

    d. Barium enema

9. A 40-year-old female presents with chronic diarrhea, abdominal pain, and weight loss over the past 2 years. She has a history of migratory arthritis and erythema nodosum. On physical exam, there are signs of malnutrition with muscle wasting. What is the most appropriate initial treatment?

    a. Mesalamine

    b. Corticosteroids

    c. Azathioprine

    d. Adalimumab

10. A 45-year-old male presents with chronic diarrhea, abdominal pain, and occasional rectal bleeding for the past 6 months. He has a history of smoking. On physical exam, there are perianal fistulas and tenderness in the left lower quadrant. What is the most likely finding on imaging?

    a. Skip lesions in the small intestine

    b. Continuous colonic involvement

    c. Diffuse thickening of the rectum

    d. Sigmoid colon strictures

11. A 50-year-old female presents with chronic diarrhea, abdominal pain, and weight loss. She has a history of anemia and osteoporosis. On physical exam, there are oral ulcers and signs of malnutrition. What is the most likely finding on colonoscopy?

    a. Continuous involvement of the colon

    b. Cobblestone appearance of the mucosa

    c. Pseudopolyps in the rectum

    d. Diffuse rectal strictures

12. A 35-year-old male presents with recurrent episodes of abdominal pain, diarrhea, and fever. He has a history of oral aphthous ulcers and occasional perianal abscesses. On physical exam, there are diffuse abdominal tenderness and palpable mass in the right lower quadrant. What is the most appropriate initial imaging test?

    a. Abdominal ultrasound

    b. CT scan of the abdomen and pelvis

    c. MRI of the small intestine

    d. Barium enema

13. A 40-year-old female presents with chronic diarrhea, abdominal pain, and weight loss over the past 2 years. She has a history of migratory arthritis and erythema nodosum. On physical exam, there are signs of malnutrition with muscle wasting. What is the most appropriate initial treatment?

    a.   Mesalamine

    b.   Corticosteroids

    c.   Azathioprine

    d.   Adalimumab

14. A 45-year-old male presents with chronic diarrhea, abdominal pain, and occasional rectal bleeding for the past 6 months. He has a history of smoking. On physical exam, there are perianal fistulas and tenderness in the left lower quadrant. What is the most likely finding on imaging?

    a.   Skip lesions in the small intestine

    b.   Continuous colonic involvement

    c.   Diffuse thickening of the rectum

    d.   Sigmoid colon strictures

15. A 50-year-old female presents with chronic diarrhea, abdominal pain, and weight loss. She has a history of anemia and osteoporosis. On physical exam, there are oral ulcers and signs of malnutrition. What is the most likely finding on colonoscopy?

    a.   Continuous involvement of the colon

    b.   Cobblestone appearance of the mucosa

    c.   Pseudopolyps in the rectum

    d.   Diffuse rectal strictures

Deep Vein Thrombosis (DVT)

1. A 55-year-old woman presents with sudden-onset swelling and pain in her left leg. On examination, the affected leg is warm, erythematous, and tender to palpation. What is the most appropriate initial diagnostic test?

   a. Doppler ultrasound

   b. D-dimer assay

   c. CT pulmonary angiography

   d. Echocardiography

2. A 65-year-old man with a history of cancer presents with dyspnea and pleuritic chest pain. He is hypotensive, tachycardic, and has crackles in both lung fields. What is the most likely diagnosis?

   a. Acute coronary syndrome

   b. Pulmonary embolism

   c. Pneumonia

   d. Aortic dissection

3. A 50-year-old woman who recently underwent surgery presents with unilateral calf pain and swelling. She has no personal or family history of clotting disorders. What is the next best step in management?

   a. Start anticoagulation therapy

   b. Perform a D-dimer assay

   c. Order bilateral lower extremity ultrasound

   d. Administer pain relief and observe

4. A 70-year-old man with atrial fibrillation presents with sudden-onset left leg pain and pallor. The left foot is cold with absent pulses and decreased sensation. What is the most likely diagnosis?

 a. Compartment syndrome

 b. Acute arterial occlusion

 c. Diabetic neuropathy

 d. Deep vein thrombosis

5. A 60-year-old woman on oral contraceptives presents with right calf swelling and tenderness. Which of the following is the most appropriate initial step in management?

 a. Immediate admission for observation

 b. Compression stockings

 c. D-dimer assay

 d. Bilateral lower extremity ultrasound

6. A 45-year-old man presents with calf pain and swelling that worsens with dorsiflexion of the foot (Homans' sign). Which of the following conditions is most likely present?

 a. Achilles tendonitis

 b. Muscle strain

 c. Deep vein thrombosis

 d. Cellulitis

7. A 55-year-old woman presents with unilateral leg pain and swelling that developed after a long flight. She has no prior history of thromboembolism. What is the next step in management?

 a. Initiate anticoagulation therapy

 b. Order a D-dimer assay

 c. Perform bilateral lower extremity ultrasound

 d. Advise elevation and compression stockings

8. A 65-year-old man with a history of congestive heart failure presents with left leg swelling and pain that worsens with prolonged standing. He has no prior history of thromboembolism. What is the most appropriate initial step in management?

    a. Compression stockings

    b. D-dimer assay

    c. Echocardiography

    d. Bilateral lower extremity ultrasound

9. A 50-year-old woman presents with acute onset dyspnea and pleuritic chest pain. She is tachycardic and hypoxic. Which of the following diagnostic tests is most appropriate initially?

    a. Pulmonary angiography

    b. Echocardiography

    c. D-dimer assay

    d. CT pulmonary angiography

10. A 60-year-old man presents with unilateral leg swelling and tenderness. He recently underwent hip replacement surgery. What is the most appropriate initial step in management?

    a. Start anticoagulation therapy

    b. Order a D-dimer assay

    c. Perform bilateral lower extremity ultrasound

    d. Monitor for progression of symptoms

11. A 45-year-old woman presents with chronic swelling and discoloration of her left leg. She reports a history of DVT treated 5 years ago. What is the most likely cause of her current symptoms?

    a. Chronic venous insufficiency

    b. Recurrent DVT

    c. Lymphedema

    d. Cellulitis

12. A 55-year-old man presents with left calf pain and swelling that developed after a long car trip. Which of the following findings on physical examination would support a diagnosis of DVT?

    a. Warmth and erythema of the calf

    b. Increased pain with plantar flexion of the foot

    c. Ulceration and hemosiderin staining

    d. Absence of tenderness on palpation

13. A 65-year-old woman with a history of smoking presents with acute onset of left leg pain and swelling. She is also experiencing hemoptysis. What is the most likely diagnosis?

    a. Acute exacerbation of chronic bronchitis

    b. Congestive heart failure exacerbation

    c. Pulmonary embolism

    d. Cellulitis

14. A 50-year-old man presents with acute right leg pain and swelling. He has a history of factor V Leiden mutation. What is the most appropriate initial step in management?

    a. D-dimer assay

    b. Echocardiography

    c. Compression stockings

    d. Bilateral lower extremity ultrasound

15. A 60-year-old woman with a history of atrial fibrillation presents with sudden-onset dyspnea and chest pain. ECG shows sinus tachycardia. What is the most appropriate next step in management?

    a. Start anticoagulation therapy

    b. Order a D-dimer assay

    c. Perform CT pulmonary angiography

    d. Monitor overnight and repeat ECG

Depression

1. Emily, a 35-year-old woman, presents with a persistent low mood, loss of interest in activities she used to enjoy, feelings of worthlessness, and decreased energy for the past 6 months. She denies any history of manic episodes. What is the most likely diagnosis?

    a. Major depressive disorder

    b. Bipolar disorder

    c. Generalized anxiety disorder

    d. Adjustment disorder

2. David, a 28-year-old man, presents with low mood, irritability, insomnia, and decreased appetite. He reports feeling hopeless and having recurrent thoughts of death or suicide. What is the initial treatment of choice?

    a. Cognitive behavioral therapy (CBT)

    b. Sertraline

    c. Benzodiazepines

    d. Exercise therapy

3. Sarah, a 40-year-old woman, has been treated with fluoxetine for depression for the past 6 weeks without improvement. What should be the next step in management?

    a. Switch to venlafaxine

    b. Add cognitive behavioral therapy (CBT)

    c. Increase the dose of fluoxetine

    d. Assess medication adherence

4. Mark, a 50-year-old man, presents with symptoms of depression, including fatigue, difficulty concentrating, and changes in appetite and sleep patterns. He also reports a history of chronic pain. Which antidepressant is often considered effective in treating both depression and chronic pain?

   a. Amitriptyline

   b. Bupropion

   c. Mirtazapine

   d. Duloxetine

5. Anna, a 25-year-old woman, presents with severe depressive symptoms, including psychomotor retardation, significant weight loss, and anhedonia. She has a family history of bipolar disorder. What is the initial concern in her management?

   a. Risk of developing psychosis

   b. Risk of treatment-emergent mania

   c. Risk of serotonin syndrome

   d. Risk of suicidal ideation

6. Matthew, a 45-year-old man, presents with symptoms of depression but also reports a history of alcohol dependence. What is the initial treatment approach?

   a. Antidepressant therapy

   b. Referral to a substance abuse program

   c. Benzodiazepine therapy

   d. Electroconvulsive therapy (ECT)

7. Rachel, a 30-year-old woman, presents with a history of recurrent depressive episodes and a strong family history of depression. She is currently pregnant. Which antidepressant is generally considered safest during pregnancy?

    a. Sertraline

    b. Fluoxetine

    c. Paroxetine

    d. Amitriptyline

8. Daniel, a 35-year-old man, presents with a history of recurrent depressive episodes and irritability. He has tried several antidepressants without sustained improvement. What is the next appropriate step in management?

    a. Augment current medication with lithium

    b. Switch to a different class of antidepressant

    c. Start psychotherapy

    d. Refer for electroconvulsive therapy (ECT)

9. Olivia, a 32-year-old woman, presents with recurrent episodes of depression and a history of postpartum depression after her first child was born. She is planning to have another child. What should be discussed in her management plan?

    a. Risk of teratogenicity with antidepressants

    b. Risk of developing psychosis

    c. Role of hormone therapy

    d. Need for continuous antidepressant treatment

10. Lucas, a 40-year-old man, presents with depressive symptoms and a history of antidepressant treatment. He is concerned about the sexual side effects of his medication. Which antidepressant is least likely to cause sexual dysfunction?

    a. Fluoxetine

    b. Bupropion

    c. Sertraline

    d. Paroxetine

11. Sophie, a 28-year-old woman, presents with symptoms of depression, including insomnia, poor appetite, and feelings of guilt. She reports that these symptoms have been present for over a year but have not significantly impaired her daily functioning. What is the most likely diagnosis?

    a. Persistent depressive disorder (dysthymia)

    b. Major depressive disorder

    c. Adjustment disorder with depressed mood

    d. Bipolar II disorder

12. Emma, a 30-year-old woman, presents with symptoms of depression, including excessive guilt, psychomotor retardation, and weight gain. She reports a history of recurrent depressive episodes and anxiety. What class of antidepressants is often considered effective for atypical depression?

    a. MAOIs (Monoamine oxidase inhibitors)

    b. SSRIs (Selective serotonin reuptake inhibitors)

    c. TCAs (Tricyclic antidepressants)

    d. SNRIs (Serotonin-norepinephrine reuptake inhibitors)

13. Peter, a 45-year-old man, presents with depressive symptoms and significant fatigue. He reports a history of chronic medical illness and is currently taking multiple medications. What antidepressant class is often chosen for its sedative effects in patients with insomnia?

    a. Bupropion

    b. Fluoxetine

    c. Mirtazapine

    d. Venlafaxine

14. Natalie, a 35-year-old woman, presents with symptoms of depression and reports a recent history of weight gain and excessive sleepiness. She has been taking a selective serotonin reuptake inhibitor (SSRI). What is the likely cause of her symptoms?

    a. SSRI-induced weight gain

    b. Treatment-resistant depression

    c. Seasonal affective disorder (SAD)

    d. Bipolar depression

15. Hannah, a 27-year-old woman, presents with symptoms of depression, including feelings of worthlessness and suicidal ideation. She has no history of previous depressive episodes. What is the initial management approach?

    a. Immediate psychiatric hospitalization

    b. Initiation of antidepressant therapy

    c. Referral for cognitive behavioral therapy (CBT)

    d. Close monitoring without intervention

Diabetes Mellitus (Type 1 and Type 2)

1. A 30-year-old female presents with polyuria, polydipsia, weight loss, and blurred vision over the past month. On examination, she appears dehydrated. Random blood glucose is 350 mg/dL. Urinalysis shows glycosuria and ketonuria. What is the most likely diagnosis?

    a. Type 1 diabetes mellitus

    b. Type 2 diabetes mellitus

    c. Gestational diabetes mellitus

    d. Latent autoimmune diabetes in adults (LADA)

2. A 55-year-old obese male presents with fatigue, polyuria, and recurrent skin infections over the past 6 months. On examination, he has acanthosis nigricans and central obesity. Fasting blood glucose is 180 mg/dL, and HbA1c is 8.5%. What is the most likely diagnosis?

    a. Type 1 diabetes mellitus

    b. Type 2 diabetes mellitus

    c. LADA

    d. Secondary diabetes

3. A 25-year-old female presents with recurrent urinary tract infections, pruritus vulvae, and polyuria. She is 20 weeks pregnant. Oral glucose tolerance test shows impaired glucose tolerance. What is the most likely diagnosis?

    a. Type 1 diabetes mellitus

    b. Type 2 diabetes mellitus

    c. Gestational diabetes mellitus

    d. LADA

4. A 40-year-old male presents with fatigue, weight gain, and slow-healing wounds over the past year. On examination, he has a blood pressure of 150/90 mmHg, central obesity, and a buffalo hump. Fasting blood glucose is 250 mg/dL. What is the most likely diagnosis?

    a. Type 1 diabetes mellitus

    b. Type 2 diabetes mellitus

    c. Cushing's syndrome

    d. Secondary diabetes

5. A 30-year-old male presents with recurrent episodes of hypoglycemia and confusion. He admits to skipping meals frequently. Random blood glucose during an episode is 45 mg/dL. What is the most likely diagnosis?

    a. Type 1 diabetes mellitus

    b. Type 2 diabetes mellitus

    c. Insulinoma

    d. Reactive hypoglycemia

6. A 50-year-old female with a history of Type 2 diabetes mellitus presents with new-onset blurred vision and floaters in her left eye. Fundoscopic examination reveals hemorrhages and cotton wool spots. What is the most likely diagnosis?

    a. Diabetic retinopathy

    b. Age-related macular degeneration

    c. Retinal detachment

    d. Cataract

7. A 35-year-old male presents with recurrent yeast infections, tingling in his hands and feet, and intermittent episodes of blurred vision. Fasting blood glucose is 200 mg/dL, and HbA1c is 9.2%. What is the most likely diagnosis?

   a. Type 1 diabetes mellitus

   b. Type 2 diabetes mellitus

   c. Gestational diabetes mellitus

   d. LADA

8. A 60-year-old female with a history of Type 2 diabetes mellitus presents with gradual onset of fatigue, nausea, and abdominal pain. On examination, she appears dehydrated, and laboratory tests show serum glucose of 400 mg/dL, serum bicarbonate of 15 mEq/L, and pH of 7.25. What is the most likely diagnosis?

   a. Diabetic ketoacidosis (DKA)

   b. Hyperosmolar hyperglycemic state (HHS)

   c. Hypoglycemia

   d. Non-ketotic hyperosmolar coma

9. A 45-year-old male with Type 1 diabetes mellitus presents with confusion and deep, rapid breathing. His blood glucose is 600 mg/dL, serum bicarbonate is 5 mEq/L, and pH is 7.10. He reports missing his insulin injections over the past two days. What is the most likely diagnosis?

   a. Diabetic ketoacidosis (DKA)

   b. Hyperosmolar hyperglycemic state (HHS)

   c. Hypoglycemia

   d. Non-ketotic hyperosmolar coma

10. A 55-year-old obese female with Type 2 diabetes mellitus presents with confusion and weakness. On examination, she is severely dehydrated. Laboratory tests show serum glucose of 800 mg/dL, serum osmolality of 320 mOsm/kg, and serum bicarbonate of 18 mEq/L. What is the most likely diagnosis?

    a. Diabetic ketoacidosis (DKA)

    b. Hyperosmolar hyperglycemic state (HHS)

    c. Hypoglycemia

    d. Non-ketotic hyperosmolar coma

11. A 25-year-old female presents with new-onset Type 1 diabetes mellitus. She is started on insulin therapy and educated about self-management. Which of the following is a short-acting insulin analogue used for mealtime coverage?

    a. Insulin glargine

    b. Insulin detemir

    c. Regular insulin

    d. Insulin lispro

12. A 60-year-old male with Type 2 diabetes mellitus complains of nocturnal hypoglycemia. He is currently on basal insulin therapy. Which of the following may help prevent nocturnal hypoglycemia?

    a. Decreasing basal insulin dose

    b. Adding a rapid-acting insulin analogue

    c. Increasing bedtime snack carbohydrate intake

    d. Switching to long-acting insulin

13. A 40-year-old female with Type 2 diabetes mellitus is started on metformin. Which of the following is a common adverse effect of metformin?

    a. Weight gain

    b. Hypoglycemia

    c. Lactic acidosis

    d. Peripheral neuropathy

14. A 55-year-old male with Type 2 diabetes mellitus is found to have microalbuminuria on routine urine testing. What is the most appropriate next step in management?

    a. Start angiotensin-converting enzyme (ACE) inhibitor or angiotensin receptor blocker (ARB)

    b. Repeat urine testing in 6 months

    c. Begin intensive insulin therapy

    d. Refer to a nephrologist

15. A 65-year-old male with Type 2 diabetes mellitus complains of tingling and burning pain in his feet that worsens at night. On examination, he has diminished sensation to light touch and monofilament testing. What is the most likely diagnosis?

    a. Diabetic ketoacidosis (DKA)

    b. Hypoglycemia

    c. Peripheral neuropathy

    d. Autonomic neuropathy

Diabetic Neuropathy

1. A 55-year-old man with type 2 diabetes mellitus presents with burning pain in both feet, worse at night.

    On examination, there is decreased sensation to light touch and pinprick in a stocking-glove distribution.

    What is the most likely type of diabetic neuropathy?

    a.   Distal symmetric polyneuropathy

    b.   Autonomic neuropathy

    c.   Mononeuropathy

    d.   Diabetic amyotrophy

2. A 60-year-old woman with type 1 diabetes mellitus has no symptoms of neuropathy. What screening test

    is recommended for early detection of diabetic neuropathy?

    a.   Nerve conduction studies

    b.   Skin biopsy

    c.   Monofilament testing

    d.   Quantitative sensory testing

3. A 65-year-old man with type 2 diabetes mellitus presents with dizziness and syncope, especially on

    standing up. What type of diabetic neuropathy is most likely responsible for these symptoms?

    a.   Distal symmetric polyneuropathy

    b.   Autonomic neuropathy

    c.   Mononeuropathy

    d.   Diabetic amyotrophy

4. A 58-year-old woman with type 2 diabetes mellitus complains of severe burning pain in both feet, worse at night, and difficulty sleeping. Which medication is first-line for managing painful diabetic neuropathy?

    a. Gabapentin

    b. Metformin

    c. Lisinopril

    d. Insulin glargine

5. A 62-year-old man with type 2 diabetes mellitus presents with a non-healing ulcer on the plantar surface of his left foot. On examination, there is decreased sensation to light touch and a palpable dorsalis pedis pulse. What is the initial management?

    a. Refer for vascular surgery consultation

    b. Start empirical antibiotics

    c. Offload pressure with a total contact cast

    d. Perform arterial Doppler ultrasound

6. A 55-year-old man with type 2 diabetes mellitus complains of sudden onset severe pain in his right wrist and weakness in hand grip strength. On examination, there is focal tenderness over the wrist and reduced sensation over the lateral hand. What is the most likely diagnosis?

    a. Carpal tunnel syndrome

    b. Diabetic foot ulcer

    c. Autonomic neuropathy

    d. Diabetic amyotrophy

7. A 60-year-old man with type 2 diabetes mellitus reports difficulty achieving and maintaining erections. He has no history of hypertension or hyperlipidemia. What type of diabetic neuropathy is associated with these symptoms?

    a. Distal symmetric polyneuropathy

    b. Autonomic neuropathy

    c. Mononeuropathy

    d. Diabetic amyotrophy

8. A 65-year-old woman with type 1 diabetes mellitus complains of early satiety, bloating, and nausea after meals. What type of diabetic neuropathy is responsible for these symptoms?

    a. Distal symmetric polyneuropathy

    b. Autonomic neuropathy

    c. Mononeuropathy

    d. Diabetic amyotrophy

9. A 70-year-old man with type 2 diabetes mellitus complains of urinary urgency and frequency. He denies dysuria or hematuria. What type of diabetic neuropathy is likely responsible for these symptoms?

    a. Distal symmetric polyneuropathy

    b. Autonomic neuropathy

    c. Mononeuropathy

    d. Diabetic amyotrophy

10. A 62-year-old man with type 2 diabetes mellitus presents with a warm, swollen, and erythematous right foot. He denies trauma or recent injury. X-ray shows midfoot collapse. What is the likely diagnosis?

    a. Diabetic foot ulcer

    b. Charcot foot

    c. Peripheral arterial disease

    d. Osteomyelitis

11. A 65-year-old woman with type 2 diabetes mellitus continues to experience severe burning pain in both feet despite starting gabapentin. What is the next appropriate step in management?

    a. Increase gabapentin dose

    b. Switch to pregabalin

    c. Initiate tricyclic antidepressants (e.g., amitriptyline)

    d. Refer to pain management specialist

12. A 68-year-old man with type 2 diabetes mellitus is advised on foot care to prevent diabetic foot ulcers. Which instruction is most appropriate?

    a. Inspect feet daily for cuts and blisters

    b. Apply moisturizer between toes daily

    c. Cut toenails straight across

    d. Soak feet in hot water daily

13. A 60-year-old woman with type 2 diabetes mellitus has no symptoms of neuropathy. What is the recommended screening interval for diabetic neuropathy?

    a. Every 6 months

    b. Annually

    c. Biennially

    d. Only if symptoms develop

14. A 65-year-old man with type 2 diabetes mellitus and severe peripheral neuropathy presents with a non-healing foot ulcer infected with Staphylococcus aureus. What intervention is most appropriate to prevent amputation?

    a. Immediate amputation below the knee

    b. Debridement and culture-directed antibiotics

    c. Hyperbaric oxygen therapy

    d. Refer for vascular surgery consultation

15. A 70-year-old man with type 2 diabetes mellitus and distal symmetric polyneuropathy asks about driving safety. What advice should be given regarding driving with diabetic neuropathy?

    a. Avoid driving altogether

    b. Limit driving to daytime hours only

    c. Regularly check blood glucose before driving

    d. Inform the local Department of Motor Vehicles (DMV)

Diabetic Retinopathy

1. A 55-year-old man with type 2 diabetes presents for an eye examination. He reports no visual symptoms but has had diabetes for 15 years. Fundus examination reveals microaneurysms and dot-blot hemorrhages. What is the most likely diagnosis?

    a. Non-proliferative diabetic retinopathy (NPDR)

    b. Proliferative diabetic retinopathy (PDR)

    c. Diabetic macular edema (DME)

    d. Retinal vein occlusion

2. A 65-year-old woman with type 1 diabetes presents with complaints of blurry vision and difficulty reading. Fundus examination reveals yellow exudates and macular edema. What is the most likely diagnosis?

    a. Non-proliferative diabetic retinopathy (NPDR)

    b. Proliferative diabetic retinopathy (PDR)

    c. Diabetic macular edema (DME)

    d. Central retinal vein occlusion

3. A 50-year-old man with poorly controlled type 2 diabetes presents with sudden onset of floaters and visual field loss. Fundus examination reveals neovascularization, vitreous hemorrhage, and fibrous proliferation. What is the most likely diagnosis?

    a. Non-proliferative diabetic retinopathy (NPDR)

    b. Proliferative diabetic retinopathy (PDR)

    c. Diabetic macular edema (DME)

    d. Retinal detachment

4. A 45-year-old woman with type 2 diabetes presents for a routine eye examination. She reports no visual symptoms. Fundus examination reveals cotton wool spots and intraretinal hemorrhages. What is the most likely diagnosis?

   a. Non-proliferative diabetic retinopathy (NPDR)

   b. Proliferative diabetic retinopathy (PDR)

   c. Diabetic macular edema (DME)

   d. Central retinal vein occlusion

5. A 60-year-old man with type 1 diabetes presents with complaints of blurred vision and metamorphopsia. Fundus examination reveals yellowish deposits at the macula. Optical coherence tomography (OCT) shows cystoid spaces within the retina. What is the most likely diagnosis?

   a. Non-proliferative diabetic retinopathy (NPDR)

   b. Proliferative diabetic retinopathy (PDR)

   c. Diabetic macular edema (DME)

   d. Central serous chorioretinopathy

6. A 55-year-old woman with type 2 diabetes presents with sudden loss of vision in her left eye. Fundus examination shows retinal hemorrhages in all four quadrants, dilated and tortuous retinal veins, and cotton wool spots. What is the most likely diagnosis?

   a. Non-proliferative diabetic retinopathy (NPDR)

   b. Proliferative diabetic retinopathy (PDR)

   c. Central retinal vein occlusion (CRVO)

   d. Hypertensive retinopathy

7. A 65-year-old man with type 2 diabetes presents with complaints of blurred vision and difficulty seeing at night. Fundus examination reveals pale optic disc, narrowed arterioles, and scattered intraretinal hemorrhages. What is the most likely diagnosis?

    a. Non-proliferative diabetic retinopathy (NPDR)

    b. Proliferative diabetic retinopathy (PDR)

    c. Diabetic macular edema (DME)

    d. Retinal artery occlusion

8. A 50-year-old woman with type 1 diabetes presents with complaints of visual distortion and difficulty reading. Fundus examination reveals lipid exudates and cystoid macular edema. What is the most likely diagnosis?

    a. Non-proliferative diabetic retinopathy (NPDR)

    b. Proliferative diabetic retinopathy (PDR)

    c. Diabetic macular edema (DME)

    d. Central retinal vein occlusion

9. A 55-year-old man with type 2 diabetes presents with complaints of sudden visual loss in his right eye. Fundus examination shows a cherry-red spot at the macula, retinal edema, and segmented blood column in a retinal artery. What is the most likely diagnosis?

    a. Non-proliferative diabetic retinopathy (NPDR)

    b. Central retinal vein occlusion (CRVO)

    c. Central retinal artery occlusion (CRAO)

    d. Proliferative diabetic retinopathy (PDR)

10. A 60-year-old woman with type 2 diabetes presents with complaints of blurred vision and difficulty reading. Fundus examination reveals scattered cotton wool spots and hard exudates. What is the most likely diagnosis?

   a. Non-proliferative diabetic retinopathy (NPDR)

   b. Proliferative diabetic retinopathy (PDR)

   c. Diabetic macular edema (DME)

   d. Branch retinal vein occlusion

11. A 65-year-old man with type 2 diabetes presents with complaints of sudden onset of floaters and decreased vision in his left eye. Fundus examination reveals vitreous hemorrhage and fibrovascular proliferation. What is the most likely diagnosis?

   a. Non-proliferative diabetic retinopathy (NPDR)

   b. Proliferative diabetic retinopathy (PDR)

   c. Central retinal vein occlusion (CRVO)

   d. Retinal detachment

12. A 55-year-old woman with type 2 diabetes presents with complaints of blurry vision and metamorphopsia. Fundus examination reveals yellowish deposits at the macula and cystoid macular edema. What is the most likely diagnosis?

   a. Non-proliferative diabetic retinopathy (NPDR)

   b. Proliferative diabetic retinopathy (PDR)

   c. Diabetic macular edema (DME)

   d. Central serous chorioretinopathy

13. A 60-year-old man with type 1 diabetes presents with complaints of sudden onset of visual field loss and floaters in his right eye. Fundus examination reveals neovascularization, vitreous hemorrhage, and fibrous proliferation. What is the most likely diagnosis?

   a. Non-proliferative diabetic retinopathy (NPDR)

   b. Proliferative diabetic retinopathy (PDR)

   c. Central retinal vein occlusion (CRVO)

   d. Retinal detachment

14. A 45-year-old man with type 2 diabetes presents for an eye examination. He reports no visual symptoms. Fundus examination reveals microaneurysms, intraretinal hemorrhages, and cotton wool spots. What is the most likely diagnosis?

   a. Non-proliferative diabetic retinopathy (NPDR)

   b. Proliferative diabetic retinopathy (PDR)

   c. Diabetic macular edema (DME)

   d. Retinal vein occlusion

15. A 55-year-old woman with type 1 diabetes presents with complaints of blurred vision and difficulty reading. Fundus examination reveals lipid exudates and cystoid macular edema. What is the most likely diagnosis?

   a. Non-proliferative diabetic retinopathy (NPDR)

   b. Proliferative diabetic retinopathy (PDR)

   c. Diabetic macular edema (DME)

   d. Central retinal vein occlusion

Dyslipidemia

1. A 55-year-old man presents with chest pain and is found to have elevated cholesterol levels on routine blood work. His total cholesterol is 280 mg/dL, LDL cholesterol is 190 mg/dL, HDL cholesterol is 40 mg/dL, and triglycerides are 150 mg/dL. What is the most appropriate initial management?

   a. Initiate high-intensity statin therapy

   b. Start fibrate therapy

   c. Begin combination therapy with a statin and ezetimibe

   d. Recommend lifestyle modifications and recheck lipid levels in 3 months

2. A 65-year-old woman with type 2 diabetes and hypertension presents for a routine follow-up. Her lipid profile shows total cholesterol of 250 mg/dL, LDL cholesterol of 180 mg/dL, HDL cholesterol of 35 mg/dL, and triglycerides of 200 mg/dL. She has no history of cardiovascular disease. What is the most appropriate next step?

   a. Start high-intensity statin therapy

   b. Add ezetimibe to her current therapy

   c. Initiate fibrate therapy

   d. Focus on lifestyle modifications and repeat lipid panel in 3 months

3. A 50-year-old man presents with acute pancreatitis. His lipid profile reveals total cholesterol of 300 mg/dL, LDL cholesterol of 200 mg/dL, HDL cholesterol of 30 mg/dL, and triglycerides of 500 mg/dL. What is the most appropriate initial management?

   a. Start high-intensity statin therapy

   b. Initiate fibrate therapy

   c. Recommend lifestyle modifications and recheck lipid levels in 6 months

   d. Start omega-3 fatty acid supplementation

4. A 45-year-old woman with a family history of premature coronary artery disease presents for a routine check-up. Her lipid profile shows total cholesterol of 220 mg/dL, LDL cholesterol of 150 mg/dL, HDL cholesterol of 45 mg/dL, and triglycerides of 120 mg/dL. What is the most appropriate next step?

   a.   Initiate moderate-intensity statin therapy

   b.   Add ezetimibe to her current therapy

   c.   Start fibrate therapy

   d.   Recommend lifestyle modifications and annual lipid panel checks

5.   A 60-year-old man with known coronary artery disease presents for follow-up. His current lipid profile reveals total cholesterol of 180 mg/dL, LDL cholesterol of 100 mg/dL, HDL cholesterol of 30 mg/dL, and triglycerides of 150 mg/dL. He is currently on atorvastatin 40 mg daily. What is the most appropriate next step?

   a.   Increase atorvastatin dose to 80 mg daily

   b.   Add ezetimibe to his current therapy

   c.   Start fibrate therapy

   d.   Continue current therapy and reassess in 6 months

6.   A 55-year-old man with type 2 diabetes presents for an annual check-up. His lipid profile shows total cholesterol of 240 mg/dL, LDL cholesterol of 160 mg/dL, HDL cholesterol of 30 mg/dL, and triglycerides of 200 mg/dL. He is currently on metformin and lisinopril. What is the most appropriate initial management?

   a.   Start high-intensity statin therapy

   b.   Add ezetimibe to his current therapy

   c.   Initiate fibrate therapy

   d.   Recommend lifestyle modifications and recheck lipid levels in 3 months

7. A 65-year-old woman presents with xanthomas on her Achilles tendons and eyelids. Her lipid profile reveals total cholesterol of 400 mg/dL, LDL cholesterol of 300 mg/dL, HDL cholesterol of 40 mg/dL, and triglycerides of 150 mg/dL. What is the most likely underlying cause of her lipid disorder?

    a. Familial hypercholesterolemia (FH)

    b. Mixed hyperlipidemia

    c. Secondary hyperlipidemia due to diabetes

    d. Drug-induced hyperlipidemia

8. A 50-year-old man presents with recurrent episodes of abdominal pain after meals. His lipid profile shows total cholesterol of 250 mg/dL, LDL cholesterol of 180 mg/dL, HDL cholesterol of 35 mg/dL, and triglycerides of 200 mg/dL. What is the most appropriate next step?

    a. Initiate high-intensity statin therapy

    b. Add ezetimibe to his current therapy

    c. Start fibrate therapy

    d. Evaluate for familial chylomicronemia syndrome

9. A 55-year-old woman with rheumatoid arthritis presents for a routine check-up. Her lipid profile shows total cholesterol of 220 mg/dL, LDL cholesterol of 150 mg/dL, HDL cholesterol of 40 mg/dL, and triglycerides of 100 mg/dL. She is currently on methotrexate and prednisone. What is the most appropriate initial management?

    a. Start moderate-intensity statin therapy

    b. Add ezetimibe to her current therapy

    c. Initiate fibrate therapy

    d. Recommend lifestyle modifications and recheck lipid levels in 6 months

10. A 60-year-old man presents with exertional chest pain. His lipid profile reveals total cholesterol of 280 mg/dL, LDL cholesterol of 200 mg/dL, HDL cholesterol of 30 mg/dL, and triglycerides of 150 mg/dL. He has a history of smoking and hypertension. What is the most appropriate next step?

    a. Initiate high-intensity statin therapy

    b. Add ezetimibe to his current therapy

    c. Start fibrate therapy

    d. Recommend lifestyle modifications and recheck lipid levels in 3 months

11. A 65-year-old woman presents with intermittent claudication. Her lipid profile shows total cholesterol of 240 mg/dL, LDL cholesterol of 160 mg/dL, HDL cholesterol of 30 mg/dL, and triglycerides of 200 mg/dL. She has a history of hypertension and peripheral arterial disease. What is the most appropriate next step?

    a. Start high-intensity statin therapy

    b. Add ezetimibe to her current therapy

    c. Initiate fibrate therapy

    d. Recommend lifestyle modifications and recheck lipid levels in 6 months

12. A 50-year-old man with type 2 diabetes presents for an annual check-up. His lipid profile shows total cholesterol of 240 mg/dL, LDL cholesterol of 150 mg/dL, HDL cholesterol of 35 mg/dL, and triglycerides of 200 mg/dL. He is currently on metformin and lisinopril. What is the most appropriate initial management?

    a. Start moderate-intensity statin therapy

    b. Add ezetimibe to his current therapy

    c. Initiate fibrate therapy

    d. Recommend lifestyle modifications and recheck lipid levels in 3 months

13. A 45-year-old man presents with xanthomas on his Achilles tendons and eyelids. His lipid profile reveals total cholesterol of 400 mg/dL, LDL cholesterol of 300 mg/dL, HDL cholesterol of 40 mg/dL, and triglycerides of 150 mg/dL. What is the most likely underlying cause of his lipid disorder?

    a. Familial hypercholesterolemia (FH)

    b. Mixed hyperlipidemia

    c. Secondary hyperlipidemia due to diabetes

    d. Drug-induced hyperlipidemia

14. A 55-year-old man with obesity and metabolic syndrome presents for a routine check-up. His lipid profile shows total cholesterol of 240 mg/dL, LDL cholesterol of 160 mg/dL, HDL cholesterol of 30 mg/dL, and triglycerides of 200 mg/dL. What is the most appropriate next step?

    a. Initiate high-intensity statin therapy

    b. Add ezetimibe to his current therapy

    c. Start fibrate therapy

    d. Recommend lifestyle modifications and recheck lipid levels in 6 months

15. A 60-year-old man with known coronary artery disease presents for follow-up. His current lipid profile reveals total cholesterol of 180 mg/dL, LDL cholesterol of 100 mg/dL, HDL cholesterol of 30 mg/dL, and triglycerides of 150 mg/dL. He is currently on atorvastatin 40 mg daily. What is the most appropriate next step?

    a. Increase atorvastatin dose to 80 mg daily

    b. Add ezetimibe to his current therapy

    c. Start fibrate therapy

    d. Continue current therapy and reassess in 6 months

Eczema

1. A 6-month-old infant presents with red, dry, and itchy patches on the cheeks and extensor surfaces of the arms and legs. The mother reports a family history of allergies. What is the most likely diagnosis?

   a. Contact dermatitis

   b. Seborrheic dermatitis

   c. Atopic dermatitis

   d. Psoriasis

2. A 25-year-old woman with a history of atopic dermatitis notices worsening of her symptoms after using scented body lotion. Which allergen is most likely exacerbating her eczema?

   a. Nickel

   b. Fragrances

   c. Latex

   d. Rubber

3. A 40-year-old man presents with chronic, itchy, scaly patches on his elbows and knees. He denies personal or family history of allergies. What is the most likely diagnosis?

   a. Atopic dermatitis

   b. Psoriasis

   c. Contact dermatitis

   d. Seborrheic dermatitis

4. A 30-year-old woman with atopic dermatitis experiences a sudden exacerbation of her symptoms with intense pruritus and erythematous patches. What is the first-line treatment for this acute flare-up?

   a. Topical corticosteroids

   b. Topical calcineurin inhibitors

   c. Oral antihistamines

   d. Moisturizers

5. A 45-year-old man with atopic dermatitis has persistent dry, scaly skin despite using emollients regularly. What additional therapy is most appropriate for his chronic eczema?

    a. Oral antihistamines

    b. Topical calcineurin inhibitors

    c. Systemic corticosteroids

    d. Phototherapy

6. A 4-year-old child presents with eczematous lesions mainly on the flexural areas (antecubital and popliteal fossae) and neck folds. What is a common complication associated with this type of eczema?

    a. Superinfection with Staphylococcus aureus

    b. Contact dermatitis from clothing

    c. Allergic reaction to food

    d. Autoimmune thyroiditis

7. A 35-year-old woman with atopic dermatitis asks about strategies to improve her skin barrier function. What recommendation is most appropriate?

    a. Apply emollients immediately after bathing

    b. Use hot water for bathing

    c. Avoid moisturizers with humectants

    d. Apply topical antifungal creams

8. A 28-year-old man with atopic dermatitis wonders if his diet affects his skin condition. What dietary recommendation is supported by evidence in managing eczema?

    a. Gluten-free diet

    b. Low-fat diet

    c. Elimination diet guided by allergy testing

    d. High-protein diet

9. A 40-year-old woman with chronic atopic dermatitis reports feeling embarrassed and self-conscious due to her skin condition. What intervention is most appropriate to address the psychosocial impact of eczema?

   a. Referral to a dermatologist

   b. Cognitive behavioral therapy (CBT)

   c. Start systemic corticosteroids

   d. Increase topical corticosteroid potency

10. A 32-year-old nurse develops eczematous lesions on her hands after frequent handwashing and glove use at work. What is the most appropriate management strategy?

   a. Use latex-free gloves

   b. Apply potent topical corticosteroids

   c. Avoid handwashing and glove use

   d. Moisturize hands with emollients regularly

11. A 50-year-old man with chronic atopic dermatitis experiences severe pruritus despite using topical corticosteroids. What medication is effective in managing refractory eczema-related pruritus?

   a. Oral antihistamines

   b. Topical calcineurin inhibitors

   c. Oral corticosteroids

   d. Phototherapy

12. A 30-year-old woman with atopic dermatitis asks if exercise affects her skin condition. What advice should be given regarding exercise in eczema management?

   a. Avoid exercise to prevent sweating

   b. Perform high-intensity exercise regularly

   c. Shower immediately after exercise

   d. Use topical corticosteroids before exercise

13. A 35-year-old woman with atopic dermatitis wants to reduce exposure to allergens that worsen her eczema. What environmental allergen is commonly associated with exacerbating eczema symptoms?

    a. Pollen

    b. Dust mites

    c. Pet dander

    d. Mold spores

14. A 40-year-old man with atopic dermatitis asks if sunlight exposure can improve his skin condition. What advice should be given regarding sun exposure in eczema management?

    a. Avoid sun exposure to prevent flare-ups

    b. Use sunscreen with high SPF daily

    c. Sunbathe for 30 minutes daily

    d. Apply topical corticosteroids before sun exposure

15. A 28-year-old pregnant woman with atopic dermatitis seeks advice on managing her eczema during pregnancy. What topical medication is considered safe for eczema treatment during pregnancy?

    a. High-potency topical corticosteroids

    b. Topical calcineurin inhibitors

    c. Coal tar preparations

    d. Salicylic acid creams

Epilepsy

1. A 25-year-old male presents to the emergency room with witnessed tonic-clonic seizures lasting 3 minutes. He has no history of seizures. Vital signs are stable postictally. What is the next step in management?

    a. Initiate antiepileptic drug (AED) therapy

    b. Perform EEG immediately

    c. Order brain MRI

    d. Discharge home with outpatient follow-up

2. A 35-year-old woman with epilepsy is stable on phenytoin therapy. She presents with complaints of double vision and unsteady gait. Neurological examination reveals nystagmus and ataxia. What is the most likely cause?

    a. Phenytoin toxicity

    b. Seizure aura

    c. Migraine headache

    d. Stress-related symptoms

3. Which of the following is a common trigger for seizures in patients with epilepsy?

    a. Regular sleep pattern

    b. Exercise

    c. Stress

    d. Antiepileptic medications

4. A 50-year-old man with epilepsy presents with breakthrough seizures despite taking carbamazepine regularly. Serum drug levels are within therapeutic range. What is the next step in management?

    a. Increase the dose of carbamazepine

    b. Switch to phenytoin

    c. Add another antiepileptic drug

    d. Discontinue carbamazepine and monitor

5. A 30-year-old pregnant woman with epilepsy is planning to conceive. Which antiepileptic drug is associated with the highest risk of neural tube defects in the fetus?

    a. Levetiracetam

    b. Lamotrigine

    c. Valproate

    d. Topiramate

6. A 45-year-old man with epilepsy presents with episodes of sudden, brief loss of awareness associated with chewing movements. What is the most likely type of seizure?

    a. Tonic-clonic seizure

    b. Absence seizure

    c. Simple partial seizure

    d. Complex partial seizure

7. A 20-year-old woman with epilepsy is started on lamotrigine. She develops a rash after a few days of therapy. What is the most appropriate management?

    a. Continue lamotrigine with close monitoring

    b. Discontinue lamotrigine and switch to levetiracetam

    c. Decrease the dose of lamotrigine

    d. Add topical corticosteroids to treat the rash

8. A 55-year-old man with epilepsy presents with new-onset confusion and agitation. His wife reports that he has been non-compliant with his antiepileptic medication. What is the most likely cause of his symptoms?

    a. Postictal state

    b. Status epilepticus

    c. Antiepileptic drug withdrawal

    d. Psychiatric illness

9. Which antiepileptic drug is considered first-line for the treatment of absence seizures?

    a. Phenytoin

    b. Carbamazepine

    c. Valproate

    d. Gabapentin

10. A 40-year-old man with epilepsy presents with sudden jerking movements of the limbs, followed by loss of consciousness and tonic-clonic movements. What is the most likely type of seizure?

    a. Myoclonic seizure

    b. Tonic seizure

    c. Absence seizure

    d. Tonic-clonic seizure

11. A 30-year-old woman with epilepsy is planning to become pregnant. She is currently on carbamazepine. What is the most appropriate counseling regarding antiepileptic drugs during pregnancy?

    a. Carbamazepine should be continued throughout pregnancy.

    b. Antiepileptic drugs should be avoided during pregnancy.

    c. Consider switching to valproate due to its effectiveness.

    d. Discuss potential risks and benefits with a healthcare provider.

12. A 50-year-old man with epilepsy presents with recurrent episodes of sudden loss of awareness, lip smacking, and automatisms. What is the most appropriate initial diagnostic test?

    a. EEG

    b. Brain MRI

    c. Lumbar puncture

    d. Serum drug levels

13. A 25-year-old woman with epilepsy experiences breakthrough seizures despite adherence to antiepileptic medications. What additional investigation is warranted?

    a. Brain MRI

    b. Routine blood tests

    c. Neuropsychological testing

    d. Genetic testing

14. A 35-year-old man with epilepsy is started on topiramate. He complains of difficulty concentrating and word-finding difficulties. What is the most likely cause?

    a. Seizure aura

    b. Psychiatric illness

    c. Topiramate side effects

    d. Underlying brain tumor

15. A 60-year-old woman with epilepsy develops a rash and fever after starting a new antiepileptic drug. What is the most concerning complication?

    a. Drug-induced hepatitis

    b. Hypersensitivity syndrome

    c. Peripheral neuropathy

    d. Cardiac arrhythmia

Erectile Dysfunction

1. A 55-year-old man presents with complaints of difficulty maintaining an erection for the past six months. He has a history of hypertension and is on antihypertensive medication. What is the most likely cause of his erectile dysfunction?

    a. Psychological factors

    b. Hypertension

    c. Medication side effects

    d. Diabetes

2. A 45-year-old male reports experiencing erectile dysfunction. He has been under significant stress at work and recently went through a divorce. What is the most likely cause of his erectile dysfunction?

    a. Cardiovascular disease

    b. Psychological factors

    c. Neurological disorder

    d. Prostate cancer

3. A 60-year-old man with a history of type 2 diabetes presents with erectile dysfunction. His blood sugar levels are poorly controlled. What is the most likely cause of his erectile dysfunction?

    a. Neuropathy

    b. Testosterone deficiency

    c. Psychological factors

    d. Venous leak

4. A 50-year-old man with erectile dysfunction is found to have low serum testosterone levels. What is the most appropriate next step in management?

    a. Start oral PDE-5 inhibitors

    b. Refer to a psychologist

    c. Start testosterone replacement therapy

    d. Advise lifestyle modifications

5. A 65-year-old man complains of erectile dysfunction. He is a heavy smoker and has a 40-pack-year smoking history. What lifestyle change could most likely improve his erectile dysfunction?

    a. Reduce alcohol intake

    b. Exercise regularly

    c. Quit smoking

    d. Reduce salt intake

6. A 38-year-old man presents with erectile dysfunction. He has no significant medical history but consumes alcohol heavily on weekends. What is the most likely cause of his erectile dysfunction?

    a. Cardiovascular disease

    b. Neuropathy

    c. Alcohol consumption

    d. Prostate cancer

7. A 70-year-old man presents with a gradual onset of erectile dysfunction. He also reports a decrease in libido and muscle mass. What is the most likely diagnosis?

    a. Hypogonadism

    b. Peyronie's disease

    c. Prostatitis

    d. Venous leak

8. A 52-year-old man with erectile dysfunction has a family history of cardiovascular disease. He reports chest pain on exertion. What is the most appropriate initial investigation?

    a. Penile Doppler ultrasound

    b. Lipid profile

    c. Exercise stress test

    d. No further investigation needed

9. A 48-year-old man with a history of prostate cancer treatment reports erectile dysfunction. What is the most likely cause of his erectile dysfunction?

    a. Neurological damage

    b. Psychological factors

    c. Radiation therapy

    d. Infection

10. A 30-year-old man complains of erectile dysfunction. He uses recreational drugs, including cocaine, regularly. What is the most likely cause of his erectile dysfunction?

    a. Endocrine disorders

    b. Drug use

    c. Depression

    d. Trauma

11. A 63-year-old man with erectile dysfunction is found to have a firm, fibrous plaque on the shaft of his penis. What is the most likely diagnosis?

    a. Peyronie's disease

    b. Penile cancer

    c. Phimosis

    d. Balanitis

12. A 55-year-old man reports erectile dysfunction and nocturia. He is diagnosed with benign prostatic hyperplasia (BPH). Which medication used to treat BPH could also help with his erectile dysfunction?

    a. Tamsulosin

    b. Finasteride

    c. Dutasteride

    d. Tadalafil

13. A 40-year-old man presents with sudden onset of erectile dysfunction. He has no medical history but reports a recent pelvic injury. What is the most likely cause of his erectile dysfunction?

    a. Psychological factors

    b. Vascular injury

    c. Endocrine disorder

    d. Neurological injury

14. A 60-year-old man with erectile dysfunction is found to have high blood pressure and hyperlipidemia. What is the most appropriate first-line treatment for his erectile dysfunction?

    a. Lifestyle modifications

    b. Oral PDE-5 inhibitors

    c. Testosterone replacement therapy

    d. Penile implants

15. A 35-year-old man presents with erectile dysfunction. He reports that he has morning erections but struggles to maintain an erection during intercourse. What is the most likely cause of his erectile dysfunction?

    a. Psychological factors

    b. Vascular disease

    c. Neurological disorder

    d. Hormonal imbalance

Fibromyalgia

1. A 45-year-old woman presents with widespread musculoskeletal pain, fatigue, and sleep disturbances for the past 6 months. She has a history of depression and anxiety. Physical examination reveals tenderness in multiple soft tissue areas. Which of the following is the most likely diagnosis?

    a. Rheumatoid arthritis

    b. Osteoarthritis

    c. Fibromyalgia

    d. Systemic lupus erythematosus

2. A 37-year-old man complains of chronic pain all over his body for the last year. He reports feeling tired all the time despite adequate sleep. His medical history includes irritable bowel syndrome. Which of the following is most likely to be elevated in this patient?

    a. Erythrocyte sedimentation rate (ESR)

    b. C-reactive protein (CRP)

    c. Antinuclear antibody (ANA)

    d. None of the above

3. A 50-year-old female with a history of fibromyalgia is seeking advice on managing her symptoms. Which of the following lifestyle modifications is recommended?

    a. Strict bed rest

    b. High-intensity interval training

    c. Regular low-impact aerobic exercise

    d. Avoidance of all physical activity

4. A patient diagnosed with fibromyalgia is experiencing significant sleep disturbances. Which of the following medications is commonly used to help with sleep in fibromyalgia patients?

    a. Metformin

    b. Amitriptyline

    c. Prednisone

    d. Methotrexate

5. A 42-year-old woman with fibromyalgia reports severe fatigue and cognitive difficulties often referred to as "fibro fog." Which of the following treatments is likely to be helpful?

    a. Glucocorticoids

    b. Opioids

    c. Cognitive-behavioral therapy (CBT)

    d. Chemotherapy

6. A patient with fibromyalgia asks about the role of diet in managing her symptoms. Which of the following dietary modifications may be beneficial?

    a. High-fat, low-carbohydrate diet

    b. Elimination of gluten and processed foods

    c. High-protein diet

    d. No specific dietary modifications are needed

7. A 55-year-old male with fibromyalgia presents with worsening pain despite pharmacological treatment. Which of the following non-pharmacological therapies might be beneficial?

    a. Transcutaneous electrical nerve stimulation (TENS)

    b. Radiation therapy

    c. Intravenous immunoglobulin (IVIG)

    d. Bone marrow transplant

8. A patient with fibromyalgia reports that her symptoms worsen with stress. Which of the following is an effective stress management technique?

    a. Ignoring the stress

    b. Yoga and mindfulness meditation

    c. Increased workload

    d. High doses of caffeine

9. A 30-year-old woman with fibromyalgia is concerned about her ability to work. Which of the following work accommodations might be beneficial?

    a. Extended periods of sitting without breaks

    b. Ergonomic workstation adjustments

    c. Increased workload

    d. No accommodations needed

10. A patient with fibromyalgia is exploring complementary therapies. Which of the following has shown some evidence of benefit in fibromyalgia?

    a. Aromatherapy

    b. Acupuncture

    c. Cryotherapy

    d. Homeopathy

11. A 47-year-old woman with fibromyalgia is experiencing depression. Which of the following medications might be helpful in treating both her fibromyalgia symptoms and depression?

    a. Duloxetine

    b. Alendronate

    c. Levothyroxine

    d. Simvastatin

12. A patient with fibromyalgia is experiencing severe morning stiffness. Which of the following interventions can help reduce morning stiffness?

    a. Drinking coffee immediately upon waking

    b. Gentle stretching exercises before getting out of bed

    c. Skipping breakfast

    d. Taking a cold shower

13. A 60-year-old male with fibromyalgia has developed gastrointestinal symptoms. Which of the following is a common comorbid condition in fibromyalgia that could explain his symptoms?

    a. Crohn's disease

    b. Irritable bowel syndrome (IBS)

    c. Peptic ulcer disease

    d. Celiac disease

14. A patient with fibromyalgia is interested in taking supplements to manage her symptoms. Which of the following supplements has some evidence supporting its use in fibromyalgia?

    a. Vitamin C

    b. Magnesium

    c. Iron

    d. Potassium

15. A 35-year-old woman with fibromyalgia reports experiencing frequent headaches. Which type of headache is commonly associated with fibromyalgia?

    a. Tension-type headaches

    b. Cluster headaches

    c. Migraine headaches

    d. Sinus headaches

Gastritis

1. A 35-year-old woman presents with burning epigastric pain that worsens after meals and improves with antacids. She reports occasional use of nonsteroidal anti-inflammatory drugs (NSAIDs). What is the most likely cause of her symptoms?

    a. Helicobacter pylori infection

    b. Autoimmune gastritis

    c. NSAID-induced gastritis

    d. Bile reflux gastritis

2. A 50-year-old man presents with nausea, vomiting, and epigastric pain that is relieved by eating. He has a history of heavy alcohol use. What is the most likely cause of his symptoms?

    a. Autoimmune gastritis

    b. Helicobacter pylori infection

    c. Alcohol-induced gastritis

    d. Chronic stress gastritis

3. A 45-year-old woman presents with epigastric pain, bloating, and early satiety. She has a history of pernicious anemia. What is the most likely cause of her symptoms?

    a. Helicobacter pylori infection

    b. Autoimmune gastritis

    c. NSAID-induced gastritis

    d. Reflux esophagitis

4. A 60-year-old man presents with epigastric pain and dark, tarry stools. He has a history of chronic renal failure and is on multiple medications. What is the most likely cause of his symptoms?

    a. Stress-related gastritis

    b. Helicobacter pylori infection

    c. Peptic ulcer disease

    d. Gastric erosions due to medication

5. A 55-year-old woman presents with epigastric pain and bloating. She reports a history of frequent use of aspirin for chronic headaches. What is the most appropriate initial step in management?

    a. Start proton pump inhibitor (PPI) therapy

    b. Perform upper endoscopy

    c. Test for Helicobacter pylori infection

    d. Discontinue aspirin

6. A 40-year-old man presents with epigastric pain and a history of untreated Helicobacter pylori infection. Which of the following is the most appropriate initial diagnostic test?

    a. Upper endoscopy with biopsy

    b. Serologic testing for H. pylori antibodies

    c. Urea breath test

    d. Stool antigen test for H. pylori

7. A 65-year-old woman presents with recurrent episodes of epigastric pain that worsen at night and are relieved by eating. She has a history of peptic ulcer disease. What is the most likely cause of her symptoms?

    a. Chronic stress gastritis

    b. NSAID-induced gastritis

    c. Reflux esophagitis

    d. Duodenitis

8. A 55-year-old man presents with epigastric pain and hematemesis. He has a history of chronic alcohol use. What is the most likely cause of his symptoms?

    a. Autoimmune gastritis

    b. Mallory-Weiss tear

    c. Peptic ulcer disease

    d. Alcoholic gastritis

9. A 50-year-old woman presents with epigastric pain that worsens with spicy foods. She denies NSAID use and has no significant medical history. What is the most likely cause of her symptoms?

    a. Helicobacter pylori infection

    b. Autoimmune gastritis

    c. Food allergy gastritis

    d. Eosinophilic gastritis

10. A 60-year-old man presents with epigastric pain, nausea, and unintentional weight loss. He has a history of chronic NSAID use for arthritis. What is the most likely cause of his symptoms?

    a. Autoimmune gastritis

    b. Peptic ulcer disease

    c. NSAID-induced gastritis

    d. Gastroesophageal reflux disease (GERD)

11. A 45-year-old woman presents with epigastric pain and nausea. She is a strict vegetarian and avoids all animal products. What is the most likely cause of her symptoms?

    a. Helicobacter pylori infection

    b. Autoimmune gastritis

    c. B12 deficiency gastritis

    d. Non-ulcer dyspepsia

12. A 55-year-old man presents with epigastric pain and coffee-ground emesis. He has a history of chronic NSAID use for osteoarthritis. What is the most likely cause of his symptoms?

    a. Peptic ulcer disease

    b. Gastric erosions due to NSAIDs

    c. Alcoholic gastritis

    d. Autoimmune gastritis

13. A 50-year-old woman presents with epigastric pain that worsens with stress. She has no significant medical history and denies NSAID use. What is the most likely cause of her symptoms?

    a. Autoimmune gastritis

    b. Chronic stress gastritis

    c. H. pylori infection

    d. GERD

14. A 65-year-old man presents with epigastric pain and black, tarry stools. He has a history of chronic NSAID use. What is the most likely cause of his symptoms?

    a. Peptic ulcer disease

    b. Esophageal varices

    c. Gastric erosions due to NSAIDs

    d. Mallory-Weiss tear

15. A 60-year-old woman presents with epigastric pain, bloating, and early satiety. She has a history of autoimmune thyroid disease. What is the most likely cause of her symptoms?

    a. H. pylori infection

    b. Autoimmune gastritis

    c. NSAID-induced gastritis

    d. Functional dyspepsia

Gastroesophageal Reflux Disease (GERD)

1. John, a 45-year-old man, presents with a burning sensation in his chest that worsens after meals and when lying down. He occasionally experiences regurgitation of sour-tasting fluid into his mouth. What is the most likely diagnosis?

   a. Peptic ulcer disease

   b. Gastroesophageal reflux disease (GERD)

   c. Esophageal cancer

   d. Gastritis

2. Emily, a 30-year-old woman, presents with a chronic cough, hoarseness, and throat clearing. She also complains of a sensation of a lump in her throat (globus sensation). What condition is most likely causing her symptoms?

   a. Allergic rhinitis

   b. Asthma

   c. Gastroesophageal reflux disease (GERD)

   d. Bronchitis

3. David, a 50-year-old man, presents with recurrent episodes of heartburn and regurgitation of sour fluid into his mouth, especially after meals and at night. He has been self-medicating with antacids for relief. What is the initial management approach?

   a. Prescription of proton pump inhibitors (PPIs)

   b. Referral for endoscopy

   c. Lifestyle modifications

   d. H2-receptor antagonists

4. Sarah, a 35-year-old woman, presents with severe, persistent heartburn that does not respond to lifestyle modifications or antacids. What is the next step in management?

    a. Initiate treatment with H2-receptor antagonists

    b. Refer for surgical consultation

    c. Prescribe proton pump inhibitors (PPIs)

    d. Perform upper endoscopy

5. James, a 40-year-old man, presents with symptoms of GERD refractory to PPI therapy. He experiences heartburn, regurgitation, and difficulty swallowing solids. What is the next appropriate step in management?

    a. Increase the dose of PPI

    b. Add prokinetic therapy

    c. Perform esophageal manometry

    d. Refer for pH monitoring

6. Jessica, a 25-year-old woman, presents with chronic GERD symptoms and a history of asthma. She has noticed worsening of her asthma symptoms recently. What is the likely explanation for this association?

    a. Allergic reaction to PPI therapy

    b. Gastroesophageal reflux causing bronchospasm

    c. Anxiety exacerbating GERD symptoms

    d. Chronic sinusitis leading to post-nasal drip

7. Anna, a 55-year-old woman, presents with persistent GERD symptoms and reports difficulty swallowing solid foods. She also experiences weight loss and occasional chest pain. What condition should be considered in her differential diagnosis?

    a. Eosinophilic esophagitis

    b. Barrett's esophagus

    c. Hiatal hernia

    d. Achalasia

8. Daniel, a 60-year-old man, presents with severe, longstanding GERD symptoms despite optimal medical therapy. He is concerned about the risks of long-term PPI use. What is a potential complication of chronic PPI use?

   a. Osteoporosis

   b. Iron-deficiency anemia

   c. Hypertension

   d. Hyperkalemia

9. Sophie, a 30-year-old woman, presents with GERD symptoms that worsen when she lies down at night. What is the most appropriate lifestyle modification to recommend?

   a. Avoiding spicy foods

   b. Eating smaller, more frequent meals

   c. Taking antacids before bedtime

   d. Elevating the head of the bed

10. Lucas, a 50-year-old man, presents with chronic GERD symptoms despite taking PPIs. He is concerned about the risk of esophageal cancer due to his longstanding symptoms. What is a premalignant condition associated with chronic GERD?

   a. Barrett's esophagus

   b. Esophageal stricture

   c. Zenker's diverticulum

   d. Mallory-Weiss tear

11. Rachel, a 45-year-old woman, presents with heartburn and regurgitation. She has been taking PPIs for the past 3 months with partial relief. What diagnostic test is recommended to evaluate the extent of esophageal damage?

    a. Upper endoscopy

    b. Barium swallow

    c. Esophageal manometry

    d. pH monitoring

12. David, a 55-year-old man, presents with severe GERD symptoms and reports a family history of esophageal cancer. What is an appropriate surveillance strategy for him?

    a. Annual upper endoscopy

    b. Biennial pH monitoring

    c. Biopsy of Barrett's esophagus every 5 years

    d. Surveillance endoscopy every 3 years

13. Sarah, a 40-year-old woman, presents with chronic GERD symptoms and persistent esophageal pain. She reports a history of NSAID use for arthritis. What is the likely cause of her symptoms?

    a. Esophageal stricture

    b. Mallory-Weiss tear

    c. Eosinophilic esophagitis

    d. NSAID-induced esophagitis

14. Jessica, a 35-year-old woman, presents with chronic GERD symptoms and dysphagia to solids. She has a history of atopic conditions. What diagnostic test is recommended to evaluate her symptoms?

    a. pH monitoring

    b. Esophageal manometry

    c. Barium swallow

    d. Upper endoscopy with biopsy

15. Anna, a 50-year-old woman, presents with severe GERD symptoms despite high-dose PPI therapy. She is interested in surgical options for definitive management. What surgical procedure is commonly performed for severe GERD?

    a. Nissen fundoplication

    b. Roux-en-Y gastric bypass

    c. Endoscopic mucosal resection

    d. Heller myotomy

Glaucoma

1. A 60-year-old male presents with gradual loss of peripheral vision in both eyes over several months. Intraocular pressure (IOP) is 26 mmHg in the right eye and 25 mmHg in the left eye. Gonioscopy reveals an open angle with normal appearing optic discs. What is the most likely diagnosis?

   a. Primary open-angle glaucoma

   b. Acute angle-closure glaucoma

   c. Normal-tension glaucoma

   d. Secondary glaucoma

2. A 45-year-old female presents with sudden onset severe eye pain, blurred vision, halos around lights, and nausea. On examination, the affected eye is red with a cloudy cornea, fixed mid-dilated pupil, and IOP of 50 mmHg. What is the most likely diagnosis?

   a. Primary open-angle glaucoma

   b. Acute angle-closure glaucoma

   c. Normal-tension glaucoma

   d. Secondary glaucoma

3. A 55-year-old male with a family history of glaucoma presents for a routine eye examination. IOP is 22 mmHg in both eyes. Optic disc examination reveals cup-to-disc ratio of 0.8 with notching and thinning of the neuroretinal rim. What is the most likely diagnosis?

   a. Primary open-angle glaucoma

   b. Acute angle-closure glaucoma

   c. Normal-tension glaucoma

   d. Secondary glaucoma

4. A 65-year-old female with controlled hypertension presents with bilateral gradual loss of peripheral vision. IOP is consistently 14 mmHg in both eyes. Optic discs show characteristic cupping with a cup-to-disc ratio of 0.7 in each eye. What is the most likely diagnosis?

    a. Primary open-angle glaucoma

    b. Acute angle-closure glaucoma

    c. Normal-tension glaucoma

    d. Secondary glaucoma

5. A 50-year-old male with diabetes mellitus presents with elevated IOP (30 mmHg) in both eyes during a routine eye examination. Optic discs show increased cupping with a cup-to-disc ratio of 0.6 in each eye. What is the most likely diagnosis?

    a. Primary open-angle glaucoma

    b. Acute angle-closure glaucoma

    c. Normal-tension glaucoma

    d. Secondary glaucoma

6. A 70-year-old female presents with difficulty seeing in dim lighting and noticing halos around lights. She denies eye pain or redness. IOP is 15 mmHg in both eyes. Pupils are equal and reactive without afferent pupillary defect. What is the most likely diagnosis?

    a. Primary open-angle glaucoma

    b. Acute angle-closure glaucoma

    c. Normal-tension glaucoma

    d. Secondary glaucoma

7. A 55-year-old male with a history of trauma to his left eye presents with chronic eye pain and decreased vision in that eye. IOP is 18 mmHg in the left eye and 15 mmHg in the right eye. Optic disc examination shows vertical elongation and optic nerve head cupping. What is the most likely diagnosis?

    a. Primary open-angle glaucoma

    b. Acute angle-closure glaucoma

    c. Normal-tension glaucoma

    d. Secondary glaucoma

8. A 60-year-old female presents with difficulty reading and blurred vision in both eyes. She has a history of hypertension and is on multiple medications. IOP is 20 mmHg in both eyes. Fundoscopy shows a cup-to-disc ratio of 0.5 with no other abnormalities. What is the most appropriate next step?

    a. Initiate treatment with topical prostaglandin analogs

    b. Order visual field testing

    c. Refer to a neurologist for further evaluation

    d. Monitor IOP every 6 months

9. A 65-year-old male presents with sudden onset severe eye pain, nausea, and vomiting. On examination, the affected eye is red with a fixed mid-dilated pupil and IOP of 55 mmHg. What is the initial management?

    a. Administer topical beta-blocker

    b. Perform immediate laser iridotomy

    c. Prescribe oral acetazolamide

    d. Refer to an ophthalmologist

10. A 55-year-old female with a family history of glaucoma presents for a routine eye examination. IOP is 24 mmHg in both eyes. Optic discs appear normal with a cup-to-disc ratio of 0.3. What is the most appropriate next step?

    a. Start treatment with topical beta-blocker

    b. Repeat IOP measurement in 3 months

    c. Perform visual field testing

    d. Prescribe oral carbonic anhydrase inhibitor

11. A 70-year-old male presents with gradual loss of peripheral vision in both eyes over the past year. IOP is 28 mmHg in the right eye and 27 mmHg in the left eye. Optic discs show marked cupping with a cup-to-disc ratio of 0.8. What is the most likely diagnosis?

    a. Primary open-angle glaucoma

    b. Acute angle-closure glaucoma

    c. Normal-tension glaucoma

    d. Secondary glaucoma

12. A 50-year-old female with Type 2 diabetes mellitus presents for a routine eye examination. IOP is 18 mmHg in both eyes. Optic discs appear normal with a cup-to-disc ratio of 0.3. What is the most appropriate next step?

    a. Start treatment with topical beta-blocker

    b. Repeat IOP measurement in 6 months

    c. Perform visual field testing

    d. Prescribe oral carbonic anhydrase inhibitor

13. A 65-year-old male presents with blurred vision and difficulty adjusting to darkness. IOP is 15 mmHg in both eyes. Fundoscopy reveals optic disc cupping with a cup-to-disc ratio of 0.7 in the left eye and 0.5 in the right eye. What is the most likely diagnosis?

    a. Primary open-angle glaucoma

    b. Acute angle-closure glaucoma

    c. Normal-tension glaucoma

    d. Secondary glaucoma

14. A 60-year-old female with hypertension presents with gradual loss of peripheral vision in both eyes. IOP is 22 mmHg in the right eye and 23 mmHg in the left eye. Optic discs show cup-to-disc ratios of 0.6 in both eyes with thinning of the neuroretinal rim. What is the most likely diagnosis?

    a. Primary open-angle glaucoma

    b. Acute angle-closure glaucoma

    c. Normal-tension glaucoma

    d. Secondary glaucoma

15. A 55-year-old male presents with a sudden headache, eye pain, and vomiting. On examination, the left eye is red with a cloudy cornea, fixed mid-dilated pupil, and IOP of 60 mmHg. What is the immediate management?

    a. Administer topical beta-blocker

    b. Perform immediate laser iridotomy

    c. Prescribe oral acetazolamide

    d. Refer to an ophthalmologist

Gout

1. A 55-year-old male presents with sudden onset severe pain and swelling in his right big toe. He has a history of hypertension and is currently taking a thiazide diuretic. On examination, the toe is erythematous and tender. His serum uric acid level is 8.5 mg/dL. Which of the following is the most likely diagnosis?

    a. Septic arthritis

    b. Pseudogout

    c. Osteoarthritis

    d. Gout

2. A 62-year-old female with a history of chronic kidney disease and hypertension presents with pain and swelling in her right knee. The joint is warm, erythematous, and tender to touch. She denies any recent trauma. Her serum uric acid level is 7.0 mg/dL. What is the most appropriate initial management for this patient?

    a. Aspiration of the joint

    b. Corticosteroid injection into the joint

    c. Nonsteroidal anti-inflammatory drugs (NSAIDs)

    d. Colchicine

3. A 40-year-old male with a history of alcohol abuse presents with severe pain in his left ankle. He reports that the pain started last night and has progressively worsened. On examination, the ankle is erythematous, warm, and swollen. His serum uric acid level is 9.8 mg/dL. What is the most appropriate initial treatment for this patient?

    a. Intravenous (IV) colchicine

    b. IV corticosteroids

    c. Oral colchicine

    d. Oral NSAIDs

4. A 68-year-old male presents with recurrent episodes of acute gouty arthritis despite allopurinol therapy. His serum uric acid level is within the normal range. Which of the following would be the next appropriate step in management?

    a. Increase allopurinol dose

    b. Initiate probenecid

    c. Initiate febuxostat

    d. Initiate pegloticase

5. A 50-year-old male presents with chronic tophaceous gout. He has multiple palpable subcutaneous nodules over his fingers, elbows, and ears. What is the most appropriate management for this patient?

    a. Oral colchicine

    b. NSAIDs

    c. Intra-articular corticosteroid injections

    d. Long-term urate-lowering therapy

6. A 45-year-old male presents with acute onset of severe pain and swelling in his left ankle. He has a history of gout and takes allopurinol daily. On examination, his ankle is erythematous, warm, and tender. His serum uric acid level is 5.5 mg/dL. Which of the following is the most likely cause of his acute flare?

    a. Dietary indiscretion

    b. Alcohol intake

    c. Non-compliance with allopurinol

    d. Recent illness

7. A 60-year-old female with hypertension and type 2 diabetes presents with acute onset of pain, redness, and swelling in her right knee. She takes metformin and lisinopril daily. Physical examination reveals an inflamed, warm, and tender knee joint. Her serum uric acid level is 6.8 mg/dL. Which of the following medications should be avoided in this patient?

    a. Colchicine

    b. Probenecid

    c. Prednisone

    d. Febuxostat

8. A 55-year-old male presents with recurrent attacks of gout despite taking allopurinol. His serum uric acid level remains elevated at 9.0 mg/dL. Which of the following would be the most appropriate next step in management?

    a. Increase allopurinol dose

    b. Switch to febuxostat

    c. Add colchicine

    d. Check for compliance with allopurinol

9. A 48-year-old male presents with acute onset of pain and swelling in his right first metatarsophalangeal joint. He has a history of hypertension and takes hydrochlorothiazide daily. His serum uric acid level is 8.2 mg/dL. Which of the following is the most appropriate initial management?

    a. Oral NSAIDs

    b. Oral colchicine

    c. Intra-articular corticosteroid injection

    d. Increase fluid intake

10. A 58-year-old male presents with tophi involving his right hand. Which of the following is the most appropriate next step in management?

    a. Initiate allopurinol

    b. Perform joint aspiration

    c. Initiate febuxostat

    d. Initiate pegloticase

11. A 65-year-old female with a history of hypertension and chronic kidney disease presents with acute pain and swelling in her left knee. She takes lisinopril daily. Her serum uric acid level is 7.5 mg/dL. Which of the following medications is contraindicated in this patient?

    a. Colchicine

    b. Allopurinol

    c. Probenecid

    d. NSAIDs

12. A 52-year-old male presents with acute gouty arthritis of the right wrist. He has a history of peptic ulcer disease. Which of the following medications is the most appropriate for initial management of his acute attack?

    a. Colchicine

    b. Allopurinol

    c. NSAIDs

    d. Corticosteroids

13. A 60-year-old male with hypertension and type 2 diabetes presents with chronic tophaceous gout involving his feet and hands. Which of the following is the most appropriate long-term management?

    a. Short-term course of colchicine

    b. Initiation of pegloticase

    c. Long-term allopurinol therapy

    d. NSAIDs for pain control

14. A 55-year-old male presents with acute gouty arthritis involving his left foot. His serum uric acid level is 9.2 mg/dL. He has a history of chronic kidney disease. Which of the following medications should be avoided in this patient?

    a.   Colchicine

    b.   Allopurinol

    c.   NSAIDs

    d.   Febuxostat

15. A 50-year-old male presents with acute onset of pain and swelling in his right knee. He has a history of gout and is currently taking allopurinol. His serum uric acid level is 5.8 mg/dL. What is the most likely cause of his acute gout flare?

    a.   Recent dietary changes

    b.   Recent alcohol intake

    c.   Non-compliance with allopurinol

    d.   Recent travel

Graves' Disease

1. A 32-year-old female presents with weight loss, palpitations, heat intolerance, and tremors. On examination, she has proptosis and a diffusely enlarged thyroid gland. Laboratory tests reveal elevated levels of free T4 and T3. Which of the following is the most likely diagnosis?

    a. Hashimoto's thyroiditis

    b. Toxic multinodular goiter

    c. Graves' disease

    d. Thyroid adenoma

2. A 45-year-old male presents with a history of weight loss, sweating, and palpitations. He also complains of frequent bowel movements and tremors in his hands. On examination, his pulse is 110 beats per minute, and he has a diffusely enlarged thyroid gland with a bruit. Which of the following is the most appropriate initial step in management?

    a. Beta-blockers

    b. Methimazole

    c. Radioactive iodine therapy

    d. Thyroidectomy

3. A 38-year-old female presents with anxiety, heat intolerance, and weight loss despite increased appetite. She has a family history of thyroid disease. On physical examination, she has a diffusely enlarged thyroid gland and lid lag. Laboratory tests reveal elevated free T4 and T3 levels with a suppressed TSH. Which of the following is the most likely diagnosis?

    a. Thyroid storm

    b. Hashimoto's thyroiditis

    c. Graves' disease

    d. Toxic adenoma

4. A 55-year-old female presents with palpitations, heat intolerance, and weight loss over the past 3 months. On examination, she has a diffusely enlarged thyroid gland, and her eyes appear prominent. Laboratory

tests reveal elevated free T4 and T3 levels with a suppressed TSH. Which of the following is the next step in management?

    a.   Start methimazole

    b.   Start levothyroxine

    c.   Order a thyroid ultrasound

    d.   Refer for radioactive iodine therapy

5. A 28-year-old male presents with a 6-month history of palpitations, sweating, heat intolerance, and weight loss. On examination, he has a diffusely enlarged thyroid gland with audible bruits over the gland. Laboratory tests show elevated free T4 and T3 with a suppressed TSH. Which of the following is the most likely cause of his symptoms?

    a.   Subacute thyroiditis

    b.   Toxic multinodular goiter

    c.   Graves' disease

    d.   Pituitary adenoma

6. A 40-year-old female presents with palpitations, heat intolerance, and weight loss over the past 2 months. On examination, her thyroid gland is diffusely enlarged and firm. She has lid lag and exophthalmos. Laboratory tests reveal elevated free T4 and T3 with a suppressed TSH. What is the most appropriate initial treatment?

    a.   Radioactive iodine therapy

    b.   Methimazole

    c.   Levothyroxine

    d.   Propranolol

7. A 35-year-old male presents with weight loss, irritability, heat intolerance, and palpitations. On examination, he has a diffusely enlarged thyroid gland. Laboratory tests reveal elevated free T4 and T3 with a suppressed TSH. Which of the following medications should be avoided initially in this patient?

    a.   Methimazole

      b.   Propranolol

      c.   Radioactive iodine

      d.   Levothyroxine

8.   A 42-year-old female presents with symptoms of palpitations, heat intolerance, and weight loss. On examination, she has a diffusely enlarged thyroid gland and exophthalmos. Laboratory tests reveal elevated free T4 and T3 with a suppressed TSH. Which of the following is the best initial test to confirm the diagnosis?

      a.   Thyroid ultrasound

      b.   Thyroid stimulating immunoglobulin (TSI)

      c.   Thyroid scan with radioactive iodine

      d.   Fine-needle aspiration (FNA) biopsy

9.   A 30-year-old female presents with symptoms of hyperthyroidism including weight loss, palpitations, and heat intolerance. On examination, she has a diffusely enlarged thyroid gland and lid lag. Laboratory tests reveal elevated free T4 and T3 with a suppressed TSH. Which of the following is a common complication associated with Graves' disease?

      a.   Hypocalcemia

      b.   Thyroid storm

      c.   Hypothyroidism

      d.   Hyperparathyroidism

10. A 50-year-old male presents with symptoms of hyperthyroidism including palpitations, weight loss, and heat intolerance. On examination, he has a diffusely enlarged thyroid gland and exophthalmos. Laboratory tests reveal elevated free T4 and T3 with a suppressed TSH. What is the most appropriate initial treatment for this patient?

   a. Methimazole

   b. Propranolol

   c. Radioactive iodine therapy

   d. Levothyroxine

11. A 36-year-old female presents with symptoms of palpitations, weight loss, and heat intolerance. On examination, she has a diffusely enlarged thyroid gland and exophthalmos. Laboratory tests reveal elevated free T4 and T3 with a suppressed TSH. Which of the following is the next step in management?

   a. Start radioactive iodine therapy

   b. Start levothyroxine

   c. Refer for thyroidectomy

   d. Start methimazole

12. A 45-year-old male presents with a 3-month history of palpitations, heat intolerance, and weight loss despite increased appetite. On examination, he has a diffusely enlarged thyroid gland with audible bruits. Laboratory tests show elevated free T4 and T3 with a suppressed TSH. Which of the following is the most likely cause of his symptoms?

   a. Subacute thyroiditis

   b. Toxic multinodular goiter

   c. Graves' disease

   d. Pituitary adenoma

13. A 40-year-old female presents with anxiety, heat intolerance, and weight loss over the past 2 months. On examination, her thyroid gland is diffusely enlarged and firm. She has lid lag and exophthalmos. Laboratory tests reveal elevated free T4 and T3 with a suppressed TSH. What is the most appropriate initial treatment?

    a. Radioactive iodine therapy

    b. Methimazole

    c. Levothyroxine

    d. Propranolol

14. A 35-year-old male presents with weight loss, irritability, heat intolerance, and palpitations. On examination, he has a diffusely enlarged thyroid gland. Laboratory tests reveal elevated free T4 and T3 with a suppressed TSH. Which of the following medications should be avoided initially in this patient?

    a. Methimazole

    b. Propranolol

    c. Radioactive iodine

    d. Levothyroxine

15. A 42-year-old female presents with symptoms of palpitations, heat intolerance, and weight loss. On examination, she has a diffusely enlarged thyroid gland and exophthalmos. Laboratory tests reveal elevated free T4 and T3 with a suppressed TSH. Which of the following is the best initial test to confirm the diagnosis?

    a. Thyroid ultrasound

    b. Thyroid stimulating immunoglobulin (TSI)

    c. Thyroid scan with radioactive iodine

    d. Fine-needle aspiration (FNA) biopsy

Heart Attack (Myocardial Infarction)

1. A 55-year-old male presents to the emergency department with sudden onset of chest pain radiating to his left arm and jaw. He is diaphoretic and nauseous. An ECG shows ST-segment elevation in leads II, III, and aVF. Troponin levels are elevated. What is the most likely diagnosis?

    a. Unstable angina

    b. Non-ST-segment elevation myocardial infarction (NSTEMI)

    c. ST-segment elevation myocardial infarction (STEMI)

    d. Aortic dissection

2. A 65-year-old female with a history of hypertension and diabetes mellitus presents with chest pain and shortness of breath for the past 2 hours. An ECG shows ST-segment depression and T-wave inversion in leads V4-V6. Troponin levels are elevated. What is the most likely diagnosis?

    a. Unstable angina

    b. Non-ST-segment elevation myocardial infarction (NSTEMI)

    c. STEMI

    d. Stable angina

3. A 50-year-old male smoker presents with chest pain that started at rest and has persisted for the past 30 minutes. An ECG shows ST-segment elevation in leads V1-V4. Troponin levels are elevated. What is the most appropriate initial management?

    a. Administer fibrinolytic therapy

    b. Immediate coronary angiography

    c. Start aspirin and heparin

    d. Administer oxygen therapy

4. A 60-year-old female presents with epigastric pain radiating to her back, nausea, and diaphoresis. An ECG shows new-onset left bundle branch block (LBBB). Troponin levels are elevated. What is the most appropriate next step?

    a. Administer fibrinolytic therapy

    b. Immediate coronary angiography

    c. Start aspirin and heparin

    d. Administer oxygen therapy

5. A 70-year-old male presents with chest pain that started 3 hours ago. He has a history of chronic kidney disease. An ECG shows ST-segment elevation in leads II, III, and aVF. Troponin levels are elevated. Which of the following medications should be avoided in this patient?

    a. Morphine

    b. Nitroglycerin

    c. Aspirin

    d. Heparin

6. A 55-year-old female presents with chest pain that started 1 hour ago. She is allergic to aspirin and has a history of hypertension. An ECG shows ST-segment elevation in leads V2-V5. Troponin levels are elevated. What is the most appropriate initial treatment?

    a. Fibrinolytic therapy

    b. Coronary angiography

    c. Beta-blocker

    d. Calcium channel blocker

7. A 65-year-old male with a history of coronary artery disease presents with chest pain that started 30 minutes ago. An ECG shows ST-segment elevation in leads II, III, and aVF. Troponin levels are elevated. Which of the following is a contraindication to fibrinolytic therapy?

    a. Age over 65 years

    b. History of hypertension

    c. History of previous myocardial infarction

    d. Intracranial hemorrhage within the past year

8. A 50-year-old female presents with chest pain that started 2 hours ago. An ECG shows ST-segment elevation in leads V1-V4. Troponin levels are elevated. What is the most appropriate initial treatment?

    a. Administer fibrinolytic therapy

    b. Immediate coronary angiography

    c. Start aspirin and heparin

    d. Administer oxygen therapy

9. A 60-year-old male smoker presents with severe chest pain that started 1 hour ago. An ECG shows ST-segment elevation in leads V2-V5. Troponin levels are elevated. What is the most appropriate initial management?

    a. Administer fibrinolytic therapy

    b. Immediate coronary angiography

    c. Start aspirin and heparin

    d. Administer oxygen therapy

10. A 55-year-old male presents with chest pain that started 2 hours ago. An ECG shows ST-segment elevation in leads II, III, and aVF. Troponin levels are elevated. Which of the following is a common complication associated with STEMI?

    a. Atrial fibrillation

    b. Ventricular tachycardia

    c. Left bundle branch block

    d. Hypertension

11. A 65-year-old female presents with chest pain that started 3 hours ago. An ECG shows ST-segment elevation in leads V2-V5. Troponin levels are elevated. Which of the following is the most appropriate initial treatment?

    a. Administer fibrinolytic therapy

    b. Immediate coronary angiography

    c. Start aspirin and heparin

    d. Administer oxygen therapy

12. A 60-year-old male smoker presents with severe chest pain that started 1 hour ago. An ECG shows ST-segment elevation in leads V2-V5. Troponin levels are elevated. What is the most appropriate initial management?

    a. Administer fibrinolytic therapy

    b. Immediate coronary angiography

    c. Start aspirin and heparin

    d. Administer oxygen therapy

13. A 55-year-old female presents with chest pain that started 2 hours ago. An ECG shows ST-segment elevation in leads V1-V4. Troponin levels are elevated. Which of the following is the most appropriate initial treatment?

    a. Administer fibrinolytic therapy

    b. Immediate coronary angiography

    c. Start aspirin and heparin

    d. Administer oxygen therapy

14. A 50-year-old male presents with chest pain that started 1 hour ago. An ECG shows ST-segment elevation in leads II, III, and aVF. Troponin levels are elevated. Which of the following medications should be avoided in this patient?

    a. Morphine

    b. Nitroglycerin

    c. Aspirin

    d. Heparin

15. A 70-year-old female presents with chest pain that started 3 hours ago. She has a history of chronic kidney disease. An ECG shows ST-segment elevation in leads II, III, and aVF. Troponin levels are elevated. Which of the following is a contraindication to fibrinolytic therapy?

    a. Age over 65 years

    b. History of hypertension

    c. History of previous myocardial infarction

    d. Intracranial hemorrhage within the past year

Hemophilia

1. A 7-year-old male presents with recurrent episodes of joint pain and swelling, particularly in the knees and ankles. There is a family history of similar symptoms in his maternal uncle. Which of the following laboratory findings is most likely in this patient?

    a. Elevated platelet count

    b. Prolonged PT (prothrombin time)

    c. Prolonged aPTT (activated partial thromboplastin time)

    d. Elevated fibrinogen levels

2. A 10-year-old boy presents with a deep muscle hematoma after minor trauma. He has no significant medical history. Which clotting factor deficiency is most likely present in this patient?

    a. Factor II

    b. Factor VII

    c. Factor VIII

    d. Factor XII

3. A 30-year-old male presents with recurrent nosebleeds since childhood. He also reports prolonged bleeding after dental extractions. Which laboratory finding would be consistent with this patient's condition?

    a. Prolonged PT

    b. Elevated platelet count

    c. Prolonged aPTT

    d. Elevated D-dimer

4. A 25-year-old male presents with swelling and pain in his right knee after a minor fall. He denies any significant medical history.Which clotting factor deficiency should be suspected?

    a. Factor II

    b. Factor V

    c. Factor VIII

    d. Factor XIII

5. A 2-year-old boy presents with excessive bleeding from his circumcision wound.Which laboratory test would be most appropriate to confirm the diagnosis?

    a. PT

    b. aPTT

    c. Platelet count

    d. Bleeding time

6. A 40-year-old man presents with recurrent episodes of spontaneous muscle and joint bleeding. He has a history of similar episodes since childhood.What is the most likely diagnosis?

    a. von Willebrand disease

    b. Factor IX deficiency

    c. Factor VIII deficiency

    d. Factor XI deficiency

7. A 15-year-old boy presents with hemarthrosis in his right ankle joint after twisting his ankle during a basketball game.Which of the following clotting factors is most likely deficient in this patient?

    a. Factor II

    b. Factor V

    c. Factor VIII

    d. Factor XIII

8. A 35-year-old woman presents with heavy menstrual bleeding and easy bruising since adolescence. What additional laboratory test is most likely to help confirm the diagnosis?

    a. Factor VIII assay

    b. Platelet aggregation studies

    c. PT

    d. Bleeding time

9. A 45-year-old man with known hemophilia presents with sudden severe headache and dizziness. What should be included in the initial evaluation of this patient?

    a. Brain MRI

    b. Factor IX assay

    c. Platelet count

    d. Skull X-ray

10. A 20-year-old man presents with extensive bruising and prolonged bleeding after minor injuries. Which of the following is the most appropriate initial test?

    a. Platelet count

    b. aPTT

    c. PT

    d. Bleeding time

11. A 8-year-old boy presents with bleeding from his gums and excessive bruising. He has no history of trauma. Which of the following is the most appropriate next step?

    a. Platelet aggregation studies

    b. aPTT

    c. PT

    d. von Willebrand factor assay

12. A 30-year-old man with hemophilia A presents with pain and swelling in his left elbow joint after a minor fall. Which treatment is most appropriate for this patient's acute joint bleed?

    a. Fibrinolytic agents

    b. Desmopressin (DDAVP)

    c. Fresh frozen plasma

    d. Recombinant factor VIII concentrate

13. A 25-year-old woman presents with heavy menstrual bleeding and epistaxis. Which of the following is the most appropriate initial test?

    a. PT

    b. aPTT

    c. Factor VIII assay

    d. Platelet count

14. A 40-year-old man with hemophilia A presents with pain and swelling in his right knee after a minor injury. Which of the following is the most appropriate treatment for this patient's acute joint bleed?

    a. Platelet transfusion

    b. Recombinant factor IX concentrate

    c. Desmopressin (DDAVP)

    d. Recombinant factor VIII concentrate

15. A 6-year-old boy presents with recurrent episodes of severe gum bleeding after minor trauma. Which of the following is the most appropriate initial test?

    a. Platelet aggregation studies

    b. aPTT

    c. PT

    d. von Willebrand factor assay

Hepatitis (A, B, C)

1. A 30-year-old male presents with jaundice, dark urine, and clay-colored stools. He reports recent travel to a developing country. Which of the following serologic markers is most likely to be positive in this patient?

    a. HBsAg

    b. HBsAb

    c. HAV IgM

    d. HCV RNA

2. A 40-year-old man presents with fatigue and abdominal discomfort for several weeks. He denies recent travel but reports multiple sexual partners and intravenous drug use. Which of the following serologic markers is most consistent with acute hepatitis B infection?

    a. HBsAg and HBcAb IgG

    b. HBsAb and HBcAb IgM

    c. HBsAg and HBeAg

    d. HBsAb and HBeAb

3. A 50-year-old woman presents with fatigue and vague right upper quadrant discomfort. She has a history of blood transfusion before 1992. Which of the following tests is most appropriate to confirm the diagnosis?

    a. HBsAg

    b. HCV RNA

    c. HAV IgM

    d. HBcAb IgM

4. A 25-year-old man presents with jaundice, nausea, and right upper quadrant pain. He recently attended a family reunion where several members had similar symptoms. Which of the following is the most appropriate next step in management?

    a. Start entecavir

    b. Administer hepatitis A vaccine

    c. Check HCV RNA

    d. Perform liver biopsy

5. A 35-year-old woman presents with nausea, vomiting, and jaundice. She denies any recent travel or sexual activity but has a history of a blood transfusion 10 years ago. Which of the following serologic markers would confirm chronic hepatitis B infection?

    a. HBsAg positive, HBeAg positive

    b. HBsAg negative, HBeAb positive

    c. HBsAb positive, HBeAb positive

    d. HBcAb IgM positive

6. A 60-year-old man presents with fatigue and weight loss. He has a history of intravenous drug use in the past. Which of the following serologic markers would confirm chronic hepatitis C infection?

    a. Anti-HAV IgM positive

    b. HCV RNA positive

    c. HBsAg positive

    d. HBcAb IgG positive

7. A 20-year-old woman presents with jaundice and dark urine. She works as a food handler in a local restaurant. Which of the following measures is most important for preventing transmission in this case?

    a. Start treatment with pegylated interferon

    b. Administer hepatitis A vaccine

    c. Avoid contact with infected individuals

    d. Improve personal hygiene practices

8. A 30-year-old man presents with malaise and dark urine. He denies any recent travel but has had multiple sexual partners and uses intravenous drugs occasionally. Which of the following serologic markers would confirm acute hepatitis B infection?

   a. HBsAg positive, HBcAb IgM positive

   b. HBsAb positive, HBeAb positive

   c. HBsAg negative, HBcAb IgG positive

   d. HBsAg positive, HBeAb positive

9. A 45-year-old man presents with fatigue and right upper quadrant discomfort. He has a history of multiple blood transfusions for treatment of thalassemia in childhood. Which of the following tests is most appropriate to confirm the diagnosis?

   a. HAV IgM

   b. HBsAg

   c. HBcAb IgM

   d. HCV RNA

10. A 28-year-old woman presents with jaundice, nausea, and anorexia. She works as a nurse in a pediatric clinic. Which of the following measures is most important for preventing transmission in this case?

   a. Administer hepatitis A vaccine

   b. Improve personal hygiene practices

   c. Avoid contact with infected individuals

   d. Initiate treatment with antiviral medications

11. A 35-year-old man presents with fatigue and right upper quadrant pain. He has a history of multiple sexual partners and intravenous drug use. Which of the following serologic markers would confirm chronic hepatitis B infection?

    a. HBsAg negative, HBeAb positive

    b. HBsAb positive, HBeAb positive

    c. HBsAg positive, HBeAg negative

    d. HBsAg positive, HBeAg positive

12. A 50-year-old man presents with fatigue and mild jaundice. He has a history of tattoos and blood transfusion during surgery. Which of the following tests is most appropriate to confirm the diagnosis?

    a. HBsAg

    b. Anti-HAV IgM

    c. HBcAb IgG

    d. HCV RNA

13. A 22-year-old woman presents with jaundice, dark urine, and right upper quadrant pain. She has no significant medical history but works as a restaurant cook. Which of the following measures is most important for preventing transmission in this case?

    a. Administer hepatitis A vaccine

    b. Improve personal hygiene practices

    c. Avoid contact with infected individuals

    d. Initiate treatment with antiviral medications

14. A 30-year-old woman presents with fatigue and right upper quadrant discomfort. She denies any recent travel but reports unprotected sexual activity with multiple partners. Which of the following serologic markers would confirm acute hepatitis B infection?

    a. HBsAb positive, HBcAb IgG positive

    b. HBsAg positive, HBcAb IgM positive

    c. HBsAg negative, HBeAb positive

    d. HBsAg positive, HBeAg positive

15. A 55-year-old man presents with fatigue and anorexia. He has a history of a blood transfusion 20 years ago for treatment of anemia. Which of the following tests is most appropriate to confirm the diagnosis?

    a. HBsAb

    b. Anti-HAV IgM

    c. HBcAb IgG

    d. HCV RNA

Herpes Simplex Virus (HSV)

1. A 28-year-old woman presents with painful vesicular lesions on her genital area. She reports that this is her first episode.What is the most likely causative agent?

    a. Herpes simplex virus type 1 (HSV-1)

    b. Herpes simplex virus type 2 (HSV-2)

    c. Varicella-zoster virus (VZV)

    d. Human papillomavirus (HPV)

2. A 35-year-old man presents with recurrent painful oral ulcers. He reports that he gets these lesions a few times a year.What is the most likely causative agent?

    a. Herpes simplex virus type 1 (HSV-1)

    b. Herpes simplex virus type 2 (HSV-2)

    c. Epstein-Barr virus (EBV)

    d. Cytomegalovirus (CMV)

3. A 25-year-old pregnant woman with no prior history of herpes presents with genital lesions at term.What is the most appropriate management strategy?

    a. Vaginal delivery with antiviral prophylaxis

    b. Cesarean section

    c. Induction of labor

    d. Wait for spontaneous resolution

4. A 42-year-old man with HIV presents with a severe, disseminated infection involving multiple organs. Biopsy of skin lesions shows multinucleated giant cells.What is the most likely diagnosis?

    a. Varicella-zoster virus (VZV) infection

    b. Cytomegalovirus (CMV) infection

    c. Herpes simplex virus (HSV) infection

    d. Epstein-Barr virus (EBV) infection

5. A 30-year-old man presents with unilateral vesicular lesions on his forehead and eye. He reports pain and blurry vision in that eye. What is the most likely diagnosis?

    a. Herpes simplex keratitis

    b. Herpes simplex encephalitis

    c. Herpes zoster ophthalmicus

    d. Bacterial conjunctivitis

6. A 22-year-old sexually active woman presents with recurrent painful genital ulcers. She has a history of cold sores. What is the most likely causative agent?

    a. Herpes simplex virus type 1 (HSV-1)

    b. Herpes simplex virus type 2 (HSV-2)

    c. Human papillomavirus (HPV)

    d. Treponema pallidum

7. A 50-year-old man presents with recurrent episodes of genital ulcers. He is diagnosed with HIV. What is the most likely complication of his condition?

    a. Meningitis

    b. Prostatitis

    c. Encephalitis

    d. Chronic ulceration

8. A 35-year-old woman with a history of genital herpes presents with flu-like symptoms and painful genital ulcers. What is the most appropriate initial management?

    a. Acyclovir

    b. Ceftriaxone

    c. Metronidazole

    d. Penicillin

9. A 28-year-old man presents with a fever, headache, and altered mental status. CSF analysis shows lymphocytic pleocytosis and elevated protein. What is the most likely diagnosis?

    a. Herpes simplex encephalitis

    b. Meningitis due to HSV-2

    c. Varicella-zoster virus encephalitis

    d. Enterovirus meningitis

10. A 40-year-old man presents with vesicular lesions on the left side of his face and neck. He reports severe pain and tingling in the area. What is the most likely diagnosis?

    a. Herpes simplex virus type 1 (HSV-1) infection

    b. Herpes simplex virus type 2 (HSV-2) infection

    c. Varicella-zoster virus (VZV) infection

    d. Epstein-Barr virus (EBV) infection

11. A 26-year-old woman presents with recurrent episodes of painful vesicular lesions on her lips. What is the most likely causative agent?

    a. Herpes simplex virus type 1 (HSV-1)

    b. Herpes simplex virus type 2 (HSV-2)

    c. Varicella-zoster virus (VZV)

    d. Human papillomavirus (HPV)

12. A 32-year-old pregnant woman with a history of genital herpes presents with vesicular lesions on her labia. What is the most appropriate management strategy?

    a. Cesarean section

    b. Topical corticosteroids

    c. Vaginal delivery with antiviral prophylaxis

    d. Induction of labor

13. A 45-year-old man with HIV presents with persistent vesicular genital lesions despite antiviral therapy. What is the most likely explanation for his condition?

    a. Acyclovir resistance

    b. Concurrent syphilis infection

    c. Herpes simplex encephalitis

    d. Cytomegalovirus (CMV) infection

14. A 60-year-old man presents with a painful rash in the T5 dermatome distribution. He reports that he had chickenpox as a child. What is the most likely diagnosis?

    a. Herpes simplex keratitis

    b. Herpes zoster (shingles)

    c. Herpes simplex encephalitis

    d. Molluscum contagiosum

15. A 30-year-old woman presents with painful vesicular lesions on her labia. She reports having similar lesions in the past. What is the most likely causative agent?

    a. Herpes simplex virus type 1 (HSV-1)

    b. Herpes simplex virus type 2 (HSV-2)

    c. Human papillomavirus (HPV)

    d. Treponema pallidum

Hypertension (High Blood Pressure)

1. A 45-year-old male presents to the clinic with a blood pressure of 160/100 mmHg. He has no significant medical history. Physical exam is unremarkable. What is the initial step in management?

    a. Start antihypertensive medication immediately

    b. Repeat blood pressure measurement in the other arm

    c. Refer for echocardiogram

    d. Recommend lifestyle modifications

2. A 60-year-old woman has been diagnosed with hypertension and started on hydrochlorothiazide. She returns to the clinic 2 weeks later complaining of muscle cramps and dizziness. Which of the following is the most appropriate next step?

    a. Increase the dose of hydrochlorothiazide

    b. Switch to a different diuretic

    c. Check serum electrolytes

    d. Add a beta-blocker

3. A 55-year-old male presents with a blood pressure of 180/110 mmHg. He has a history of type 2 diabetes and chronic kidney disease. Which antihypertensive medication is most beneficial in this patient?

    a. Amlodipine

    b. Losartan

    c. Metoprolol

    d. Lisinopril

4. A 35-year-old female presents with a blood pressure of 140/90 mmHg. She has no other medical problems. What is the first-line antihypertensive agent for this patient?

    a. Hydrochlorothiazide

    b. Amlodipine

    c. Metoprolol

    d. Enalapril

5. A 50-year-old male has a blood pressure of 160/100 mmHg on initial visit. He is otherwise healthy with no other medical problems. What is the appropriate next step?

    a. Recheck blood pressure in 2 weeks

    b. Start lifestyle modifications

    c. Refer for echocardiogram

    d. Initiate antihypertensive medication

6. A 65-year-old male presents with a blood pressure of 160/100 mmHg. He has a history of benign prostatic hyperplasia (BPH) and uses tamsulosin. Which antihypertensive agent is most appropriate for this patient?

    a. Amlodipine

    b. Lisinopril

    c. Metoprolol

    d. Terazosin

7. A 40-year-old female presents with a blood pressure of 140/90 mmHg. She has a history of migraine headaches. Which antihypertensive agent is contraindicated in this patient?

    a. Amlodipine

    b. Metoprolol

    c. Lisinopril

    d. Propranolol

8. A 55-year-old male presents with a blood pressure of 160/100 mmHg. He has a history of gout. Which antihypertensive agent should be avoided in this patient?

    a. Losartan

    b. Amlodipine

    c. Hydrochlorothiazide

    d. Metoprolol

9. A 70-year-old female presents with a blood pressure of 180/110 mmHg. She has chronic obstructive pulmonary disease (COPD). Which antihypertensive agent is most appropriate for this patient?

    a. Amlodipine

    b. Lisinopril

    c. Metoprolol

    d. Losartan

10. A 65-year-old male presents with a blood pressure of 150/90 mmHg. He has a history of coronary artery disease (CAD). Which antihypertensive agent is most beneficial for this patient?

    a. Atenolol

    b. Amlodipine

    c. Lisinopril

    d. Hydrochlorothiazide

11. A 50-year-old male presents with a blood pressure of 140/90 mmHg. He has a history of heart failure with reduced ejection fraction (HFrEF). Which antihypertensive agent is most appropriate for this patient?

    a. Amlodipine

    b. Metoprolol

    c. Lisinopril

    d. Spironolactone

12. A 45-year-old female presents with a blood pressure of 160/100 mmHg. She is pregnant. Which antihypertensive agent is most appropriate for this patient?

    a. Atenolol

    b. Methyldopa

    c. Lisinopril

    d. Amlodipine

13. A 60-year-old male presents with a blood pressure of 180/110 mmHg. He has a history of hyperkalemia. Which antihypertensive agent should be avoided in this patient?

    a. Lisinopril

    b. Amlodipine

    c. Metoprolol

    d. Losartan

14. A 55-year-old male presents with a blood pressure of 160/100 mmHg. He has a history of benign prostatic hyperplasia (BPH). Which antihypertensive agent is most appropriate for this patient?

    a. Atenolol

    b. Tamsulosin

    c. Lisinopril

    d. Verapamil

15. A 65-year-old female presents with a blood pressure of 150/90 mmHg. She has a history of osteoporosis. Which antihypertensive agent is most appropriate for this patient?

    a. Hydrochlorothiazide

    b. Amlodipine

    c. Metoprolol

    d. Lisinopril

Hyperthyroidism

1. A 32-year-old female presents with palpitations, weight loss, and heat intolerance. She reports increased appetite and occasional tremors. Physical examination reveals a diffusely enlarged thyroid gland with a bruit. Laboratory tests show TSH < 0.01 mIU/L (normal range 0.4-4.0 mIU/L), free T4 > 3.5 ng/dL (normal range 0.8-1.8 ng/dL), and positive thyroid peroxidase antibodies. What is the most likely diagnosis?

    a. Subacute thyroiditis

    b. Graves' disease

    c. Toxic multinodular goiter

    d. Hashimoto's thyroiditis

2. A 55-year-old male presents with weight loss, anxiety, and heat intolerance. On examination, there is a palpable thyroid nodule. Laboratory tests show TSH < 0.01 mIU/L (normal range 0.4-4.0 mIU/L), free T4 > 3.5 ng/dL (normal range 0.8-1.8 ng/dL), and an ultrasound confirms a solitary thyroid nodule. What is the most likely diagnosis?

    a. Subacute thyroiditis

    b. Toxic multinodular goiter

    c. Graves' disease

    d. Follicular adenoma

3. A 40-year-old female presents with weight loss, increased appetite, and anxiety. She has a history of postpartum thyroiditis two years ago. Laboratory tests show TSH < 0.01 mIU/L (normal range 0.4-4.0 mIU/L), free T4 > 3.5 ng/dL (normal range 0.8-1.8 ng/dL), and elevated thyroid peroxidase antibodies. What is the most likely diagnosis?

    a. Graves' disease

    b. Toxic multinodular goiter

    c. Hashimoto's thyroiditis

    d. Subacute thyroiditis

4. A 28-year-old male presents with palpitations, weight loss, and heat intolerance. He is a smoker and has a family history of autoimmune diseases. On examination, there is a diffusely enlarged thyroid gland without tenderness. Laboratory tests show TSH < 0.01 mIU/L (normal range 0.4-4.0 mIU/L), free T4 > 3.5 ng/dL (normal range 0.8-1.8 ng/dL), and positive thyroid peroxidase antibodies. What is the most likely diagnosis?

   a. Subacute thyroiditis

   b. Graves' disease

   c. Toxic multinodular goiter

   d. Hashimoto's thyroiditis

5. A 60-year-old female presents with palpitations, weight loss, and heat intolerance. She has a history of a rapidly growing neck mass over the past 6 months. Physical examination reveals a firm, non-tender, and non-mobile mass in the right lobe of the thyroid gland. Laboratory tests show TSH < 0.01 mIU/L (normal range 0.4-4.0 mIU/L), free T4 > 3.5 ng/dL (normal range 0.8-1.8 ng/dL), and a thyroid ultrasound confirms a solid nodule with microcalcifications. What is the most likely diagnosis?

   a. Follicular adenoma

   b. Subacute thyroiditis

   c. Papillary thyroid carcinoma

   d. Toxic multinodular goiter

6. A 45-year-old female presents with palpitations, weight loss, and heat intolerance. She has a diffuse, nontender goiter. Laboratory tests show TSH < 0.01 mIU/L (normal range 0.4-4.0 mIU/L), free T4 > 3.5 ng/dL (normal range 0.8-1.8 ng/dL), and a radioactive iodine uptake scan reveals diffuse uptake throughout the thyroid gland. What is the most likely diagnosis?

   a. Graves' disease

   b. Toxic multinodular goiter

   c. Subacute thyroiditis

   d. Hashimoto's thyroiditis

7. A 38-year-old male presents with weight loss, tremors, and heat intolerance. He has a history of autoimmune disorders and takes medications for rheumatoid arthritis. Laboratory tests show TSH < 0.01 mIU/L (normal range 0.4-4.0 mIU/L), free T4 > 3.5 ng/dL (normal range 0.8-1.8 ng/dL), and thyroid ultrasound reveals diffuse thyroid enlargement with a hypoechoic pattern. What is the most likely diagnosis?

   a. Graves' disease

   b. Subacute thyroiditis

   c. Toxic multinodular goiter

   d. Hashimoto's thyroiditis

8. A 55-year-old female presents with palpitations, weight loss, and heat intolerance. She has a history of chronic iodine deficiency and is not taking any medications. Physical examination reveals a diffusely enlarged thyroid gland with a bruit. Laboratory tests show TSH < 0.01 mIU/L (normal range 0.4-4.0 mIU/L), free T4 > 3.5 ng/dL (normal range 0.8-1.8 ng/dL), and a radioactive iodine uptake scan confirms diffuse uptake. What is the most likely diagnosis?

   a. Toxic multinodular goiter

   b. Graves' disease

   c. Subacute thyroiditis

   d. Hashimoto's thyroiditis

9. A 65-year-old male presents with palpitations, weight loss, and heat intolerance. He has a history of chronic lithium therapy for bipolar disorder. Physical examination reveals a diffusely enlarged thyroid gland without tenderness. Laboratory tests show TSH < 0.01 mIU/L (normal range 0.4-4.0 mIU/L), free T4 > 3.5 ng/dL (normal range 0.8-1.8 ng/dL), and a thyroid ultrasound reveals a heterogeneous echotexture. What is the most likely diagnosis?

   a. Graves' disease

   b. Toxic multinodular goiter

   c. Hashimoto's thyroiditis

   d. Iodine-induced hyperthyroidism

10. A 50-year-old female presents with palpitations, weight loss, and heat intolerance. She has a history of undergoing neck radiation therapy for Hodgkin lymphoma 30 years ago. Physical examination reveals a diffusely enlarged thyroid gland with a bruit. Laboratory tests show TSH < 0.01 mIU/L (normal range 0.4-4.0 mIU/L), free T4 > 3.5 ng/dL (normal range 0.8-1.8 ng/dL), and a radioactive iodine uptake scan confirms diffuse uptake. What is the most likely diagnosis?

   a. Graves' disease

   b. Toxic multinodular goiter

   c. Radiation-induced thyroiditis

   d. Hashimoto's thyroiditis

11. A 35-year-old female presents with palpitations, weight loss, and heat intolerance. She has a history of having a baby 6 months ago. Physical examination reveals a diffusely enlarged thyroid gland without tenderness. Laboratory tests show TSH < 0.01 mIU/L (normal range 0.4-4.0 mIU/L), free T4 > 3.5 ng/dL (normal range 0.8-1.8 ng/dL), and positive thyroid peroxidase antibodies. What is the most likely diagnosis?

    a. Graves' disease

    b. Postpartum thyroiditis

    c. Toxic multinodular goiter

    d. Hashimoto's thyroiditis

12. A 45-year-old male presents with palpitations, weight loss, and heat intolerance. He has a history of being treated for Hodgkin lymphoma with radioactive iodine therapy 10 years ago. Physical examination reveals a diffusely enlarged thyroid gland with a bruit. Laboratory tests show TSH < 0.01 mIU/L (normal range 0.4-4.0 mIU/L), free T4 > 3.5 ng/dL (normal range 0.8-1.8 ng/dL), and a radioactive iodine uptake scan confirms diffuse uptake. What is the most likely diagnosis?

    a. Graves' disease

    b. Toxic multinodular goiter

    c. Radiation-induced thyroiditis

    d. Hashimoto's thyroiditis

13. A 30-year-old female presents with palpitations, weight loss, and heat intolerance. She has a history of recent upper respiratory tract infection. Physical examination reveals a diffusely enlarged thyroid gland that is tender to palpation. Laboratory tests show TSH < 0.01 mIU/L (normal range 0.4-4.0 mIU/L), free T4 > 3.5 ng/dL (normal range 0.8-1.8 ng/dL), and an elevated erythrocyte sedimentation rate. What is the most likely diagnosis?

    a. Graves' disease

    b. Subacute thyroiditis

    c. Toxic multinodular goiter

    d. Hashimoto's thyroiditis

14. A 55-year-old female presents with palpitations, weight loss, and heat intolerance. She has a history of taking amiodarone for the past 5 years due to atrial fibrillation. Physical examination reveals a diffusely enlarged thyroid gland without tenderness. Laboratory tests show TSH < 0.01 mIU/L (normal range 0.4-4.0 mIU/L), free T4 > 3.5 ng/dL (normal range 0.8-1.8 ng/dL), and a thyroid ultrasound reveals a heterogeneous echotexture. What is the most likely diagnosis?

    a. Graves' disease

    b. Amiodarone-induced thyrotoxicosis

    c. Toxic multinodular goiter

    d. Hashimoto's thyroiditis

15. A 40-year-old female presents with palpitations, weight loss, and heat intolerance. She has a history of recent upper respiratory tract infection. Physical examination reveals a diffusely enlarged thyroid gland that is tender to palpation. Laboratory tests show TSH < 0.01 mIU/L (normal range 0.4-4.0 mIU/L), free T4 > 3.5 ng/dL (normal range 0.8-1.8 ng/dL), and an elevated erythrocyte sedimentation rate. What is the most likely diagnosis?

   a. Graves' disease

   b. Subacute thyroiditis

   c. Toxic multinodular goiter

   d. Hashimoto's thyroiditis

Hypothyroidism

1. A 35-year-old female presents with fatigue, weight gain, and constipation. On examination, she has dry skin, coarse hair, and bradycardia. Her TSH level is elevated and free T4 is decreased. What is the most likely diagnosis?

    a. Hyperthyroidism

    b. Hypothyroidism

    c. Thyroiditis

    d. Thyroid cancer

2. A 50-year-old male presents with memory loss, depression, and lethargy. Physical examination reveals a puffy face, dry skin, and slow reflexes. Laboratory tests show an elevated TSH level and decreased free T4. What is the most likely diagnosis?

    a. Hyperthyroidism

    b. Hypothyroidism

    c. Thyroiditis

    d. Thyroid cancer

3. A 28-year-old female presents with weight loss, anxiety, and palpitations. Physical examination reveals a diffusely enlarged thyroid gland. Laboratory tests show a low TSH level and elevated free T4. What is the most likely diagnosis?

    a. Hyperthyroidism

    b. Hypothyroidism

    c. Thyroiditis

    d. Thyroid cancer

4. A 45-year-old female presents with fatigue, cold intolerance, and weight gain. Physical examination reveals dry skin, brittle hair, and slow movements. Laboratory tests show an elevated TSH level and normal free T4. What is the most likely diagnosis?

    a. Primary hypothyroidism

    b. Secondary hypothyroidism

    c. Hashimoto's thyroiditis

    d. Subacute thyroiditis

5. A 60-year-old male presents with fatigue, constipation, and muscle cramps. Physical examination reveals a puffy face and dry skin. Laboratory tests show an elevated TSH level and normal free T4. What is the most likely diagnosis?

    a. Primary hypothyroidism

    b. Secondary hypothyroidism

    c. Hashimoto's thyroiditis

    d. Subacute thyroiditis

6. A 25-year-old female presents with fatigue, hair loss, and weight gain. Physical examination reveals dry skin and brittle hair. Laboratory tests show an elevated TSH level and positive anti-thyroid peroxidase antibodies. What is the most likely diagnosis?

    a. Primary hypothyroidism

    b. Secondary hypothyroidism

    c. Hashimoto's thyroiditis

    d. Subacute thyroiditis

7. A 35-year-old male presents with fatigue, weight gain, and cold intolerance. Physical examination reveals dry skin and bradycardia. Laboratory tests show an elevated TSH level and decreased free T4. He has a history of pituitary surgery. What is the most likely diagnosis?

    a. Primary hypothyroidism

    b. Secondary hypothyroidism

    c. Hashimoto's thyroiditis

    d. Subacute thyroiditis

8. A 30-year-old female presents with neck pain, fever, and a tender thyroid gland. She has a recent upper respiratory tract infection. Laboratory tests show an elevated TSH level and low free T4. What is the most likely diagnosis?

    a. Primary hypothyroidism

    b. Secondary hypothyroidism

    c. Hashimoto's thyroiditis

    d. Subacute thyroiditis

9. A 40-year-old female presents with a painless, firm thyroid nodule. Physical examination is otherwise unremarkable. Laboratory tests show a low TSH level and normal free T4. What is the most likely diagnosis?

    a. Primary hypothyroidism

    b. Secondary hypothyroidism

    c. Thyroid cancer

    d. Subacute thyroiditis

10. A 25-year-old female presents with a neck mass, hoarseness, and difficulty swallowing. Physical examination reveals a fixed, hard thyroid nodule. Laboratory tests show an elevated TSH level and normal free T4. What is the most likely diagnosis?

   a. Primary hypothyroidism

   b. Secondary hypothyroidism

   c. Thyroid cancer

   d. Subacute thyroiditis

11. A 55-year-old male presents with weight loss, heat intolerance, and palpitations. Physical examination reveals exophthalmos and a diffusely enlarged thyroid gland. Laboratory tests show a low TSH level and elevated free T4. What is the most likely diagnosis?

   a. Primary hypothyroidism

   b. Secondary hypothyroidism

   c. Hashimoto's thyroiditis

   d. Graves' disease

12. A 45-year-old female presents with a neck mass and difficulty breathing. Physical examination reveals a large, fixed thyroid mass. Laboratory tests show a low TSH level and normal free T4. What is the most likely diagnosis?

   a. Primary hypothyroidism

   b. Secondary hypothyroidism

   c. Thyroid cancer

   d. Subacute thyroiditis

13. A 60-year-old male presents with fatigue, constipation, and cold intolerance. Physical examination reveals dry skin and bradycardia. Laboratory tests show a low TSH level and normal free T4. He has a history of pituitary adenoma treated with surgery. What is the most likely diagnosis?

    a. Primary hypothyroidism

    b. Secondary hypothyroidism

    c. Hashimoto's thyroiditis

    d. Subacute thyroiditis

14. A 35-year-old female presents with fatigue, weight gain, and constipation. Physical examination reveals dry skin, coarse hair, and bradycardia. Laboratory tests show an elevated TSH level and normal free T4. What is the most likely diagnosis?

    a. Primary hypothyroidism

    b. Secondary hypothyroidism

    c. Hashimoto's thyroiditis

    d. Subacute thyroiditis

15. A 50-year-old male presents with memory loss, depression, and lethargy. Physical examination reveals a puffy face, dry skin, and slow reflexes. Laboratory tests show an elevated TSH level and decreased free T4. What is the most likely diagnosis?

    a. Primary hypothyroidism

    b. Secondary hypothyroidism

    c. Hashimoto's thyroiditis

    d. Subacute thyroiditis

Insomnia

1. A 45-year-old male presents with difficulty falling asleep, frequent awakenings during the night, and early morning awakenings. He reports feeling tired and irritable during the day. He denies alcohol or drug use.Which of the following is the most likely diagnosis?

   a. Restless Legs Syndrome

   b. Obstructive Sleep Apnea

   c. Primary Insomnia

   d. Depression

   e. Shift Work Sleep Disorder

2. A 30-year-old female presents with difficulty falling asleep. She states that she feels tired but wired at bedtime, often worrying about work and family responsibilities.Which of the following is the most appropriate initial management?

   a. Lorazepam

   b. Zolpidem

   c. Cognitive Behavioral Therapy for Insomnia (CBT-I)

   d. Amitriptyline

   e. Melatonin

3. A 55-year-old male presents with a history of chronic insomnia. He takes zolpidem nightly but still has difficulty sleeping.What is the most appropriate next step in management?

   a. Increase the dose of zolpidem

   b. Switch to lorazepam

   c. Add eszopiclone

   d. Perform a sleep study

   e. Start CBT-I

4. A 65-year-old female presents with difficulty falling asleep and staying asleep. She wakes up multiple times during the night to use the bathroom. Which of the following is the most likely contributing factor to her insomnia?

    a. Anxiety disorder

    b. Nocturia

    c. Sleep apnea

    d. Restless Legs Syndrome

    e. Depression

5. A 40-year-old male presents with difficulty maintaining sleep. He sleeps for 4-5 hours a night and wakes up feeling unrefreshed. What is the most likely diagnosis?

    a. Obstructive Sleep Apnea

    b. Restless Legs Syndrome

    c. Primary Insomnia

    d. Depression

    e. Circadian Rhythm Sleep Disorder

6. A 50-year-old female presents with difficulty falling asleep. She works rotating shifts and has trouble adjusting to different sleep schedules. Which of the following is the most likely diagnosis?

    a. Obstructive Sleep Apnea

    b. Restless Legs Syndrome

    c. Primary Insomnia

    d. Depression

    e. Shift Work Sleep Disorder

7. A 25-year-old male presents with excessive daytime sleepiness. He has a history of loud snoring and is often awakened by gasping for air. What is the most likely diagnosis?

    a. Insomnia Disorder

    b. Narcolepsy

    c. Obstructive Sleep Apnea

    d. Restless Legs Syndrome

    e. Delayed Sleep Phase Disorder

8. A 35-year-old female presents with difficulty falling asleep and frequent awakenings during the night. She reports an overwhelming urge to move her legs at night. What is the most likely diagnosis?

    a. Insomnia Disorder

    b. Narcolepsy

    c. Obstructive Sleep Apnea

    d. Restless Legs Syndrome

    e. Delayed Sleep Phase Disorder

9. A 60-year-old male presents with difficulty falling asleep. He has a history of chronic low back pain and often takes pain medications at bedtime. Which of the following is the most likely contributing factor to his insomnia?

    a. Anxiety disorder

    b. Nocturia

    c. Chronic pain

    d. Restless Legs Syndrome

    e. Sleep apnea

10. A 20-year-old female presents with difficulty falling asleep. She often stays up until 3 AM despite trying to go to bed earlier. What is the most likely diagnosis?

    a. Insomnia Disorder

    b. Narcolepsy

    c. Delayed Sleep Phase Disorder

    d. Restless Legs Syndrome

    e. Anxiety disorder

11. A 70-year-old male presents with difficulty staying asleep. He wakes up frequently during the night and often wakes up early in the morning. What is the most likely diagnosis?

    a. Insomnia Disorder

    b. Narcolepsy

    c. Obstructive Sleep Apnea

    d. Restless Legs Syndrome

    e. Advanced Sleep Phase Disorder

12. A 40-year-old male presents with difficulty falling asleep. He reports feeling stressed about work and often drinks alcohol at night to help him relax. Which of the following is the most appropriate initial management?

    a. Zolpidem

    b. Lorazepam

    c. Amitriptyline

    d. Melatonin

    e. Cognitive Behavioral Therapy for Insomnia (CBT-I)

13. A 55-year-old female presents with excessive daytime sleepiness. She reports vivid dreams and sudden loss of muscle tone during emotional situations.What is the most likely diagnosis?

    a. Insomnia Disorder

    b. Narcolepsy

    c. Obstructive Sleep Apnea

    d. Restless Legs Syndrome

    e. Parasomnia

14. A 30-year-old male presents with difficulty falling asleep. He reports a family history of similar sleep problems and describes his sleep as light and easily disrupted.What is the most likely diagnosis?

    a. Insomnia Disorder

    b. Narcolepsy

    c. Obstructive Sleep Apnea

    d. Restless Legs Syndrome

    e. Familial Advanced Sleep Phase Disorder

15. A 50-year-old female presents with difficulty falling asleep. She is worried about her husband's recent illness and feels anxious at night.Which of the following is the most appropriate initial management?

    a. Lorazepam

    b. Zolpidem

    c. Cognitive Behavioral Therapy for Insomnia (CBT-I)

    d. Amitriptyline

    e. Melatonin

Irritable Bowel Syndrome (IBS)

1. A 34-year-old female presents with complaints of abdominal pain and bloating. She reports that her symptoms improve after defecation and worsen with stress. She has noticed alternating constipation and diarrhea over the past few months. On examination, there is no tenderness or organomegaly. Which of the following is the most likely diagnosis?

    a. Acute appendicitis

    b. Irritable Bowel Syndrome (IBS)

    c. Crohn's disease

    d. Celiac disease

2. A 45-year-old male presents with chronic abdominal pain, bloating, and constipation. He has no significant weight loss or rectal bleeding. On examination, there is no tenderness or palpable masses. Which of the following diagnostic tests would be most appropriate to perform initially?

    a. Colonoscopy

    b. Abdominal ultrasound

    c. Stool culture

    d. Rome IV criteria questionnaire

3. A 28-year-old female complains of recurrent diarrhea, abdominal cramping, and bloating. She has noted these symptoms for several months, which are not associated with any specific triggers. Her physical examination is unremarkable. Which of the following is the most appropriate initial management?

    a. High-fiber diet

    b. Loperamide (Imodium)

    c. Amitriptyline

    d. Behavioral therapy

4. A 32-year-old male presents with complaints of chronic abdominal pain and constipation. He has a history of anxiety and stress. His symptoms are relieved by defecation. What is the most appropriate initial management?

    a. Start a selective serotonin reuptake inhibitor (SSRI)

    b. Refer to a gastroenterologist for colonoscopy

    c. Prescribe loperamide (Imodium)

    d. Trial of a low-FODMAP diet

5. A 38-year-old female presents with symptoms of bloating, abdominal pain, and alternating diarrhea and constipation. She reports that her symptoms have worsened recently due to increased stress at work. On examination, there is no tenderness or organomegaly. What is the most likely diagnosis?

    a. Crohn's disease

    b. Diverticulitis

    c. Irritable Bowel Syndrome (IBS)

    d. Celiac disease

6. A 25-year-old male presents with abdominal pain and diarrhea. His symptoms have been present for several months. On examination, he has mild abdominal tenderness, but no masses or organomegaly. Stool studies are negative for infection. What is the most likely diagnosis?

    a. Crohn's disease

    b. Ulcerative colitis

    c. Irritable Bowel Syndrome (IBS)

    d. Diverticulitis

7. A 30-year-old female presents with chronic abdominal pain, bloating, and diarrhea. Her symptoms are worse during menstruation. Physical examination is unremarkable. What is the next best step in management?

    a. Refer for colonoscopy

    b. Trial of antispasmodic medication

    c. Trial of a low-FODMAP diet

    d. Start a tricyclic antidepressant

8. A 40-year-old male presents with chronic abdominal pain and constipation. He reports that his symptoms are often relieved by defecation. Physical examination is unremarkable. What is the most appropriate initial management?

    a. Trial of lubiprostone (Amitiza)

    b. Trial of loperamide (Imodium)

    c. Trial of rifaximin (Xifaxan)

    d. Trial of a low-FODMAP diet

9. A 35-year-old female presents with recurrent episodes of diarrhea and bloating. She reports that her symptoms often occur after consuming dairy products. Physical examination is unremarkable. What is the most appropriate initial management?

    a. Trial of a low-FODMAP diet

    b. Trial of loperamide (Imodium)

    c. Trial of rifaximin (Xifaxan)

    d. Refer for colonoscopy

10. A 50-year-old female presents with chronic abdominal pain and alternating diarrhea and constipation. Her symptoms are worse during stressful periods at work. Physical examination is unremarkable. What is the most appropriate initial management?

    a. Trial of a tricyclic antidepressant

    b. Trial of a selective serotonin reuptake inhibitor (SSRI)

    c. Trial of antispasmodic medication

    d. Cognitive-behavioral therapy (CBT)

11. A 42-year-old male presents with chronic abdominal pain, bloating, and constipation. He reports that his symptoms are often triggered by certain foods, such as onions and garlic. Physical examination is unremarkable. What is the most appropriate initial management?

    a. Trial of a low-FODMAP diet

    b. Trial of loperamide (Imodium)

    c. Trial of lubiprostone (Amitiza)

    d. Trial of rifaximin (Xifaxan)

12. A 38-year-old female presents with chronic abdominal pain and alternating diarrhea and constipation. Her symptoms have been present for several years and have not responded to dietary changes. Physical examination is unremarkable. What is the most appropriate initial management?

    a. Trial of antispasmodic medication

    b. Trial of loperamide (Imodium)

    c. Trial of lubiprostone (Amitiza)

    d. Cognitive-behavioral therapy (CBT)

13. A 32-year-old male presents with chronic abdominal pain and diarrhea. His symptoms have been present for several months. Physical examination is unremarkable. Stool studies are negative for infection. What is the most appropriate initial management?

    a. Trial of loperamide (Imodium)

    b. Trial of rifaximin (Xifaxan)

    c. Trial of a low-FODMAP diet

    d. Trial of a selective serotonin reuptake inhibitor (SSRI)

14. A 40-year-old female presents with chronic abdominal pain and bloating. Her symptoms are worse during menstruation. Physical examination is unremarkable. What is the next best step in management?

    a. Trial of a low-FODMAP diet

    b. Trial of lubiprostone (Amitiza)

    c. Start a tricyclic antidepressant

    d. Refer for colonoscopy

15. A 35-year-old male presents with recurrent episodes of diarrhea and bloating. He reports that his symptoms often occur after consuming dairy products. Physical examination is unremarkable. What is the most appropriate initial management?

    a. Trial of a low-FODMAP diet

    b. Trial of loperamide (Imodium)

    c. Trial of rifaximin (Xifaxan)

    d. Refer for colonoscopy

Malaria

1. A 35-year-old traveler presents with fever, chills, and sweats, which have been occurring every 48 hours for the past week. On examination, he has a temperature of 39°C (102.2°F). Blood smear examination shows the presence of Plasmodium vivax. What is the most appropriate treatment?

    a. Chloroquine

    b. Artemether-lumefantrine

    c. Atovaquone-proguanil

    d. Doxycycline

2. A 25-year-old returned traveler presents with fever, headache, and myalgias. On examination, she has hepatosplenomegaly. Blood smear examination reveals Plasmodium falciparum. Which of the following is the most appropriate initial treatment?

    a. Quinine plus doxycycline

    b. Artemether-lumefantrine

    c. Chloroquine

    d. Primaquine

3. A 30-year-old pregnant female presents with fever and malaise. She has recently returned from a region with endemic malaria. Blood smear examination confirms Plasmodium falciparum infection. What is the most appropriate treatment?

    a. Quinine plus clindamycin

    b. Artemether-lumefantrine

    c. Chloroquine

    d. Atovaquone-proguanil

4. A 40-year-old traveler presents with fever, nausea, and vomiting. Blood smear examination reveals the presence of Plasmodium malariae. What is the most appropriate treatment?

    a. Chloroquine

    b. Artemether-lumefantrine

    c. Atovaquone-proguanil

    d. Primaquine

5. A 22-year-old traveler presents with fever and confusion. Blood smear examination shows the presence of Plasmodium falciparum. He is hypotensive and has evidence of acute kidney injury. What is the most appropriate initial management?

    a. Artesunate plus doxycycline

    b. Intravenous quinine

    c. Artemether-lumefantrine

    d. Chloroquine

6. A 45-year-old returned traveler presents with fever, jaundice, and hemoglobinuria. Blood smear examination reveals Plasmodium falciparum. What is the most appropriate treatment?

    a. Artemether-lumefantrine

    b. Primaquine

    c. Quinine plus doxycycline

    d. Artesunate plus clindamycin

7. A 28-year-old returned traveler presents with fever and severe headache. Blood smear examination reveals Plasmodium knowlesi infection. What is the most appropriate treatment?

    a. Chloroquine

    b. Quinine plus doxycycline

    c. Artemether-lumefantrine

    d. Atovaquone-proguanil

8. A 35-year-old returned traveler presents with fever, chills, and jaundice. Blood smear examination reveals Plasmodium vivax. He has a history of glucose-6-phosphate dehydrogenase (G6PD) deficiency. What is the most appropriate treatment?

    a. Chloroquine

    b. Artemether-lumefantrine

    c. Primaquine

    d. Atovaquone-proguanil

9. A 30-year-old returned traveler presents with fever, headache, and muscle pain. Blood smear examination reveals Plasmodium ovale. What is the most appropriate treatment?

    a. Chloroquine

    b. Artemether-lumefantrine

    c. Atovaquone-proguanil

    d. Primaquine

10. A 25-year-old traveler presents with fever, chills, and headache. Blood smear examination reveals Plasmodium falciparum. She is planning to travel to an area where chloroquine-resistant P. falciparum is endemic. What is the most appropriate prophylaxis?

    a. Mefloquine

    b. Atovaquone-proguanil

    c. Doxycycline

    d. Primaquine

11. A 40-year-old returned traveler presents with fever and headache. Blood smear examination reveals Plasmodium malariae. What is the most appropriate treatment?

    a. Artemether-lumefantrine

    b. Chloroquine

    c. Doxycycline

    d. Primaquine

12. A 35-year-old returned traveler presents with fever and jaundice. Blood smear examination reveals Plasmodium falciparum. He is hemodynamically stable. What is the most appropriate treatment?

    a. Artemether-lumefantrine

    b. Intravenous quinine

    c. Quinine plus doxycycline

    d. Atovaquone-proguanil

13. A 30-year-old pregnant female presents with fever and malaise. She has recently returned from a region with endemic malaria. Blood smear examination confirms Plasmodium vivax infection. What is the most appropriate treatment?

    a. Quinine plus clindamycin

    b. Artemether-lumefantrine

    c. Chloroquine

    d. Atovaquone-proguanil

14. A 25-year-old returned traveler presents with fever, chills, and headache. Blood smear examination reveals Plasmodium falciparum. She has no significant medical history. What is the most appropriate treatment?

    a. Chloroquine

    b. Artemether-lumefantrine

    c. Quinine plus doxycycline

    d. Atovaquone-proguanil

15. A 35-year-old returned traveler presents with fever, chills, and headache. Blood smear examination reveals Plasmodium falciparum. He is hypotensive and has evidence of acute kidney injury. What is the most appropriate initial management?

    a. Artesunate plus doxycycline

    b. Intravenous quinine

    c. Artemether-lumefantrine

    d. Chloroquine

Menopause

1. A 52-year-old woman presents with irregular menstrual cycles over the past year. She reports hot flashes, night sweats, and mood swings. What is the most likely diagnosis?

    a. Premenstrual syndrome (PMS)

    b. Polycystic ovarian syndrome (PCOS)

    c. Menopause

    d. Ovarian cancer

2. A 48-year-old woman complains of vaginal dryness, painful intercourse, and urinary urgency. She still has regular menstrual cycles. What is the most likely cause of her symptoms?

    a. Ovarian cyst

    b. Premature ovarian failure

    c. Menopause

    d. Pelvic inflammatory disease (PID)

3. A 55-year-old woman presents with concerns about her risk of osteoporosis and heart disease. She reports hot flashes and mood changes. What is the most appropriate counseling regarding her risks?

    a. No increased risk of osteoporosis or heart disease

    b. Increased risk of osteoporosis but not heart disease

    c. Increased risk of heart disease but not osteoporosis

    d. Increased risk of both osteoporosis and heart disease

4. A 52-year-old woman has not had a menstrual period for 10 months. She is experiencing hot flashes, night sweats, and difficulty sleeping. What is the best initial management for her symptoms?

    a. Hormone replacement therapy (HRT)

    b. Selective serotonin reuptake inhibitors (SSRIs)

    c. Non-hormonal therapies (e.g., gabapentin)

    d. Lifestyle modifications (e.g., regular exercise)

5. A 53-year-old woman with menopause-related symptoms is considering hormone replacement therapy (HRT). She has a history of breast cancer. What is the most appropriate recommendation regarding HRT?

    a. Start estrogen therapy

    b. Start combination estrogen-progestin therapy

    c. Avoid HRT due to the history of breast cancer

    d. Use estrogen patch only

6. A 50-year-old woman is concerned about weight gain and mood changes since entering menopause. She has noticed increased abdominal fat. What metabolic changes commonly occur in menopause?

    a. Increased insulin sensitivity

    b. Decreased total cholesterol levels

    c. Decreased abdominal fat distribution

    d. Increased risk of metabolic syndrome

7. A 54-year-old woman presents with symptoms of dry, itchy skin and painful joints. She has not had a menstrual period for 14 months. What is the most likely cause of her symptoms?

    a. Rheumatoid arthritis

    b. Menopause-related changes

    c. Psoriasis

    d. Systemic lupus erythematosus (SLE)

8. A 56-year-old woman presents with bothersome vaginal atrophy and dyspareunia. She has been postmenopausal for 5 years. What is the most appropriate treatment for her symptoms?

    a. Oral estrogen therapy

    b. Vaginal estrogen cream

    c. Progestin-only pill

    d. Transdermal estrogen patch

9. A 52-year-old woman presents with moderate to severe hot flashes and night sweats. She is concerned about hormone therapy due to potential side effects. What non-hormonal therapy is recommended for her symptoms?

    a. Clonidine

    b. Gabapentin

    c. Both A and B

    d. All of the above

10. A 48-year-old woman with a history of migraines presents with severe hot flashes and night sweats. She has been in menopause for 2 years. What is the most appropriate therapy for her menopausal symptoms?

    a. Estrogen patch

    b. Venlafaxine

    c. Progesterone cream

    d. St. John's wort

11. A 50-year-old woman is concerned about her bone health after menopause. She has never had a fracture and has no significant medical history. What is the most appropriate initial screening test for osteoporosis?

    a. Dual-energy X-ray absorptiometry (DXA) scan

    b. Bone mineral density (BMD) test

    c. Serum calcium level

    d. Fracture risk assessment

12. A 54-year-old woman is concerned about her increased risk of cardiovascular disease after menopause. She has a family history of heart disease. What is the most significant cardiovascular risk factor in menopausal women?

    a. Obesity

    b. Hypertension

    c. Dyslipidemia

    d. Smoking

13. A 56-year-old woman presents with sleep disturbances, hot flashes, and palpitations. She has been menopausal for 3 years. What is the most likely cause of her palpitations?

    a. Anxiety

    b. Thyroid dysfunction

    c. Hormonal fluctuations

    d. Arrhythmia

14. A 52-year-old woman is concerned about her risk of breast cancer after menopause. She has a family history of breast cancer. What is the most accurate statement regarding breast cancer risk in menopausal women?

    a. Decreased risk due to decreased estrogen levels

    b. No change in risk compared to premenopausal women

    c. Increased risk due to decreased estrogen levels

    d. Increased risk only in women with a family history of breast cancer

15. A 53-year-old woman is experiencing bothersome vaginal symptoms since entering menopause. She prefers non-hormonal therapy. What non-hormonal therapy is recommended for vaginal symptoms in menopausal women?

    a. Topical lidocaine

    b. Vaginal lubricants

    c. Oral clonidine

    d. Selective estrogen receptor modulators (SERMs)

Migraine Headaches

1. A 30-year-old woman presents with severe headache, nausea, and sensitivity to light. The headache is throbbing in nature and worsens with physical activity. What is the most likely diagnosis?

    a. Tension-type headache

    b. Migraine headache

    c. Cluster headache

    d. Sinus headache

2. A 25-year-old male presents with unilateral throbbing headache accompanied by nausea and vomiting. He also reports seeing zigzag lines before the headache starts. What is the most likely diagnosis?

    a. Tension-type headache

    b. Migraine with aura

    c. Cluster headache

    d. Sinus headache

3. A 40-year-old woman presents with recurrent headaches that are severe, unilateral, and associated with ipsilateral lacrimation and rhinorrhea. What is the most likely diagnosis?

    a. Tension-type headache

    b. Migraine headache

    c. Cluster headache

    d. Sinus headache

4. A 35-year-old man presents with sudden onset of severe headache that he describes as the worst headache of his life. He has neck stiffness and photophobia. What is the most likely diagnosis?

    a. Migraine headache

    b. Cluster headache

    c. Subarachnoid hemorrhage

    d. Sinus headache

5. A 50-year-old woman with a history of migraines presents with a headache associated with aura. She also reports temporary visual impairment in one eye and difficulty speaking during the aura phase. What type of aura is most likely?

    a. Visual

    b. Sensory

    c. Motor

    d. Language

6. A 28-year-old woman presents with severe headache, nausea, and vomiting. She reports that her headaches often occur around her menstrual cycle. What is the most likely type of migraine?

    a. Migraine with aura

    b. Chronic migraine

    c. Menstrual migraine

    d. Abdominal migraine

7. A 45-year-old man presents with recurrent, brief, stabbing headaches that occur multiple times a day over several weeks. Each headache episode lasts 15 minutes to 3 hours and is associated with restlessness and agitation. What is the most likely diagnosis?

    a. Tension-type headache

    b. Migraine headache

    c. Cluster headache

    d. Sinus headache

8. A 32-year-old woman presents with episodic headaches that are bilateral, pressing in quality, and not associated with nausea or vomiting. She has experienced these headaches for the past 6 months. What is the most likely diagnosis?

    a. Tension-type headache

    b. Migraine headache

    c. Cluster headache

    d. Sinus headache

9. A 22-year-old man presents with recurrent episodes of headache that occur after heavy alcohol consumption. The headache is unilateral and lasts for several hours. What is the most likely diagnosis?

    a. Tension-type headache

    b. Migraine headache

    c. Cluster headache

    d. Sinus headache

10. A 38-year-old woman presents with recurrent headaches that last for 4-72 hours, and are unilateral, pulsating, and associated with nausea and photophobia. She has a family history of similar headaches. What is the most likely diagnosis?

    a. Tension-type headache

    b. Migraine headache

    c. Cluster headache

    d. Sinus headache

11. A 25-year-old woman presents with recurrent headaches that last for 30 minutes to 7 days, occurring on ≥15 days per month for >3 months. What is the most likely diagnosis?

    a. Tension-type headache

    b. Migraine headache

    c. Chronic migraine

    d. Cluster headache

12. A 60-year-old man presents with unilateral headache, red eye, and drooping eyelid. The headache is excruciating and occurs at the same time every day for several weeks. What is the most likely diagnosis?

    a. Tension-type headache

    b. Migraine headache

    c. Cluster headache

    d. Sinus headache

13. A 45-year-old woman presents with episodic headache that starts with aura, including visual disturbances and sensory symptoms, followed by a throbbing headache, nausea, and sensitivity to light. What is the most likely diagnosis?

    a. Tension-type headache

    b. Migraine headache

    c. Cluster headache

    d. Sinus headache

14. A 55-year-old man presents with headache and facial pain, which worsens when bending over. He also has nasal congestion and discharge. What is the most likely diagnosis?

    a. Tension-type headache

    b. Migraine headache

    c. Cluster headache

    d. Sinus headache

15. A 40-year-old woman presents with headache, nausea, and vomiting, which typically occur during her menstrual cycle. The headache is severe and throbbing, and she has a family history of similar headaches. What is the most likely diagnosis?

    a. Tension-type headache

    b. Migraine headache

    c. Cluster headache

    d. Sinus headache

Multiple Sclerosis (MS)

1. A 30-year-old female presents with bilateral optic neuritis, numbness in her legs, and difficulty walking for the past month. MRI shows multiple demyelinating lesions in the brain and spinal cord. What is the most likely diagnosis?

    a. Guillain-Barré Syndrome

    b. Myasthenia Gravis

    c. Multiple Sclerosis (MS)

    d. Amyotrophic Lateral Sclerosis (ALS)

2. A 25-year-old male presents with worsening weakness and difficulty with coordination over the past year. His symptoms fluctuate and worsen with heat exposure. MRI shows demyelinating plaques in the brainstem and spinal cord. What is the most likely diagnosis?

    a. Myasthenia Gravis

    b. Amyotrophic Lateral Sclerosis (ALS)

    c. Multiple Sclerosis (MS)

    d. Parkinson's Disease

3. A 40-year-old woman presents with episodes of slurred speech, double vision, and difficulty walking that last for a few weeks before resolving. These episodes have occurred intermittently over the past year. What is the most likely diagnosis?

    a. Myasthenia Gravis

    b. Guillain-Barré Syndrome

    c. Multiple Sclerosis (MS)

    d. Parkinson's Disease

4. A 30-year-old man with known MS presents with acute worsening of motor function and sensation in the lower limbs over the past 24 hours. On examination, he has spasticity and hyperreflexia in the legs. What is the most appropriate immediate management?

    a. High-dose corticosteroids

    b. IV immunoglobulin (IVIG)

    c. Plasmapheresis

    d. Physical therapy

5. A 35-year-old woman with MS is planning a pregnancy. What is the most appropriate advice regarding disease-modifying therapy (DMT)?

    a. Continue the current DMT during pregnancy

    b. Discontinue DMT before conception

    c. Switch to a different DMT known to be safer during pregnancy

    d. Start a new DMT to prevent relapses during pregnancy

6. A 28-year-old male presents with unilateral facial weakness and numbness, along with double vision. Symptoms have been worsening over the past week. MRI shows demyelinating lesions in the pons and cerebellum. What is the most likely diagnosis?

    a. Stroke

    b. Transverse Myelitis

    c. Multiple Sclerosis (MS)

    d. Myasthenia Gravis

7. A 45-year-old woman with MS complains of fatigue, muscle weakness, and difficulty with coordination. Examination reveals intention tremor and scanning speech. What area of the CNS is most likely affected?

    a. Basal ganglia

    b. Cerebellum

    c. Frontal lobes

    d. Brainstem

8. A 50-year-old man with MS presents with urinary urgency, frequency, and occasional incontinence. What is the most likely cause of his symptoms?

   a. Urinary tract infection (UTI)

   b. Bladder cancer

   c. Neurogenic bladder

   d. Benign prostatic hyperplasia (BPH)

9. A 32-year-old woman with MS is started on interferon beta-1a. What is the mechanism of action of this medication in treating MS?

   a. Decreases pro-inflammatory cytokine production

   b. Enhances acetylcholine release at the neuromuscular junction

   c. Inhibits B-cell maturation

   d. Stimulates myelination of axons

10. A 38-year-old man with relapsing-remitting MS has been stable on dimethyl fumarate (Tecfidera) for the past year. He presents with a severe and sudden increase in symptoms. MRI shows new active lesions in the brain. What is the most appropriate next step in management?

    a. Increase the dose of dimethyl fumarate

    b. Switch to a different disease-modifying therapy

    c. Add corticosteroids

    d. Initiate physical therapy

11. A 45-year-old woman with MS presents with spasticity and muscle spasms that are interfering with her daily activities. What is the most appropriate treatment?

    a. Physical therapy

    b. Baclofen

    c. Methotrexate

    d. Acetaminophen

12. A 55-year-old man with progressive MS has developed significant cognitive impairment and emotional lability. What is the most likely area of the CNS affected?

    a. Basal ganglia

    b. Hippocampus

    c. Frontal lobes

    d. Temporal lobes

13. A 30-year-old woman with MS has been experiencing severe itching and burning pain in her legs for the past month. She describes it as a band-like sensation around her abdomen. What is the term for this symptom?

    a. Neuralgia

    b. Lhermitte's sign

    c. Hyperalgesia

    d. Dysesthesia

14. A 40-year-old man with MS is found to have low vitamin D levels during a routine evaluation. What is the most appropriate recommendation regarding vitamin D supplementation?

    a. Start high-dose vitamin D supplementation

    b. Do not supplement with vitamin D

    c. Encourage sun exposure

    d. Recommend a balanced diet

15. A 35-year-old woman with relapsing-remitting MS is considering pregnancy. What is the most appropriate advice regarding disease activity during pregnancy?

    a. Disease activity tends to worsen during pregnancy

    b. Disease activity tends to improve during pregnancy

    c. Disease activity remains stable during pregnancy

    d. Pregnancy has no effect on disease activity

Narcotic Addiction

1. A 28-year-old woman presents to the emergency room with pinpoint pupils, respiratory depression, and a history of heroin use. What is the initial management for this patient?

    a. Naloxone administration

    b. Methadone maintenance therapy

    c. Referral to a psychiatrist

    d. NSAIDs for pain relief

2. A 35-year-old man with a history of chronic opioid use presents for outpatient management. What is the first-line treatment for opioid use disorder?

    e. Buprenorphine

    f. Naltrexone

    g. Clonidine

    h. Benzodiazepines

3. A 40-year-old woman with a history of heroin addiction is interested in treatment for her addiction. Which medication is an opioid antagonist used for relapse prevention?

    a. Naloxone

    b. Buprenorphine

    c. Methadone

    d. Naltrexone

4. A 25-year-old man presents with withdrawal symptoms including dilated pupils, agitation, and anxiety after stopping heroin use. What is the most appropriate initial treatment for opioid withdrawal?

    a. Naloxone

    b. Buprenorphine

    c. Methadone

    d. Clonidine

5. A 30-year-old woman with a history of opioid use disorder is pregnant. What is the recommended treatment for opioid use disorder during pregnancy?

    a. Naloxone

    b. Methadone

    c. Naltrexone

    d. Buprenorphine

6. A 45-year-old man is being treated for opioid use disorder with methadone. What is the primary benefit of methadone maintenance therapy?

    a. Rapid detoxification

    b. Reduction in cravings and withdrawal symptoms

    c. Antagonism of opioid receptors

    d. Long-term sobriety without relapse

7. A 55-year-old woman is interested in quitting opioids after a long history of addiction. Which medication can be used to help prevent relapse after detoxification?

    a. Naloxone

    b. Buprenorphine

    c. Methadone

    d. Naltrexone

8. A 32-year-old man presents with chronic opioid use and hepatitis C infection. Which medication is suitable for managing opioid use disorder in this patient?

    a. Buprenorphine

    b. Methadone

    c. Naltrexone

    d. Clonidine

9. A 40-year-old woman with chronic pain and opioid use disorder is being considered for treatment. What is an advantage of buprenorphine over methadone?

    a. Higher risk of overdose

    b. Lower risk of respiratory depression

    c. Longer duration of action

    d. Availability only in specialized clinics

10. A 50-year-old man is seeking treatment for opioid use disorder after multiple failed attempts at detoxification. Which medication is associated with improved retention in treatment programs?

    a. Naloxone

    b. Buprenorphine

    c. Methadone

    d. Naltrexone

11. A 35-year-old woman with opioid use disorder is interested in a medication that can be prescribed by her primary care physician. Which medication is suitable for office-based treatment of opioid use disorder?

    a. Naloxone

    b. Buprenorphine

    c. Methadone

    d. Clonidine

12. A 45-year-old man with opioid use disorder is in a stable recovery phase. What is the goal of maintenance therapy with buprenorphine?

    a. Rapid detoxification

    b. Long-term abstinence without medications

    c. Reduction in opioid cravings and withdrawal symptoms

    d. Monthly injections for sustained release

13. A 30-year-old woman with opioid use disorder and depression is seeking treatment. Which medication is contraindicated in patients with severe depression?

   a. Naloxone

   b. Buprenorphine

   c. Methadone

   d. Naltrexone

14. A 55-year-old man with chronic opioid use disorder is interested in a medication that helps prevent relapse and is not addictive. Which medication fits this description?

   a. Naloxone

   b. Buprenorphine

   c. Methadone

   d. Naltrexone

15. A 40-year-old woman is undergoing treatment for opioid use disorder with methadone. What is an important consideration regarding methadone treatment?

   a. Daily visits to the clinic for administration

   b. Rapid detoxification

   c. Use of methadone during pregnancy

   d. Availability in primary care settings

Narcolepsy

1. A 25-year-old female presents with a history of excessive daytime sleepiness and sudden loss of muscle tone triggered by emotions. She reports having vivid dreams upon falling asleep. What is the most likely diagnosis?

   a. Obstructive sleep apnea

   b. Narcolepsy

   c. Restless legs syndrome

   d. Insomnia

2. A 30-year-old male complains of excessive daytime sleepiness despite getting 8 hours of sleep per night. He denies cataplexy, but reports experiencing vivid dreams and hallucinations upon falling asleep. What is the next step in management?

   a. Initiate modafinil

   b. Prescribe a tricyclic antidepressant

   c. Recommend cognitive behavioral therapy

   d. Refer for polysomnography

3. A 35-year-old female presents with excessive daytime sleepiness and episodes of cataplexy triggered by laughter. She has no other significant medical history. What is the most appropriate initial treatment?

   a. Modafinil

   b. Sodium oxybate

   c. Methylphenidate

   d. Clonazepam

4. A 40-year-old male with narcolepsy is started on modafinil but continues to experience excessive daytime sleepiness. What is the next appropriate step in management?

   a. Increase the dose of modafinil

   b. Add an SSRI

   c. Prescribe methylphenidate

d. Switch to armodafinil

5. A 45-year-old female with narcolepsy presents with persistent insomnia despite adequate treatment of daytime sleepiness. What is the most appropriate next step in management?

    a. Increase the dose of modafinil

    b. Prescribe trazodone

    c. Add a selective serotonin reuptake inhibitor (SSRI)

    d. Consider sodium oxybate

6. A 50-year-old male with narcolepsy and cataplexy presents with refractory symptoms despite treatment with modafinil and sodium oxybate. What is the next appropriate step in management?

    a. Increase the dose of sodium oxybate

    b. Add an antidepressant

    c. Prescribe methylphenidate

    d. Consider pitolisant

7. A 55-year-old female with narcolepsy has been stable on modafinil for several years. She presents with new-onset cataplexy. What is the most appropriate next step in management?

    a. Increase the dose of modafinil

    b. Add an antidepressant

    c. Prescribe sodium oxybate

    d. Switch to armodafinil

8. A 60-year-old male presents with excessive daytime sleepiness, cataplexy, and hypnagogic hallucinations. He has a history of hypertension. Which medication should be avoided in this patient?

    a. Modafinil

    b. Armodafinil

    c. Methylphenidate

    d. Sodium oxybate

9. A 65-year-old female with narcolepsy presents with severe daytime sleepiness and has a history of chronic kidney disease (CKD). Which medication should be avoided in this patient?

    a. Modafinil

    b. Armodafinil

    c. Methylphenidate

    d. Sodium oxybate

10. A 70-year-old male with narcolepsy presents with excessive daytime sleepiness and a history of liver disease. Which medication should be avoided in this patient?

    a. Modafinil

    b. Armodafinil

    c. Methylphenidate

    d. Sodium oxybate

11. A 45-year-old female presents with excessive daytime sleepiness and a history of anxiety disorder. Which medication is most appropriate for this patient?

    a. Modafinil

    b. Armodafinil

    c. Methylphenidate

    d. Sodium oxybate

12. A 50-year-old male presents with excessive daytime sleepiness and a history of depression. Which medication is most appropriate for this patient?

    a. Modafinil

    b. Armodafinil

    c. Methylphenidate

    d. Sodium oxybate

13. A 55-year-old female presents with excessive daytime sleepiness and a history of bipolar disorder. Which medication is most appropriate for this patient?

    a. Modafinil

    b. Armodafinil

    c. Methylphenidate

    d. Sodium oxybate

14. A 60-year-old male presents with excessive daytime sleepiness and a history of substance use disorder. Which medication is most appropriate for this patient?

    a. Modafinil

    b. Armodafinil

    c. Methylphenidate

    d. Sodium oxybate

15. A 65-year-old female presents with excessive daytime sleepiness and a history of glaucoma. Which medication should be avoided in this patient?

    a. Modafinil

    b. Armodafinil

    c. Methylphenidate

    d. Sodium oxybate

Nephrotic Syndrome

1. A 45-year-old male presents with swelling around his eyes, legs, and ankles, and frothy urine. Lab tests show hypoalbuminemia, hyperlipidemia, and proteinuria (>3.5 g/day). What is the most likely diagnosis?

   a. Acute kidney injury

   b. Nephrotic syndrome

   c. Chronic kidney disease

   d. Urinary tract infection

2. A 30-year-old female presents with sudden onset of nephrotic syndrome. She has a history of recent upper respiratory tract infection. Urinalysis shows proteinuria and hematuria. What is the most likely diagnosis?

   a. Minimal change disease

   b. Focal segmental glomerulosclerosis (FSGS)

   c. Membranous nephropathy

   d. IgA nephropathy

3. A 50-year-old male presents with nephrotic syndrome. Renal biopsy shows diffuse effacement of podocyte foot processes. What is the most likely diagnosis?

   a. Minimal change disease

   b. Focal segmental glomerulosclerosis (FSGS)

   c. Membranous nephropathy

   d. IgA nephropathy

4. A 35-year-old female presents with nephrotic syndrome. Renal biopsy shows granular immune complex deposits along the basement membrane. What is the most likely diagnosis?

   a. Minimal change disease

   b. Focal segmental glomerulosclerosis (FSGS)

   c. Membranous nephropathy

   d. IgA nephropathy

5. A 40-year-old male presents with nephrotic syndrome. Renal biopsy shows segmental sclerosis and hyalinosis of glomeruli. What is the most likely diagnosis?

    a. Minimal change disease

    b. Focal segmental glomerulosclerosis (FSGS)

    c. Membranous nephropathy

    d. IgA nephropathy

6. A 55-year-old male presents with nephrotic syndrome. Renal biopsy shows mesangial hypercellularity and IgA deposits. What is the most likely diagnosis?

    a. Minimal change disease

    b. Focal segmental glomerulosclerosis (FSGS)

    c. Membranous nephropathy

    d. IgA nephropathy

7. A 45-year-old female presents with nephrotic syndrome. She has a history of hepatitis B. Renal biopsy shows immune complex deposition in a diffuse granular pattern. What is the most likely diagnosis?

    a. Minimal change disease

    b. Focal segmental glomerulosclerosis (FSGS)

    c. Membranous nephropathy

    d. IgA nephropathy

8. A 40-year-old female presents with nephrotic syndrome. She has a history of solid tumor malignancy. Renal biopsy shows thickening of the glomerular basement membrane. What is the most likely diagnosis?

    a. Minimal change disease

    b. Focal segmental glomerulosclerosis (FSGS)

    c. Membranous nephropathy

    d. Secondary amyloidosis

9. A 50-year-old male presents with nephrotic syndrome. Renal biopsy shows apple-green birefringence under polarized light. What is the most likely diagnosis?

    a. Minimal change disease

    b. Focal segmental glomerulosclerosis (FSGS)

    c. Membranous nephropathy

    d. Secondary amyloidosis

10. A 55-year-old female presents with nephrotic syndrome. She has a history of rheumatoid arthritis. Renal biopsy shows deposition of amyloid fibrils. What is the most likely diagnosis?

    a. Minimal change disease

    b. Focal segmental glomerulosclerosis (FSGS)

    c. Membranous nephropathy

    d. Secondary amyloidosis

11. A 45-year-old male presents with nephrotic syndrome. Renal biopsy shows deposition of monoclonal immunoglobulin light chains. What is the most likely diagnosis?

    a. Minimal change disease

    b. Focal segmental glomerulosclerosis (FSGS)

    c. Membranous nephropathy

    d. Light chain cast nephropathy

12. A 50-year-old female presents with nephrotic syndrome. She has a history of diabetes mellitus. Renal biopsy shows nodular mesangial expansion and thickened glomerular basement membrane. What is the most likely diagnosis?

    a. Minimal change disease

    b. Focal segmental glomerulosclerosis (FSGS)

    c. Membranous nephropathy

    d. Diabetic nephropathy

13. A 55-year-old male presents with nephrotic syndrome. He has a history of hepatitis C. Renal biopsy shows membranoproliferative glomerulonephritis (MPGN) pattern. What is the most likely diagnosis?

    a. Minimal change disease

    b. Focal segmental glomerulosclerosis (FSGS)

    c. Membranous nephropathy

    d. Hepatitis C-associated glomerulonephritis

14. A 60-year-old female presents with nephrotic syndrome. Renal biopsy shows a diffuse proliferative pattern with wire-loop lesions. What is the most likely diagnosis?

    a. Minimal change disease

    b. Focal segmental glomerulosclerosis (FSGS)

    c. Membranous nephropathy

    d. Lupus nephritis

15. A 65-year-old male presents with nephrotic syndrome. Renal biopsy shows deposition of Congo red-positive material. What is the most likely diagnosis?

    a. Minimal change disease

    b. Focal segmental glomerulosclerosis (FSGS)

    c. Membranous nephropathy

    d. Amyloidosis

Obsessive-Compulsive Disorder (OCD)

1. A 30-year-old woman presents with recurrent intrusive thoughts about contamination and cleanliness. She feels compelled to wash her hands multiple times a day. What is the most likely diagnosis?

    a. Major depressive disorder

    b. Generalized anxiety disorder

    c. Obsessive-compulsive disorder (OCD)

    d. Panic disorder

2. A 25-year-old man presents with obsessions about harming his family, despite having no history of violent behavior. He avoids his family members due to fear of acting on these thoughts. What is the most likely diagnosis?

    a. Bipolar disorder

    b. Post-traumatic stress disorder (PTSD)

    c. Obsessive-compulsive disorder (OCD)

    d. Schizophrenia

3. A 35-year-old woman is excessively focused on symmetry and orderliness. She spends several hours each day arranging and rearranging items in her home to achieve a perfect order. What is the most likely diagnosis?

    a. Obsessive-compulsive disorder (OCD)

    b. Social anxiety disorder

    c. Hoarding disorder

    d. Body dysmorphic disorder

4. A 40-year-old man presents with a fear of germs and contamination. He avoids public places and refuses to shake hands or touch door handles. He compulsively washes his hands dozens of times a day. What is the most likely diagnosis?

    a. Hypochondriasis

    b. Obsessive-compulsive disorder (OCD)

    c. Panic disorder

    d. Social anxiety disorder

5. A 30-year-old woman has intrusive thoughts about accidentally leaving appliances on and causing a fire. Despite checking them repeatedly, she still worries excessively. What is the most likely diagnosis?

    a. Obsessive-compulsive disorder (OCD)

    b. Post-traumatic stress disorder (PTSD)

    c. Generalized anxiety disorder

    d. Panic disorder

6. A 25-year-old man feels compelled to count steps whenever he walks on a sidewalk. He believes something bad will happen if he doesn't count correctly. What is the most likely diagnosis?

    a. Obsessive-compulsive disorder (OCD)

    b. Schizophrenia

    c. Attention-deficit/hyperactivity disorder (ADHD)

    d. Major depressive disorder

7. A 35-year-old woman experiences intrusive thoughts about harm coming to her family if she doesn't perform rituals, such as tapping objects a certain number of times. What is the most likely diagnosis?

    a. Obsessive-compulsive disorder (OCD)

    b. Bipolar disorder

    c. Borderline personality disorder

    d. Panic disorder

8. A 40-year-old man has obsessive thoughts about whether he locked his door, even after checking it multiple times. He returns home multiple times to re-check. What is the most likely diagnosis?

   a. Generalized anxiety disorder

   b. Obsessive-compulsive disorder (OCD)

   c. Panic disorder

   d. Social anxiety disorder

9. A 30-year-old woman spends hours each day cleaning her house, fearing contamination and germs. She feels intense distress if her cleaning routine is interrupted. What is the most likely diagnosis?

   a. Major depressive disorder

   b. Obsessive-compulsive disorder (OCD)

   c. Panic disorder

   d. Post-traumatic stress disorder (PTSD)

10. A 25-year-old man is preoccupied with unwanted thoughts about being contaminated by germs. He avoids touching objects in public places and spends several hours washing his hands each day. What is the most likely diagnosis?

    a. Obsessive-compulsive disorder (OCD)

    b. Hypochondriasis

    c. Panic disorder

    d. Social anxiety disorder

11. A 35-year-old woman has an intense fear of accidentally harming others. She avoids sharp objects and feels compelled to perform rituals to prevent harm. What is the most likely diagnosis?

    a. Obsessive-compulsive disorder (OCD)

    b. Post-traumatic stress disorder (PTSD)

    c. Schizophrenia

    d. Bipolar disorder

12. A 40-year-old man has intrusive thoughts about contamination and feels compelled to wash his hands until they bleed. He experiences anxiety if he tries to resist the urge to wash. What is the most likely diagnosis?

    a. Obsessive-compulsive disorder (OCD)

    b. Social anxiety disorder

    c. Panic disorder

    d. Generalized anxiety disorder

13. A 30-year-old woman feels compelled to repeat certain words silently until they "feel right." She spends hours each day performing these mental rituals. What is the most likely diagnosis?

    a. Obsessive-compulsive disorder (OCD)

    b. Generalized anxiety disorder

    c. Major depressive disorder

    d. Panic disorder

14. A 25-year-old man experiences intrusive thoughts about his house being burglarized. He checks the locks repeatedly before leaving home, which makes him late for work. What is the most likely diagnosis?

    a. Obsessive-compulsive disorder (OCD)

    b. Panic disorder

    c. Generalized anxiety disorder

    d. Major depressive disorder

15. A 35-year-old woman has persistent thoughts about her hands being contaminated by touching others. She avoids shaking hands and washes her hands excessively. What is the most likely diagnosis?

    a. Major depressive disorder

    b. Obsessive-compulsive disorder (OCD)

    c. Panic disorder

    d. Post-traumatic stress disorder (PTSD)

Osteoarthritis

1. A 60-year-old female presents with chronic pain and stiffness in her hands, worse in the mornings and improving throughout the day. On examination, there are Heberden's nodes present.What is the most likely diagnosis?

    a. Rheumatoid arthritis

    b. Osteoarthritis

    c. Gout

    d. Systemic lupus erythematosus

    e. Psoriatic arthritis

2. A 70-year-old male presents with knee pain that worsens with activity and improves with rest. He does not have significant morning stiffness. On examination, there is crepitus and tenderness over the knee joint.What is the most likely diagnosis?

    a. Rheumatoid arthritis

    b. Osteoarthritis

    c. Gout

    d. Ankylosing spondylitis

    e. Septic arthritis

3. A 55-year-old female presents with pain and swelling in the base of her thumb, worse when she grasps objects. She has no history of trauma to the area.What is the most likely diagnosis?

    a. Rheumatoid arthritis

    b. Osteoarthritis

    c. Gout

    d. Systemic lupus erythematosus

    e. Psoriatic arthritis

4. A 65-year-old male presents with chronic low back pain and stiffness, worse in the mornings and after prolonged sitting or standing. There is no radiation of pain into the legs. What is the most likely diagnosis?

    a. Rheumatoid arthritis

    b. Osteoarthritis

    c. Ankylosing spondylitis

    d. Systemic lupus erythematosus

    e. Psoriatic arthritis

5. A 60-year-old female presents with knee pain that is worse with climbing stairs and after prolonged walking. She notes that her knee joints are stiff after sitting for a while and then improve after she starts moving. What is the most likely diagnosis?

    a. Rheumatoid arthritis

    b. Osteoarthritis

    c. Gout

    d. Systemic lupus erythematosus

    e. Psoriatic arthritis

6. A 70-year-old male presents with chronic hip pain that worsens with weight-bearing activities and improves with rest. On examination, there is limited range of motion and crepitus in the affected hip joint. What is the most likely diagnosis?

    a. Rheumatoid arthritis

    b. Osteoarthritis

    c. Gout

    d. Ankylosing spondylitis

    e. Septic arthritis

7. A 55-year-old female presents with pain and swelling in multiple joints, including the wrists and hands. She reports morning stiffness lasting more than an hour. On examination, there are symmetric joint involvement and rheumatoid nodules. What is the most likely diagnosis?

    a. Rheumatoid arthritis

    b. Osteoarthritis

    c. Gout

    d. Systemic lupus erythematosus

    e. Psoriatic arthritis

8. A 60-year-old male presents with pain and stiffness in his fingers, worse in the mornings and improving throughout the day. On examination, there are no systemic symptoms, but Heberden's nodes are present. What is the most likely diagnosis?

    a. Rheumatoid arthritis

    b. Osteoarthritis

    c. Gout

    d. Systemic lupus erythematosus

    e. Psoriatic arthritis

9. A 65-year-old female presents with chronic pain and stiffness in her hands and knees. She notes that the pain worsens with activity and improves with rest. On examination, there are Heberden's and Bouchard's nodes. What is the most likely diagnosis?

    a. Rheumatoid arthritis

    b. Osteoarthritis

    c. Gout

    d. Systemic lupus erythematosus

    e. Psoriatic arthritis

10. A 50-year-old male presents with chronic pain and swelling in his knees. He notes that the pain is worse with climbing stairs and after prolonged walking. On examination, there is crepitus and tenderness over the knee joints. What is the most likely diagnosis?

    a. Rheumatoid arthritis

    b. Osteoarthritis

    c. Gout

    d. Ankylosing spondylitis

    e. Septic arthritis

11. A 60-year-old female presents with pain and swelling in her big toe. She notes that the pain started suddenly and is very intense, making it difficult to walk. What is the most likely diagnosis?

    a. Rheumatoid arthritis

    b. Osteoarthritis

    c. Gout

    d. Systemic lupus erythematosus

    e. Psoriatic arthritis

12. A 70-year-old male presents with chronic low back pain and stiffness, worse in the mornings and after prolonged sitting or standing. There is no radiation of pain into the legs. What is the most likely diagnosis?

    a. Rheumatoid arthritis

    b. Osteoarthritis

    c. Ankylosing spondylitis

    d. Systemic lupus erythematosus

    e. Psoriatic arthritis

13. A 55-year-old female presents with pain and swelling in multiple joints, including the wrists and hands. She reports morning stiffness lasting more than an hour. On examination, there are symmetric joint involvement and rheumatoid nodules. What is the most likely diagnosis?

    a.   Rheumatoid arthritis

    b.   Osteoarthritis

    c.   Gout

    d.   Systemic lupus erythematosus

    e.   Psoriatic arthritis

14. A 60-year-old male presents with pain and stiffness in his fingers, worse in the mornings and improving throughout the day. On examination, there are no systemic symptoms, but Heberden's nodes are present. What is the most likely diagnosis?

    a.   Rheumatoid arthritis

    b.   Osteoarthritis

    c.   Gout

    d.   Systemic lupus erythematosus

    e.   Psoriatic arthritis

15. A 65-year-old female presents with chronic pain and stiffness in her hands and knees. She notes that the pain worsens with activity and improves with rest. On examination, there are Heberden's and Bouchard's nodes. What is the most likely diagnosis?

    a.   Rheumatoid arthritis

    b.   Osteoarthritis

    c.   Gout

    d.   Systemic lupus erythematosus

    e.   Psoriatic arthritis

Osteoporosis

1. A 65-year-old postmenopausal woman presents with a history of multiple fragility fractures over the past few years. She has no other significant medical history. What is the most likely diagnosis for this patient?

    a. Osteomalacia

    b. Osteoarthritis

    c. Osteoporosis

    d. Paget's disease

2. A 70-year-old man presents with acute-onset severe back pain after lifting a heavy object. He has a history of chronic steroid use for his asthma. What is the most likely cause of his back pain?

    a. Spinal stenosis

    b. Vertebral compression fracture

    c. Disc herniation

    d. Spondylolisthesis

3. A 60-year-old woman presents with height loss of 2 inches over the past few years and a stooped posture. She has no significant medical history. What is the most likely diagnosis for this patient?

    a. Osteoarthritis

    b. Osteoporosis

    c. Rheumatoid arthritis

    d. Ankylosing spondylitis

4. A 75-year-old man presents with sudden-onset pain and swelling in his right hip after a minor fall. He has a history of chronic kidney disease. What is the most appropriate next step in management?

    a. Start bisphosphonate therapy

    b. Perform hip arthroscopy

    c. Administer vitamin D supplementation

    d. Order a hip X-ray

5. A 55-year-old woman presents with chronic lower back pain and a history of several fragility fractures in the past year. She is otherwise healthy. Which of the following diagnostic tests is most appropriate for confirming osteoporosis in this patient?

    a. MRI of the lumbar spine

    b. Dual-energy X-ray absorptiometry (DXA) scan

    c. Bone scan

    d. CT scan of the spine

6. A 68-year-old woman presents with a history of hip fracture 6 months ago. She is concerned about her risk of future fractures. Which of the following medications is most appropriate for reducing the risk of future fractures in this patient?

    a. Ibuprofen

    b. Alendronate

    c. Paracetamol

    d. Benzodiazepines

7. A 70-year-old man presents with gradual onset of back pain and height loss. He has no significant medical history. Which of the following findings is most likely on imaging studies?

    a. Osteophytes

    b. Vertebral compression fractures

    c. Joint space narrowing

    d. Subchondral cysts

8. A 65-year-old woman with a history of osteoporosis presents with acute right hip pain after a fall. What is the most appropriate initial management for this patient?

    a. Perform hip arthroscopy

    b. Start teriparatide therapy

    c. Administer intravenous bisphosphonates

    d. Order a hip X-ray

9. A 70-year-old woman presents with chronic lower back pain and height loss. She has no significant medical history. Which of the following treatments is most appropriate for this patient?

    a. NSAIDs for pain relief

    b. Corticosteroids

    c. Calcium and vitamin D supplementation

    d. Teriparatide

10. A 60-year-old woman presents with a history of wrist and hip fractures over the past year. She has no other significant medical history. Which of the following laboratory tests is most appropriate for evaluating secondary causes of osteoporosis?

    a. Serum calcium

    b. Thyroid function tests

    c. Liver function tests

    d. Complete blood count

11. A 75-year-old man presents with sudden-onset severe back pain after lifting a heavy object. He has a history of chronic steroid use for his rheumatoid arthritis. What is the most likely cause of his back pain?

    a. Vertebral compression fracture

    b. Osteoarthritis

    c. Disc herniation

    d. Spinal stenosis

12. A 70-year-old woman presents with acute right hip pain after a fall. She has a history of chronic kidney disease. What is the most appropriate next step in management?

    a. Start bisphosphonate therapy

    b. Perform hip arthroscopy

    c. Administer vitamin D supplementation

    d. Order a hip X-ray

13. A 65-year-old man presents with height loss of 2 inches over the past few years and a stooped posture. He has no significant medical history. Which of the following findings is most likely on physical examination?

    a.   Decreased range of motion in the hip

    b.   Forward flexion of the spine

    c.   Knee effusion

    d.   Swelling in the wrists

14. A 60-year-old woman presents with chronic lower back pain and a history of several fragility fractures in the past year. She is otherwise healthy. Which of the following diagnostic tests is most appropriate for confirming osteoporosis in this patient?

    a.   MRI of the lumbar spine

    b.   Dual-energy X-ray absorptiometry (DXA) scan

    c.   Bone scan

    d.   CT scan of the spine

15. A 55-year-old woman presents with chronic lower back pain and a history of several fragility fractures in the past year. She is otherwise healthy. Which of the following medications is most appropriate for reducing the risk of future fractures in this patient?

    a.   NSAIDs

    b.   Alendronate

    c.   Paracetamol

    d.   Benzodiazepines

Panic Disorder

1. A 30-year-old woman presents to the emergency room with palpitations, sweating, and a sensation of impending doom. She reports similar episodes over the past month. What is the most likely diagnosis?

    a. Acute myocardial infarction

    b. Panic disorder

    c. Generalized anxiety disorder

    d. Hyperthyroidism

2. A 25-year-old man presents with recurrent episodes of sweating, trembling, shortness of breath, and fear of losing control. He is otherwise healthy. What is the most likely diagnosis?

    a. Panic disorder

    b. Social anxiety disorder

    c. Obsessive-compulsive disorder

    d. Post-traumatic stress disorder

3. A 35-year-old woman presents with recurrent episodes of palpitations, chest pain, and dizziness. She worries excessively about her health and often seeks reassurance from her family. What is the most likely diagnosis?

    a. Panic disorder

    b. Hypochondriasis

    c. Social anxiety disorder

    d. Generalized anxiety disorder

4. A 40-year-old man presents with recurrent episodes of sweating, trembling, and a feeling of impending doom. He has no significant medical history. Which of the following is the most appropriate initial treatment for this patient?

    a. Sertraline

    b. Cognitive-behavioral therapy (CBT)

    c. Lorazepam

    d. Escitalopram

5. A 30-year-old woman presents to her primary care physician with recurrent episodes of chest pain, palpitations, and shortness of breath. She fears she might have a heart condition. What is the most likely diagnosis?

    a. Panic disorder

    b. Acute coronary syndrome

    c. Generalized anxiety disorder

    d. Mitral valve prolapse

6. A 25-year-old man presents with recurrent episodes of sweating, trembling, shortness of breath, and a fear of dying. His symptoms occur suddenly and peak within minutes. What is the most likely diagnosis?

    a. Panic disorder

    b. Social anxiety disorder

    c. Obsessive-compulsive disorder

    d. Post-traumatic stress disorder

7. A 35-year-old woman presents with recurrent episodes of palpitations, chest pain, and dizziness. She has been worried about her health and frequently visits the emergency room.What is the most likely diagnosis?

   a. Panic disorder

   b. Hypochondriasis

   c. Social anxiety disorder

   d. Generalized anxiety disorder

8. A 40-year-old man presents with recurrent episodes of sweating, trembling, and a feeling of impending doom. He has no significant medical history.Which of the following is the most appropriate initial treatment for this patient?

   a. Sertraline

   b. Cognitive-behavioral therapy (CBT)

   c. Lorazepam

   d. Escitalopram

9. A 30-year-old woman presents to her primary care physician with recurrent episodes of chest pain, palpitations, and shortness of breath. She fears she might have a heart condition.What is the most likely diagnosis?

   a. Panic disorder

   b. Acute coronary syndrome

   c. Generalized anxiety disorder

   d. Mitral valve prolapse

10. A 25-year-old man presents with recurrent episodes of sweating, trembling, shortness of breath, and a fear of dying. His symptoms occur suddenly and peak within minutes. What is the most likely diagnosis?

   a. Panic disorder

   b. Social anxiety disorder

   c. Obsessive-compulsive disorder

   d. Post-traumatic stress disorder

11. A 35-year-old woman presents with recurrent episodes of palpitations, chest pain, and dizziness. She has been worried about her health and frequently visits the emergency room. What is the most likely diagnosis?

   a. Panic disorder

   b. Hypochondriasis

   c. Social anxiety disorder

   d. Generalized anxiety disorder

12. A 40-year-old man presents with recurrent episodes of sweating, trembling, and a feeling of impending doom. He has no significant medical history. Which of the following is the most appropriate initial treatment for this patient?

   a. Sertraline

   b. Cognitive-behavioral therapy (CBT)

   c. Lorazepam

   d. Escitalopram

13. A 30-year-old woman presents to her primary care physician with recurrent episodes of chest pain, palpitations, and shortness of breath. She fears she might have a heart condition. What is the most likely diagnosis?

    a.   Panic disorder

    b.   Acute coronary syndrome

    c.   Generalized anxiety disorder

    d.   Mitral valve prolapse

14. A 25-year-old man presents with recurrent episodes of sweating, trembling, shortness of breath, and a fear of dying. His symptoms occur suddenly and peak within minutes. What is the most likely diagnosis?

    a.   Panic disorder

    b.   Social anxiety disorder

    c.   Obsessive-compulsive disorder

    d.   Post-traumatic stress disorder

15. A 35-year-old woman presents with recurrent episodes of palpitations, chest pain, and dizziness. She has been worried about her health and frequently visits the emergency room. What is the most likely diagnosis?

    a.   Panic disorder

    b.   Hypochondriasis

    c.   Social anxiety disorder

    d.   Generalized anxiety disorder

Parkinson's Disease

1. A 65-year-old man presents with a resting tremor in his right hand that started six months ago. He also complains of stiffness in his right arm and leg, which improves with movement. What is the most likely diagnosis?

    a. Essential tremor

    b. Parkinson's disease

    c. Multiple sclerosis

    d. Huntington's disease

2. A 70-year-old woman presents with slowness of movement, stiffness, and difficulty with balance. Her symptoms have progressively worsened over the past year. What is the most likely pathology underlying her symptoms?

    a. Degeneration of the basal ganglia

    b. Degeneration of the cerebellum

    c. Degeneration of the motor cortex

    d. Degeneration of the hippocampus

3. A 60-year-old man presents with tremor, muscle rigidity, and slow movement. His symptoms are more pronounced on the right side of his body. What is the classic triad of symptoms seen in Parkinson's disease?

    a. Tremor, rigidity, and bradykinesia

    b. Tremor, ataxia, and dyskinesia

    c. Ataxia, rigidity, and dysarthria

    d. Bradykinesia, ataxia, and dystonia

4. A 65-year-old woman presents with a tremor in her right hand that improves with action and worsens at rest. She has a family history of similar symptoms in her father. What is the most likely diagnosis?

    a. Parkinson's disease

    b. Essential tremor

    c. Huntington's disease

    d. Alzheimer's disease

5. A 70-year-old man presents with a resting tremor, muscle rigidity, and bradykinesia. He also experiences freezing episodes while walking. Which of the following is a common motor complication in Parkinson's disease characterized by a sudden inability to move?

    a. Freezing of gait

    b. Chorea

    c. Dystonia

    d. Bradykinesia

6. A 60-year-old man presents with progressive difficulty with balance, stiffness, and slowness of movement. He has noticed a slight tremor in his left hand for the past year. What is the initial pharmacological treatment for this patient's symptoms?

    a. Levodopa

    b. Donepezil

    c. Propranolol

    d. Haloperidol

7. A 65-year-old woman presents with a resting tremor in her right hand, muscle stiffness, and slowness of movement. She has noticed that her symptoms worsen when she is stressed. Which of the following is a non-motor symptom commonly associated with Parkinson's disease?

    a. Dysphagia

    b. Hyperactivity

    c. Tachycardia

    d. Hypertension

8. A 70-year-old man presents with a resting tremor in his right hand, muscle rigidity, and slowness of movement. His symptoms have gradually worsened over the past two years. Which of the following is a potential side effect of long-term levodopa therapy?

    a. Dyskinesia

    b. Hypotension

    c. Constipation

    d. Insomnia

9. A 60-year-old woman presents with a resting tremor in her left hand, muscle stiffness, and slowness of movement. She has difficulty with balance and has fallen twice in the past month. Which of the following imaging modalities is most helpful in diagnosing Parkinson's disease?

    a. Magnetic resonance imaging (MRI)

    b. Computed tomography (CT)

    c. Single-photon emission computed tomography (SPECT)

    d. Positron emission tomography (PET)

10. A 65-year-old man presents with a resting tremor in his right hand, muscle rigidity, and slowness of movement. He also complains of a decreased ability to smell and vivid dreams. Which of the following is a common non-motor symptom associated with Parkinson's disease?

    a. Diarrhea

    b. Urinary retention

    c. Hyposmia

    d. Hypertension

11. A 70-year-old woman presents with a resting tremor in her right hand, muscle stiffness, and slowness of movement. She also experiences pain in her right shoulder. Which of the following is a common non-motor symptom associated with Parkinson's disease?

    a. Constipation

    b. Hypertension

    c. Hyperactivity

    d. Tachycardia

12. A 60-year-old man presents with progressive difficulty with balance, stiffness, and slowness of movement. He has noticed a slight tremor in his left hand for the past year. What is the initial pharmacological treatment for this patient's symptoms?

    a. Levodopa

    b. Donepezil

    c. Propranolol

    d. Haloperidol

13. A 65-year-old woman presents with a resting tremor in her right hand, muscle stiffness, and slowness of movement. She has noticed that her symptoms worsen when she is stressed. Which of the following is a non-motor symptom commonly associated with Parkinson's disease?

    a. Dysphagia

    b. Hyperactivity

    c. Tachycardia

    d. Hypertension

14. A 70-year-old man presents with a resting tremor in his right hand, muscle rigidity, and slowness of movement. His symptoms have gradually worsened over the past two years. Which of the following is a potential side effect of long-term levodopa therapy?

    a. Dyskinesia

    b. Hypotension

    c. Constipation

    d. Insomnia

15. A 60-year-old woman presents with a resting tremor in her left hand, muscle stiffness, and slowness of movement. She has difficulty with balance and has fallen twice in the past month. Which of the following imaging modalities is most helpful in diagnosing Parkinson's disease?

    a. Magnetic resonance imaging (MRI)

    b. Computed tomography (CT)

    c. Single-photon emission computed tomography (SPECT)

    d. Positron emission tomography (PET)

Peptic Ulcer Disease

1. A 45-year-old male presents with burning epigastric pain that improves with food intake and worsens with fasting. He has a history of NSAID use for chronic back pain. Which of the following is the most likely diagnosis?

    a. Acute pancreatitis

    b. Peptic ulcer disease (PUD)

    c. Gastroesophageal reflux disease (GERD)

    d. Gallstone pancreatitis

2. A 30-year-old female presents with epigastric pain that worsens at night and is relieved by antacids. She has no significant medical history. Which of the following is the most appropriate initial diagnostic test?

    a. Esophagogastroduodenoscopy (EGD)

    b. Helicobacter pylori serology

    c. Abdominal ultrasound

    d. Barium swallow

3. A 50-year-old male presents with epigastric pain that improves with food intake and is associated with nausea and bloating. He has a history of smoking and alcohol use. Which of the following is the most likely cause of his symptoms?

    a. Gastric adenocarcinoma

    b. Duodenal ulcer

    c. Pancreatitis

    d. Gastroesophageal reflux disease (GERD)

4. A 55-year-old female presents with epigastric pain that is worse on an empty stomach and improves with food intake. She has no significant medical history. Which of the following medications is the most appropriate initial treatment?

    a. Proton pump inhibitor (PPI)

    b. H2 receptor antagonist (H2RA)

    c. Sucralfate

    d. Antacid

5. A 40-year-old male presents with epigastric pain that worsens after meals and is associated with unintentional weight loss. Upper endoscopy reveals a gastric ulcer with irregular borders. Which of the following is the most appropriate next step in management?

    a. Biopsy of the ulcer

    b. Treatment with a PPI

    c. Helicobacter pylori testing

    d. Surgical consultation

6. A 35-year-old male presents with recurrent epigastric pain and has a history of chronic NSAID use. Upper endoscopy reveals multiple small ulcers in the duodenum. Which of the following is the most appropriate next step in management?

    a. Start treatment with a PPI

    b. Perform a urea breath test for H. pylori

    c. Discontinue NSAID use

    d. Refer for surgical consultation

7. A 60-year-old male presents with epigastric pain that worsens at night and is relieved by food intake. Upper endoscopy reveals a duodenal ulcer with an adherent clot. What is the most appropriate initial management?

    a. Perform endoscopic hemostasis

    b. Start treatment with a PPI

    c. Immediate surgical consultation

    d. Transfuse packed red blood cells

8. A 50-year-old female presents with epigastric pain and hematemesis. She is hemodynamically stable. Upper endoscopy reveals a bleeding gastric ulcer. What is the most appropriate initial management?

    a. Perform endoscopic hemostasis

    b. Start treatment with a PPI

    c. Immediate surgical consultation

    d. Transfuse packed red blood cells

9. A 45-year-old male presents with severe epigastric pain that radiates to the back. He is vomiting and has a distended abdomen. Imaging reveals a perforated duodenal ulcer. What is the most appropriate initial management?

    a. Immediate surgical consultation

    b. Start treatment with a PPI

    c. Perform endoscopic hemostasis

    d. Start broad-spectrum antibiotics

10. A 55-year-old male presents with epigastric pain that is relieved by food intake. He has a history of smoking and alcohol use. Upper endoscopy reveals an ulcer in the gastric antrum. Which of the following is the most appropriate next step in management?

    a. Perform H. pylori testing

    b. Start treatment with a PPI

    c. Refer for surgical consultation

    d. Repeat endoscopy in 6 months

11. A 60-year-old female presents with epigastric pain and nausea. She has a history of chronic NSAID use. Upper endoscopy reveals a gastric ulcer with a visible vessel. What is the most appropriate initial management?

    a. Perform endoscopic hemostasis

    b. Start treatment with a PPI

    c. Immediate surgical consultation

    d. Discontinue NSAID use

12. A 65-year-old male presents with epigastric pain that is worse on an empty stomach. He has a history of smoking and alcohol use. Upper endoscopy reveals a duodenal ulcer. Which of the following is the most appropriate initial treatment?

    a. Start treatment with a PPI

    b. Perform H. pylori testing

    c. Refer for surgical consultation

    d. Discontinue NSAID use

13. A 55-year-old male presents with severe epigastric pain and hematemesis. He is hemodynamically unstable. Imaging reveals a bleeding gastric ulcer. What is the most appropriate initial management?

    a. Immediate surgical consultation

    b. Perform endoscopic hemostasis

    c. Start treatment with a PPI

    d. Transfuse packed red blood cells

14. A 50-year-old male presents with epigastric pain that is worse on an empty stomach. He has a history of chronic NSAID use. Upper endoscopy reveals multiple duodenal ulcers. Which of the following is the most appropriate next step in management?

    a. Perform H. pylori testing

    b. Start treatment with a PPI

    c. Refer for surgical consultation

    d. Discontinue NSAID use

15. A 45-year-old female presents with epigastric pain that improves with food intake. She has no significant medical history. Which of the following medications is the most appropriate initial treatment?

    a. Proton pump inhibitor (PPI)

    b. H2 receptor antagonist (H2RA)

    c. Sucralfate

    d. Antacid

Peripheral Arterial Disease (PAD)

1. A 65-year-old male smoker presents with cramping leg pain that occurs with walking and resolves with rest. Physical examination reveals diminished pedal pulses. What is the most likely diagnosis?

    a. Deep vein thrombosis (DVT)

    b. Peripheral Arterial Disease (PAD)

    c. Chronic venous insufficiency

    d. Buerger's disease

2. A 72-year-old woman with diabetes and hypertension presents with pain in her left foot at rest. On examination, her left foot is cool to touch and appears pale. What is the most likely cause of her symptoms?

    a. Diabetic neuropathy

    b. Diabetic foot ulcer

    c. Peripheral Arterial Disease (PAD)

    d. Osteomyelitis

3. A 60-year-old man presents with non-healing ulcers on his right foot. He reports a history of smoking and diabetes. What is the most likely cause of his non-healing ulcers?

    a. Diabetic foot ulcer

    b. Neuropathic ulcer

    c. Peripheral Arterial Disease (PAD)

    d. Venous stasis ulcer

4. A 68-year-old woman presents with sudden onset of pain, pallor, and paralysis of her left leg. Her left foot is cold to touch. What is the most likely diagnosis?

    a. Acute arterial thrombosis

    b. Venous thromboembolism

    c. Diabetic neuropathy

    d. Osteomyelitis

5. A 70-year-old man with PAD presents with an ulcer on his left great toe. The ulcer is well-demarcated with no signs of infection.What is the most appropriate initial management of this patient's ulcer?

    a. Debridement and topical antibiotics

    b. Compression therapy

    c. Surgical revascularization

    d. Offloading and wound care

6. A 62-year-old man presents with calf pain that worsens with elevation and improves with dangling his legs over the bedside.What physical examination finding is likely present in this patient?

    a. Hair loss on legs

    b. Pitting edema

    c. Diminished pedal pulses

    d. Cyanotic discoloration of toes

7. A 58-year-old woman with PAD presents with persistent leg pain at rest and non-healing ulcers on both feet.What is the most appropriate next step in management?

    a. Start cilostazol therapy

    b. Perform angiography with possible intervention

    c. Start dual antiplatelet therapy

    d. Refer for amputation evaluation

8. A 65-year-old man with PAD presents with intermittent claudication. He asks about exercise recommendations.What is the most appropriate exercise recommendation for this patient?

    a. High-intensity interval training

    b. Avoid exercise to prevent worsening of symptoms

    c. Supervised exercise program (e.g., walking program)

    d. Weightlifting and resistance training

9. A 70-year-old woman with PAD presents with progressive pain in her left leg that is worse at night and improves with dependency. What is the most likely diagnosis?

    a. Diabetic neuropathy

    b. Restless legs syndrome

    c. Arterial insufficiency

    d. Sciatica

10. A 66-year-old man with PAD is found to have decreased ankle-brachial index (ABI) on examination. What does a decreased ABI indicate in this patient?

    a. Venous insufficiency

    b. Diabetic neuropathy

    c. Arterial insufficiency

    d. Osteoarthritis

11. A 63-year-old man with PAD presents with acute onset of numbness and weakness in his right leg. What is the most likely cause of his symptoms?

    a. Ischemic stroke

    b. Peripheral neuropathy

    c. Acute arterial thrombosis

    d. Deep vein thrombosis (DVT)

12. A 69-year-old woman with PAD presents with severe leg pain, pallor, and paralysis in her left leg. There is absence of distal pulses. What is the most appropriate initial management of this patient?

    a. Start anticoagulation therapy

    b. Perform immediate surgical revascularization

    c. Apply a warming blanket to the affected leg

    d. Refer for amputation evaluation

13. A 67-year-old man with PAD presents with severe pain in his right leg. On examination, his right foot is cyanotic, cold, and pulseless. What is the most likely cause of his symptoms?

    a. Acute arterial thrombosis

    b. Diabetic foot ulcer

    c. Cellulitis

    d. Deep vein thrombosis (DVT)

14. A 71-year-old man with PAD presents with worsening intermittent claudication. He is currently on aspirin therapy. What is the most appropriate next step in management?

    a. Increase aspirin dose

    b. Add clopidogrel to aspirin therapy

    c. Start cilostazol therapy

    d. Refer for amputation evaluation

15. A 64-year-old woman with PAD is started on cilostazol therapy. She develops palpitations and dizziness. What is the most appropriate next step in management?

    a. Discontinue cilostazol

    b. Switch to aspirin therapy

    c. Add beta-blocker therapy

    d. Perform an ECG

Pneumonia

1. A 65-year-old man presents with sudden onset fever, productive cough with purulent sputum, and pleuritic chest pain. On auscultation, coarse crackles are heard in the right lower lung field. What is the most likely diagnosis?

    1. Bronchitis

    2. Pneumonia

    3. Asthma exacerbation

    4. Pulmonary embolism

2. A 50-year-old woman presents with fever, non-productive cough, and pleuritic chest pain. She has a history of systemic lupus erythematosus (SLE). Her chest X-ray shows patchy infiltrates in the left lower lobe. What is the most likely diagnosis?

    1. Bronchitis

    2. Pneumonia

    3. Pulmonary embolism

    4. Tuberculosis

3. An 80-year-old man presents with confusion, fever, and cough with yellowish sputum. On examination, decreased breath sounds and dullness to percussion are noted over the right lower lung field. What is the most likely diagnosis?

    1. Bronchitis

    2. Pneumonia

    3. Pulmonary embolism

    4. Lung cancer

4. A 25-year-old woman presents with sudden onset high fever, chills, and pleuritic chest pain. She has a history of sickle cell disease. Her chest X-ray shows a wedge-shaped infiltrate in the left lower lobe. What is the most likely diagnosis?

    1. Bronchitis

    2. Pneumonia

    3. Pulmonary embolism

    4. Lung abscess

5. A 60-year-old man presents with cough, shortness of breath, and greenish foul-smelling sputum. His chest X-ray shows a cavitary lesion with an air-fluid level. What is the most likely diagnosis?

    1. Bronchitis

    2. Pneumonia

    3. Pulmonary embolism

    4. Lung abscess

6. A 45-year-old woman presents with fever, cough, and shortness of breath. She has a history of rheumatoid arthritis treated with methotrexate. Her chest X-ray shows bilateral interstitial infiltrates. What is the most likely diagnosis?

    1. Bronchitis

    2. Pneumonia

    3. Pulmonary embolism

    4. Pneumocystis pneumonia

7. A 70-year-old man presents with cough, dyspnea, and a low-grade fever. His chest X-ray shows a right middle lobe infiltrate and a small pleural effusion. What is the most likely diagnosis?

    1. Bronchitis

    2. Pneumonia

    3. Pulmonary embolism

    4. Lung cancer

8. A 55-year-old woman presents with a cough productive of rusty-colored sputum, fever, and pleuritic chest pain. On examination, there are crackles heard over the right lower lung field. What is the most likely diagnosis?

   1. Bronchitis
   2. Pneumonia
   3. Pulmonary embolism
   4. Lung cancer

9. A 30-year-old man presents with sudden onset sharp chest pain and shortness of breath. He has a history of recent leg surgery. His chest X-ray shows a wedge-shaped infiltrate in the right lower lobe. What is the most likely diagnosis?

   1. Bronchitis
   2. Pneumonia
   3. Pulmonary embolism
   4. Lung cancer

10. A 65-year-old woman presents with cough, fever, and pleuritic chest pain. Her chest X-ray shows a right lower lobe infiltrate with an air-fluid level. What is the most likely diagnosis?

    1. Bronchitis
    2. Pneumonia
    3. Pulmonary embolism
    4. Lung abscess

11. A 40-year-old man presents with a cough that is productive of foul-smelling sputum. He has a history of poor dentition. On examination, decreased breath sounds and dullness to percussion are noted over the right lower lung field. What is the most likely diagnosis?

    1. Bronchitis

    2. Pneumonia

    3. Pulmonary embolism

    4. Lung abscess

12. A 55-year-old woman presents with a cough, fever, and dyspnea. She is a smoker and has chronic obstructive pulmonary disease (COPD). Her chest X-ray shows hyperinflation and scattered infiltrates. What is the most likely diagnosis?

    1. Bronchitis

    2. Pneumonia

    3. Pulmonary embolism

    4. Exacerbation of COPD

13. A 28-year-old woman presents with fever, cough, and chest pain. She recently traveled to Southeast Asia. Her chest X-ray shows patchy infiltrates. What is the most likely diagnosis?

    1. Bronchitis

    2. Pneumonia

    3. Pulmonary embolism

    4. Tuberculosis

14. A 60-year-old man presents with cough, fever, and dyspnea. His chest X-ray shows a cavitary lesion in the left upper lobe with an air-fluid level. What is the most likely diagnosis?

    1. Bronchitis

    2. Pneumonia

    3. Pulmonary embolism

    4. Lung abscess

15. A 50-year-old man presents with fever, cough, and hemoptysis. His chest X-ray shows a coin lesion in the left upper lobe. What is the most likely diagnosis?

    1. Bronchitis

    2. Pneumonia

    3. Pulmonary embolism

    4. Lung cancer

Post-Traumatic Stress Disorder (PTSD)

1. A 30-year-old military veteran presents with intrusive memories, nightmares, and flashbacks of combat experiences. He avoids crowds and loud noises. What is the most likely diagnosis?

    a. Generalized Anxiety Disorder

    b. Major Depressive Disorder

    c. Post-Traumatic Stress Disorder (PTSD)

    d. Panic Disorder

2. A 25-year-old woman was involved in a car accident 6 months ago. She now experiences distressing dreams, emotional numbness, and difficulty concentrating. What is the most likely diagnosis?

    a. Adjustment Disorder

    b. Panic Disorder

    c. Post-Traumatic Stress Disorder (PTSD)

    d. Social Anxiety Disorder

3. A 40-year-old man presents with persistent irritability, difficulty sleeping, and exaggerated startle response after witnessing a violent crime. What is the most appropriate initial management?

    a. Benzodiazepines

    b. Cognitive-behavioral therapy (CBT)

    c. Antidepressants

    d. Supportive therapy

4. A 35-year-old woman reports feeling detached from others, emotional numbness, and an inability to experience positive emotions since being sexually assaulted 2 years ago. What is the term for this symptom?

    a. Depersonalization

    b. Derealization

    c. Dissociation

    d. Anhedonia

5. A 28-year-old man with PTSD has been having nightmares and intrusive memories of his military service in Iraq. He is started on prazosin. What is the mechanism of action of this medication?

    a. Selective serotonin reuptake inhibition

    b. Alpha-1 adrenergic receptor antagonism

    c. GABA agonism

    d. Norepinephrine reuptake inhibition

6. A 45-year-old woman with PTSD has been avoiding reminders of her traumatic experience. What is the term for this symptom?

    a. Anhedonia

    b. Avoidance

    c. Hypervigilance

    d. Flashbacks

7. A 32-year-old man who witnessed a fatal accident has been experiencing intrusive thoughts, flashbacks, and irritability for the past month. What is the most appropriate initial intervention?

    a. Benzodiazepines

    b. Trauma-focused cognitive-behavioral therapy (CBT)

    c. Antipsychotic medication

    d. Selective serotonin reuptake inhibitor (SSRI)

8. A 35-year-old woman with PTSD has been having difficulty concentrating, exaggerated startle response, and difficulty sleeping since a severe earthquake 6 months ago. What is the term for this cluster of symptoms?

    a. Hyperarousal

    b. Intrusion

    c. Negative alterations in mood or cognitions

    d. Avoidance

9. A 40-year-old man with PTSD has started experiencing recurrent episodes of feeling detached from his surroundings, as if in a dream, since his traumatic event. What is the term for this symptom?

   a. Depersonalization

   b. Derealization

   c. Dissociation

   d. Anhedonia

10. A 30-year-old woman with PTSD has been having difficulty remembering aspects of her traumatic experience. What is the term for this symptom?

   a. Amnesia

   b. Avoidance

   c. Intrusion

   d. Dissociation

11. A 35-year-old man with PTSD has been avoiding talking about his traumatic experience and refuses to visit the place where it occurred. What is the term for this symptom?

   a. Anhedonia

   b. Avoidance

   c. Hypervigilance

   d. Flashbacks

12. A 28-year-old woman with PTSD has been experiencing recurrent, distressing memories and nightmares about her abusive childhood. What is the most appropriate treatment?

   a. Benzodiazepines

   b. Antipsychotic medication

   c. Trauma-focused cognitive-behavioral therapy (CBT)

   d. Selective serotonin reuptake inhibitor (SSRI)

13. A 45-year-old man with PTSD is started on sertraline (Zoloft). What is the mechanism of action of this medication in treating PTSD?

    a. Blocks alpha-1 adrenergic receptors

    b. Selective serotonin reuptake inhibition

    c. GABA agonism

    d. Norepinephrine reuptake inhibition

14. A 30-year-old woman with PTSD is experiencing significant nightmares that disrupt her sleep. What medication is commonly used to reduce nightmares in PTSD?

    a. Amitriptyline

    b. Prazosin

    c. Olanzapine

    d. Risperidone

15. A 35-year-old man with PTSD is experiencing severe anxiety and avoidance behaviors related to his traumatic experience. What is the most appropriate initial therapy?

    a. Dialectical behavior therapy (DBT)

    b. Prolonged exposure therapy (PE)

    c. Eye movement desensitization and reprocessing (EMDR)

    d. Supportive therapy

Premenstrual Syndrome (PMS)

1. A 28-year-old woman presents with irritability, mood swings, and breast tenderness that worsen in the days leading up to her menstrual period. What is the most likely diagnosis?

    a. Premenstrual syndrome (PMS)

    b. Dysmenorrhea

    c. Endometriosis

    d. Menopause

2. A 30-year-old woman reports feeling bloated, experiencing headaches, and having difficulty sleeping for several days before her period starts. Which symptom is not typically associated with PMS?

    a. Bloating

    b. Headaches

    c. Breast tenderness

    d. Hot flashes

3. A 25-year-old woman is experiencing severe mood swings, anxiety, and depression during the luteal phase of her menstrual cycle. Which is the most appropriate initial management?

    a. Selective serotonin reuptake inhibitors (SSRIs)

    b. Oral contraceptive pills (OCPs)

    c. Nonsteroidal anti-inflammatory drugs (NSAIDs)

    d. Behavioral therapies

4. A 35-year-old woman complains of feeling fatigued, having trouble concentrating, and being overly emotional for a few days before her period each month. Which is the most appropriate next step in management?

    a. Behavioral therapy

    b. Hormonal therapy

    c. Cognitive behavioral therapy (CBT)

    d. Symptom diary

5. A 40-year-old woman with a history of PMS presents with severe emotional symptoms and asks for additional treatment options. What is a second-line treatment for severe PMS symptoms?

    a. Calcium supplementation

    b. Diuretics

    c. SSRIs

    d. Vitamin D supplementation

6. A 30-year-old woman has been diagnosed with PMS. She is concerned about weight gain and fluid retention before her period. Which treatment option is least likely to exacerbate weight gain and fluid retention?

    a. Behavioral therapy

    b. Calcium supplementation

    c. Diuretics

    d. Exercise

7. A 28-year-old woman reports feeling irritable and anxious for several days before her period each month. She is otherwise healthy. Which physical symptom is most commonly associated with PMS?

    a. Headaches

    b. Lower back pain

    c. Nausea

    d. Palpitations

8. A 35-year-old woman presents with severe irritability, crying spells, and difficulty concentrating during the luteal phase of her menstrual cycle. What is the first-line pharmacologic treatment for these symptoms?

    a. SSRIs

    b. OCPs

    c. NSAIDs

    d. Calcium supplementation

9. A 32-year-old woman has been diagnosed with PMS. She asks if changes in diet could help alleviate her symptoms. Which dietary recommendation is supported for managing PMS symptoms?

    a. Increased caffeine intake

    b. High-fat diet

    c. Low-salt diet

    d. High-sugar diet

10. A 40-year-old woman with severe PMS symptoms is concerned about the impact on her work and personal relationships. What is the most appropriate next step?

    a. Refer for psychotherapy

    b. Prescribe diuretics

    c. Initiate SSRIs

    d. Recommend calcium supplementation

11. A 28-year-old woman experiences severe breast tenderness, bloating, and irritability before her period each month. What is the initial step in diagnosing PMS?

    a. Complete blood count (CBC)

    b. Thyroid function tests

    c. Symptom diary

    d. Pelvic ultrasound

12. A 35-year-old woman presents with symptoms of PMS, including mood swings, fatigue, and food cravings. What is the first-line non-pharmacologic treatment for these symptoms?

    a. Exercise

    b. Acupuncture

    c. Meditation

    d. Herbal supplements

14. A 30-year-old woman with severe PMS symptoms asks about the effectiveness of herbal supplements for symptom relief. Which herbal supplement has evidence supporting its use for PMS symptoms?

    a. St. John's wort

    b. Evening primrose oil

    c. Ginseng

    d. Ginkgo biloba

15. A 40-year-old woman is considering starting oral contraceptive pills (OCPs) for the management of her PMS symptoms. How do OCPs help alleviate PMS symptoms?

    a. By reducing estrogen levels

    b. By stabilizing hormone levels

    c. By increasing serotonin levels

    d. By promoting ovulation

Prostate Cancer

1. A 65-year-old male presents with lower urinary tract symptoms (LUTS), including frequency, nocturia, and hesitancy. Digital rectal examination (DRE) reveals an enlarged prostate with a firm nodule. PSA level is 10 ng/mL. What is the next step in management?

   a. Start alpha-blocker therapy

   b. Repeat PSA measurement in 3 months

   c. Perform transrectal ultrasound-guided biopsy

   d. Refer to urology for cystoscopy

2. A 55-year-old male presents for a routine health check-up. He has no urinary symptoms. PSA level is 2 ng/mL. What is the next step in management?

   a. Perform transrectal ultrasound-guided biopsy

   b. Repeat PSA measurement in 1 year

   c. Start alpha-blocker therapy

   d. Refer to urology for cystoscopy

3. A 70-year-old male presents with bone pain and elevated alkaline phosphatase. PSA level is 60 ng/mL. DRE reveals a palpable prostate nodule. What is the next step in management?

   a. Perform transrectal ultrasound-guided biopsy

   b. Start androgen deprivation therapy

   c. Refer to oncology for chemotherapy

   d. Order a bone scan

4. A 60-year-old male with a history of prostate cancer treated with radical prostatectomy presents with rising PSA levels 2 years after surgery. The PSA doubling time is 6 months. What is the next step in management?

    a. Perform transrectal ultrasound-guided biopsy

    b. Start androgen deprivation therapy

    c. Monitor PSA every 3 months

    d. Perform a bone scan

5. A 50-year-old male presents with lower urinary tract symptoms. PSA level is 4 ng/mL. DRE reveals a suspicious nodule in the left lobe. MRI of the prostate shows a lesion suspicious for prostate cancer. What is the next step in management?

    a. Perform transrectal ultrasound-guided biopsy

    b. Start alpha-blocker therapy

    c. Repeat PSA measurement in 6 months

    d. Refer to urology for cystoscopy

6. A 65-year-old male presents with back pain and lower extremity weakness. MRI shows metastatic lesions in the lumbar spine. PSA level is 200 ng/mL. What is the next step in management?

    a. Perform transrectal ultrasound-guided biopsy

    b. Start androgen deprivation therapy

    c. Refer to radiation oncology for spine radiation

    d. Order a bone scan

7. A 55-year-old male with a family history of prostate cancer presents for screening. PSA level is 3.5 ng/mL. DRE is normal. What is the next step in management?

    a. Perform transrectal ultrasound-guided biopsy

    b. Repeat PSA measurement in 1 year

    c. Start alpha-blocker therapy

    d. Refer to urology for cystoscopy

8. A 70-year-old male presents with difficulty in starting urination and weak urinary stream. PSA level is 15 ng/mL. DRE reveals a palpable nodule in the right lobe. What is the next step in management?

   a. Perform transrectal ultrasound-guided biopsy

   b. Start alpha-blocker therapy

   c. Repeat PSA measurement in 3 months

   d. Refer to urology for cystoscopy

9. A 60-year-old male presents with PSA level of 6 ng/mL and a normal DRE. He is concerned about prostate cancer. What is the next step in management?

   a. Perform transrectal ultrasound-guided biopsy

   b. Start alpha-blocker therapy

   c. Repeat PSA measurement in 6 months

   d. Refer to urology for cystoscopy

10. A 55-year-old male presents with lower urinary tract symptoms. PSA level is 3 ng/mL. DRE reveals a small nodule in the left lobe. What is the next step in management?

    a. Perform transrectal ultrasound-guided biopsy

    b. Start alpha-blocker therapy

    c. Repeat PSA measurement in 1 year

    d. Refer to urology for cystoscopy

11. A 65-year-old male presents with elevated PSA level of 12 ng/mL and a normal DRE. He has multiple comorbidities. What is the next step in management?

    a. Perform transrectal ultrasound-guided biopsy

    b. Start androgen deprivation therapy

    c. Monitor PSA every 6 months

    d. Refer to urology for cystoscopy

12. A 70-year-old male presents with hematuria and urinary retention. PSA level is 25 ng/mL. DRE reveals an irregular prostate contour. What is the next step in management?

    a. Perform transrectal ultrasound-guided biopsy

    b. Start alpha-blocker therapy

    c. Repeat PSA measurement in 3 months

    d. Refer to urology for cystoscopy

13. A 60-year-old male presents with elevated PSA level of 8 ng/mL and a normal DRE. He is otherwise healthy. What is the next step in management?

    a. Perform transrectal ultrasound-guided biopsy

    b. Start androgen deprivation therapy

    c. Monitor PSA every 6 months

    d. Refer to urology for cystoscopy

14. A 55-year-old male presents with elevated PSA level of 6 ng/mL and a normal DRE. He is concerned about prostate cancer. What is the next step in management?

    a. Perform transrectal ultrasound-guided biopsy

    b. Start alpha-blocker therapy

    c. Repeat PSA measurement in 6 months

    d. Refer to urology for cystoscopy

15. A 65-year-old male presents with elevated PSA level of 10 ng/mL and a normal DRE. He has a strong family history of prostate cancer. What is the next step in management?

    a. Perform transrectal ultrasound-guided biopsy

    b. Start androgen deprivation therapy

    c. Monitor PSA every 6 months

    d. Refer to urology for cystoscopy

Psoriasis

1. A 32-year-old female presents with well-demarcated, erythematous plaques with silvery scales on her elbows and knees. She reports itching and occasional bleeding from scratching. What is the most likely diagnosis?

    a. Atopic dermatitis

    b. Psoriasis

    c. Seborrheic dermatitis

    d. Contact dermatitis

2. A 45-year-old male presents with scaly, erythematous plaques with silvery scales on his scalp and in the intergluteal cleft. He also has nail pitting and onycholysis. What is the most likely diagnosis?

    a. Tinea corporis

    b. Psoriasis

    c. Seborrheic dermatitis

    d. Pityriasis rosea

3. A 28-year-old female presents with well-demarcated, erythematous plaques with silvery scales on her elbows and knees. On examination, there are also small pustules within the plaques. What is the most likely diagnosis?

    a. Pityriasis rosea

    b. Guttate psoriasis

    c. Atopic dermatitis

    d. Seborrheic dermatitis

4. A 50-year-old male presents with thick, silver-white scales covering sharply demarcated, erythematous plaques on his knees and elbows. On examination, there is involvement of the scalp with adherent scales. What is the most likely diagnosis?

   a. Psoriasis

   b. Tinea corporis

   c. Seborrheic dermatitis

   d. Contact dermatitis

5. A 35-year-old female presents with a new onset of red, scaly plaques on her palms and soles. She reports that these plaques are itchy and painful, and they have gradually worsened over the past few weeks. What is the most likely diagnosis?

   a. Palmoplantar eczema

   b. Psoriasis

   c. Tinea manuum and pedis

   d. Lichen planus

6. A 55-year-old male presents with well-demarcated, erythematous plaques with silvery scales on his knees and elbows. He has a history of hypertension and type 2 diabetes mellitus. What is the most appropriate initial management?

   a. Topical corticosteroids

   b. Oral corticosteroids

   c. Methotrexate

   d. Phototherapy

7. A 40-year-old female presents with widespread, erythematous plaques with thick, adherent, silvery scales covering her entire body surface area. She reports severe itching and pain. What is the most appropriate initial management?

    a. Topical corticosteroids

    b. Methotrexate

    c. Cyclosporine

    d. Biologic therapy

8. A 30-year-old male presents with well-demarcated, erythematous plaques with silvery scales on his knees and elbows. He is concerned about the aesthetic appearance of his skin. What is the most appropriate initial management?

    a. Topical corticosteroids

    b. Phototherapy

    c. Calcineurin inhibitors

    d. Oral retinoids

9. A 45-year-old female presents with well-demarcated, erythematous plaques with silvery scales on her elbows and knees. She is pregnant and concerned about potential risks of treatment to her baby. What is the most appropriate initial management?

    a. Topical corticosteroids

    b. Phototherapy

    c. Calcineurin inhibitors

    d. Oral retinoids

10. A 55-year-old male presents with well-demarcated, erythematous plaques with silvery scales on his knees and elbows. He has a history of hepatitis B infection. What is the most appropriate initial management?

    a. Topical corticosteroids

    b. Methotrexate

    c. Cyclosporine

    d. Biologic therapy

11. A 35-year-old female presents with red, scaly plaques on her scalp, accompanied by severe itching. She also has involvement of the external ear canal with a silvery scale and pinpoint bleeding. What is the most likely diagnosis?

    a. Seborrheic dermatitis

    b. Psoriasis

    c. Atopic dermatitis

    d. Lichen simplex chronicus

12. A 40-year-old male presents with red, scaly plaques on his face, particularly involving the nasolabial folds and eyebrows. He also has involvement of the scalp with thick, adherent scales. What is the most likely diagnosis?

    a. Atopic dermatitis

    b. Seborrheic dermatitis

    c. Psoriasis

    d. Rosacea

13. A 45-year-old female presents with well-demarcated, erythematous plaques with silvery scales on her elbows and knees. She has a history of HIV infection. What is the most appropriate initial management?

    a. Topical corticosteroids

    b. Methotrexate

    c. Cyclosporine

    d. Biologic therapy

14. A 50-year-old male presents with thick, silver-white scales covering sharply demarcated, erythematous plaques on his knees and elbows. He has a history of chronic alcohol use disorder. What is the most appropriate initial management?

   a. Topical corticosteroids

   b. Methotrexate

   c. Acitretin

   d. Phototherapy

15. A 35-year-old female presents with red, scaly plaques on her scalp and elbows, accompanied by joint pain and swelling of her fingers and toes. She has a history of rheumatoid arthritis. What is the most likely diagnosis?

   a. Psoriasis

   b. Rheumatoid arthritis

   c. Gout

   d. Reactive arthritis

Pulmonary Embolism

1. A 55-year-old woman presents to the emergency department with sudden onset of pleuritic chest pain, dyspnea, and hemoptysis. She had surgery for a fractured femur two weeks ago. What is the most likely diagnosis?

    a. Acute coronary syndrome

    b. Pulmonary embolism

    c. Pneumothorax

    d. Aortic dissection

2. A 60-year-old man with a history of atrial fibrillation and recent hospitalization for pneumonia presents with sudden onset of chest pain, dyspnea, and tachycardia. What is the most appropriate initial diagnostic test for this patient?

    a. Chest X-ray

    b. D-dimer assay

    c. Electrocardiogram (ECG)

    d. CT pulmonary angiography (CTPA)

3. A 45-year-old woman presents with sudden onset of shortness of breath and pleuritic chest pain after a long flight. She has no significant medical history. What is the most likely diagnosis?

    a. Pneumonia

    b. Pulmonary embolism

    c. Acute myocardial infarction

    d. Anxiety attack

4. A 65-year-old man with a history of cancer presents with sudden onset of dyspnea, pleuritic chest pain, and syncope. What is the most appropriate initial diagnostic test for this patient?

    a. Chest X-ray

    b. D-dimer assay

    c. Electrocardiogram (ECG)

    d. CT pulmonary angiography (CTPA)

5. A 50-year-old woman presents with sudden onset of dyspnea, chest pain, and tachycardia. She has been taking oral contraceptives for the past 10 years. What is the most likely diagnosis?

    a. Acute myocardial infarction

    b. Pulmonary embolism

    c. Pneumonia

    d. Aortic dissection

6. A 70-year-old man presents with sudden onset of dyspnea, chest pain, and tachypnea. He has a history of hip replacement surgery one week ago. What is the most likely diagnosis?

    a. Pulmonary embolism

    b. Pneumothorax

    c. Acute myocardial infarction

    d. Aortic dissection

7. A 55-year-old woman presents with sudden onset of dyspnea, pleuritic chest pain, and hypoxemia. She recently underwent knee replacement surgery. What is the most appropriate initial management for this patient?

    a. Administer oxygen and monitor closely

    b. Start anticoagulation therapy

    c. Perform urgent percutaneous coronary intervention (PCI)

    d. Transfer to the intensive care unit (ICU)

8. A 65-year-old man presents with sudden onset of dyspnea and pleuritic chest pain. He has a history of atrial fibrillation and takes warfarin. What is the most appropriate next step in management?

    a. Start heparin therapy

    b. Perform echocardiography

    c. Obtain a D-dimer assay

    d. Discontinue warfarin

9. A 50-year-old woman presents with sudden onset of dyspnea, chest pain, and tachycardia. She has a history of recent major surgery. What is the most appropriate initial diagnostic test for this patient?

    a. Chest X-ray

    b. D-dimer assay

    c. Electrocardiogram (ECG)

    d. CT pulmonary angiography (CTPA)

10. A 60-year-old man presents with sudden onset of dyspnea, pleuritic chest pain, and hemoptysis. He recently underwent surgery for a fractured hip. What is the most likely diagnosis?

    a. Acute coronary syndrome

    b. Pulmonary embolism

    c. Pneumothorax

    d. Aortic dissection

11. A 55-year-old woman presents with sudden onset of dyspnea, chest pain, and hypoxemia. She has been immobile due to a recent stroke. What is the most likely diagnosis?

    a. Pulmonary embolism

    b. Pneumothorax

    c. Acute myocardial infarction

    d. Aortic dissection

12. A 70-year-old man presents with sudden onset of dyspnea, chest pain, and tachypnea. He has a history of cancer. What is the most appropriate initial diagnostic test for this patient?

    a.   Chest X-ray

    b.   D-dimer assay

    c.   Electrocardiogram (ECG)

    d.   CT pulmonary angiography (CTPA)

13. A 65-year-old woman presents with sudden onset of dyspnea, chest pain, and tachycardia. She has a history of lupus and takes hydroxychloroquine. What is the most likely diagnosis?

    a.   Acute coronary syndrome

    b.   Pulmonary embolism

    c.   Pneumonia

    d.   Aortic dissection

14. A 50-year-old woman presents with sudden onset of dyspnea, chest pain, and tachycardia. She is currently pregnant. What is the most appropriate initial management for this patient?

    a.   Administer oxygen and monitor closely

    b.   Start anticoagulation therapy

    c.   Perform urgent percutaneous coronary intervention (PCI)

    d.   Transfer to the intensive care unit (ICU)

15. A 60-year-old man presents with sudden onset of dyspnea, chest pain, and tachypnea. He has a history of chronic obstructive pulmonary disease (COPD). What is the most appropriate initial diagnostic test for this patient?

    a.   Chest X-ray

    b.   D-dimer assay

    c.   Electrocardiogram (ECG)

    d.   CT pulmonary angiography (CTPA)

Rheumatoid Arthritis

1. A 45-year-old woman presents with symmetrical joint pain, swelling, and stiffness in her hands that is worse in the mornings and improves with activity. She has noticed small nodules under her skin. What is the most likely diagnosis?

    a. Osteoarthritis

    b. Rheumatoid arthritis

    c. Systemic lupus erythematosus (SLE)

    d. Gout

2. A 60-year-old man presents with joint pain and stiffness that is worse in the mornings and improves with activity. He has a history of hypertension and diabetes. Which of the following laboratory findings is most specific for rheumatoid arthritis?

    a. Anti-cyclic citrullinated peptide (anti-CCP) antibodies

    b. Rheumatoid factor (RF)

    c. Elevated erythrocyte sedimentation rate (ESR)

    d. Positive antinuclear antibodies (ANA)

3. A 55-year-old woman presents with fatigue, joint pain, and morning stiffness that lasts for more than an hour. She also has dry eyes and dry mouth. Which autoantibody is commonly associated with both rheumatoid arthritis and Sjögren's syndrome?

    a. Anti-cyclic citrullinated peptide (anti-CCP) antibodies

    b. Rheumatoid factor (RF)

    c. Antinuclear antibodies (ANA)

    d. Anti-Ro (SSA) antibodies

4. A 50-year-old man presents with symmetrical joint pain and swelling in his hands and feet. On examination, there are subcutaneous nodules over the extensor surfaces of his forearms. What is the pathophysiological mechanism underlying rheumatoid nodules?

    a. Deposition of urate crystals

    b. Proliferation of synovial cells

    c. Granulomatous inflammation

    d. Fibrinoid necrosis of small vessels

5. A 65-year-old woman presents with symmetrical joint pain and stiffness that is worse in the mornings and improves with activity. She also has a history of chronic obstructive pulmonary disease (COPD). Which of the following is a common extra-articular manifestation of rheumatoid arthritis in this patient?

    a. Nodular vasculitis

    b. Ocular inflammation

    c. Pulmonary nodules

    d. Rheumatoid nodules

6. A 55-year-old man presents with fatigue, weight loss, and morning stiffness in his hands. On examination, there is joint swelling and tenderness in multiple joints. Which of the following is the most appropriate initial test to assess disease activity and monitor response to treatment in this patient?

    a. Anti-cyclic citrullinated peptide (anti-CCP) antibodies

    b. Rheumatoid factor (RF)

    c. C-reactive protein (CRP)

    d. Serum creatinine

7. A 60-year-old woman presents with joint pain and stiffness that is worse in the mornings and improves with activity. She has a history of chronic kidney disease. Which of the following medications is contraindicated in this patient due to her renal impairment?

    a. Methotrexate

    b. Hydroxychloroquine

    c. Sulfasalazine

    d. Prednisone

8. A 65-year-old man presents with symmetrical joint pain and swelling in his hands and feet. He has a history of diabetes and hypertension. Which imaging modality is most appropriate to confirm the diagnosis of rheumatoid arthritis in this patient?

    a. X-ray

    b. MRI

    c. Ultrasound

    d. CT scan

9. A 50-year-old woman presents with fatigue, morning stiffness, and joint pain that worsens with rest. She has a history of bilateral wrist pain and swelling. Which of the following is a common radiographic finding in rheumatoid arthritis?

    a. Subchondral cysts

    b. Osteophytes

    c. Heberden's nodes

    d. Bouchard's nodes

10. A 60-year-old man presents with joint pain and swelling in his hands and feet. He also complains of dry eyes and a dry mouth. On examination, there are small nodules under his skin.Which of the following autoantibodies is commonly found in patients with rheumatoid arthritis and Sjögren's syndrome?

    a.   Anti-cyclic citrullinated peptide (anti-CCP) antibodies

    b.   Rheumatoid factor (RF)

    c.   Anti-Ro (SSA) antibodies

    d.   Anti-DNA antibodies

11. A 55-year-old woman presents with joint pain, swelling, and stiffness that is worse in the mornings and improves with activity. She has a family history of rheumatoid arthritis.Which of the following is a common environmental risk factor for developing rheumatoid arthritis?

    a.   Obesity

    b.   Smoking

    c.   Sedentary lifestyle

    d.   Alcohol consumption

12. A 65-year-old man presents with joint pain and morning stiffness that lasts for more than an hour. He has a history of hypertension and diabetes.Which of the following joints is commonly involved in rheumatoid arthritis?

    a.   Proximal interphalangeal (PIP) joints

    b.   Distal interphalangeal (DIP) joints

    c.   Hip joints

    d.   Sacroiliac joints

13. A 50-year-old woman presents with joint pain and swelling that is worse in the mornings and improves with activity. She also has a history of chronic obstructive pulmonary disease (COPD). Which of the following extra-articular manifestations is commonly associated with rheumatoid arthritis?

    a. Uveitis

    b. Psoriasis

    c. Osteomyelitis

    d. Rheumatoid nodules

14. A 60-year-old man presents with joint pain, swelling, and stiffness that is worse in the mornings and improves with activity. He has a history of chronic kidney disease. Which of the following medications is contraindicated in this patient due to his renal impairment?

    a. Methotrexate

    b. Hydroxychloroquine

    c. Sulfasalazine

    d. Prednisone

15. A 55-year-old woman presents with joint pain, swelling, and morning stiffness in her hands. She has a history of depression and anxiety. Which of the following is a common comorbidity associated with rheumatoid arthritis in this patient?

    a. Hypothyroidism

    b. Asthma

    c. Irritable bowel syndrome (IBS)

    d. Depression

Rosacea

1. A 35-year-old woman presents with facial redness that worsens after sun exposure. She also has small, red, pus-filled bumps on her nose and cheeks.What is the most likely diagnosis?

    a. Acne vulgaris

    b. Rosacea

    c. Seborrheic dermatitis

    d. Atopic dermatitis

2. A 50-year-old man presents with persistent redness on his cheeks and nose. He notices that his skin appears to be thicker than before.Which subtype of rosacea is most likely affecting this patient?

    a. Erythematotelangiectatic rosacea

    b. Papulopustular rosacea

    c. Phymatous rosacea

    d. Ocular rosacea

3. A 45-year-old woman presents with facial redness, flushing, and telangiectasias. She reports that her symptoms worsen with emotional stress.Which subtype of rosacea is most likely affecting this patient?

    a. Erythematotelangiectatic rosacea

    b. Papulopustular rosacea

    c. Phymatous rosacea

    d. Ocular rosacea

4. A 55-year-old man presents with facial redness, papules, and pustules on his cheeks and nose. He also complains of burning and stinging sensations.Which subtype of rosacea is most likely affecting this patient?

    a. Erythematotelangiectatic rosacea

    b. Papulopustular rosacea

    c. Phymatous rosacea

    d. Ocular rosacea

5. A 60-year-old woman presents with red, irritated eyes and eyelid swelling. She also reports that her skin on her cheeks and nose is red and sensitive. What is the most likely diagnosis?

    a. Blepharitis

    b. Conjunctivitis

    c. Ocular rosacea

    d. Allergic conjunctivitis

6. A 50-year-old woman presents with redness, flushing, and persistent red bumps on her face. She also has small visible blood vessels. Which of the following factors is a common trigger for rosacea symptoms in this patient?

    a. Sun exposure

    b. Cold weather

    c. Emotional stress

    d. All of the above

7. A 45-year-old woman presents with persistent redness on her face, especially on her cheeks and nose. She reports that her skin feels sensitive and warm. Which of the following treatments is most appropriate as first-line therapy for this patient?

    a. Topical corticosteroids

    b. Topical metronidazole

    c. Oral antibiotics

    d. Oral isotretinoin

8. A 55-year-old man presents with thickened, bumpy skin on his nose and cheeks. He notices that his nose has become larger in size over the past few years. What is the most likely complication of untreated or severe phymatous rosacea?

    a. Ocular damage

    b. Permanent facial scarring

    c. Permanent telangiectasias

    d. Skin cancer

9. A 60-year-old woman presents with red, irritated eyes and eyelid swelling. She also reports flushing and persistent redness on her cheeks and nose. Which subtype of rosacea is most likely affecting this patient?

    a. Erythematotelangiectatic rosacea

    b. Papulopustular rosacea

    c. Phymatous rosacea

    d. Ocular rosacea

10. A 55-year-old man presents with facial redness and small, red, pus-filled bumps on his cheeks and nose. His symptoms are exacerbated by spicy foods and alcohol. Which of the following triggers is most likely exacerbating this patient's rosacea symptoms?

    a. Cold weather

    b. Emotional stress

    c. Spicy foods

    d. Excessive sun exposure

11. A 50-year-old woman presents with facial redness and persistent red bumps on her cheeks and nose. She reports that her symptoms worsen with emotional stress. Which subtype of rosacea is most likely affecting this patient?

    a. Erythematotelangiectatic rosacea

    b. Papulopustular rosacea

    c. Phymatous rosacea

    d. Ocular rosacea

12. A 45-year-old woman presents with persistent redness and small, pus-filled bumps on her face. She reports that her symptoms are worse in the mornings. Which of the following treatments is most appropriate as first-line therapy for this patient?

    a. Oral antibiotics

    b. Topical corticosteroids

    c. Oral isotretinoin

    d. Topical metronidazole

13. A 55-year-old man presents with thickened, bumpy skin on his nose and cheeks. He notices that his nose has become larger in size over the past few years. What is the most likely complication of untreated or severe phymatous rosacea?

    a. Ocular damage

    b. Permanent facial scarring

    c. Permanent telangiectasias

    d. Skin cancer

14. A 60-year-old woman presents with red, irritated eyes and eyelid swelling. She also reports flushing and persistent redness on her cheeks and nose. Which subtype of rosacea is most likely affecting this patient?

    a. Erythematotelangiectatic rosacea

    b. Papulopustular rosacea

    c. Phymatous rosacea

    d. Ocular rosacea

15. A 55-year-old man presents with facial redness, papules, and pustules on his cheeks and nose. He also complains of burning and stinging sensations. Which subtype of rosacea is most likely affecting this patient?

    a. Erythematotelangiectatic rosacea

    b. Papulopustular rosacea

    c. Phymatous rosacea

    d. Ocular rosacea

Schizophrenia

1. A 22-year-old male presents with auditory hallucinations, disorganized speech, and social withdrawal. He reports that he hears voices commenting on his actions. What is the most likely diagnosis?

    a. Bipolar disorder

    b. Schizophrenia

    c. Major depressive disorder

    d. Generalized anxiety disorder

2. A 30-year-old female presents with delusions of persecution and disorganized behavior. She believes that her neighbors are plotting against her and has started hoarding food in her apartment. What is the most likely diagnosis?

    a. Schizoaffective disorder

    b. Schizophreniform disorder

    c. Delusional disorder

    d. Schizophrenia

3. A 25-year-old male presents with a history of social withdrawal, odd beliefs, and magical thinking. He believes that he has special powers and can communicate with aliens through his thoughts. What is the most likely diagnosis?

    a. Brief psychotic disorder

    b. Schizotypal personality disorder

    c. Delusional disorder

    d. Schizophrenia

4. A 35-year-old male presents with auditory hallucinations, paranoid delusions, and flat affect. He believes that the government is monitoring his thoughts through a chip implanted in his brain. What is the most appropriate initial treatment?

    a. Haloperidol

    b. Lorazepam

    c. Fluoxetine

    d. Lithium

5. A 28-year-old female presents with disorganized speech, flat affect, and social withdrawal. She has been experiencing these symptoms for the past 6 months. What is the most likely diagnosis?

    a. Schizophrenia, paranoid type

    b. Schizophrenia, disorganized type

    c. Schizophrenia, catatonic type

    d. Schizophrenia, residual type

6. A 40-year-old male presents with bizarre motor behaviors, including repetitive movements and mutism. He has been maintaining a rigid posture for hours. What is the most likely diagnosis?

    a. Schizophrenia, paranoid type

    b. Schizophrenia, disorganized type

    c. Schizophrenia, catatonic type

    d. Schizophrenia, residual type

7. A 32-year-old male presents with a first episode of psychosis, including auditory hallucinations and delusions of grandeur. His symptoms have been present for the past month. What is the most appropriate next step in management?

    a. Start antipsychotic medication

    b. Refer for cognitive behavioral therapy (CBT)

    c. Start mood stabilizer medication

    d. Admit to the psychiatric hospital

8. A 45-year-old female with a history of schizophrenia presents with worsening negative symptoms, including avolition and social withdrawal. She has been compliant with her medication. What is the most appropriate next step in management?

    a. Increase the dose of the current antipsychotic medication

    b. Switch to a different class of antipsychotic medication

    c. Refer for electroconvulsive therapy (ECT)

    d. Start psychotherapy

9. A 50-year-old male with a history of schizophrenia presents with acute agitation and aggression. He is refusing to take his medication. What is the most appropriate initial management?

    a. Start an antipsychotic medication

    b. Administer lorazepam

    c. Refer for involuntary hospitalization

    d. Start cognitive behavioral therapy (CBT)

10. A 55-year-old female with a history of schizophrenia presents with auditory hallucinations and paranoid delusions. She is non-adherent to her medication. What is the most appropriate next step in management?

    a. Increase the dose of the current antipsychotic medication

    b. Switch to a long-acting injectable antipsychotic medication

    c. Refer for psychotherapy

    d. Discharge with outpatient follow-up

11. A 60-year-old male with a history of schizophrenia presents with visual hallucinations and paranoid delusions. He has been compliant with his medication. What is the most appropriate next step in management?

      a. Increase the dose of the current antipsychotic medication

      b. Refer for cognitive behavioral therapy (CBT)

      c. Add a mood stabilizer medication

      d. Perform neuroimaging studies

12. A 65-year-old female with a history of schizophrenia presents with worsening disorganized speech and social withdrawal. She has been compliant with her medication. What is the most appropriate next step in management?

      a. Refer for electroconvulsive therapy (ECT)

      b. Switch to a different class of antipsychotic medication

      c. Start cognitive remediation therapy

      d. Increase the dose of the current antipsychotic medication

13. A 70-year-old male with a history of schizophrenia presents with bizarre motor behaviors and echolalia. He has been non-adherent to his medication. What is the most appropriate next step in management?

      a. Switch to a long-acting injectable antipsychotic medication

      b. Refer for cognitive behavioral therapy (CBT)

      c. Start an anticholinergic medication

      d. Discharge with outpatient follow-up

14. A 55-year-old female with a history of schizophrenia presents with auditory hallucinations and persecutory delusions. She has been compliant with her medication. What is the most appropriate next step in management?

    a. Increase the dose of the current antipsychotic medication

    b. Add a mood stabilizer medication

    c. Refer for cognitive behavioral therapy (CBT)

    d. Perform neuroimaging studies

15. A 60-year-old male with a history of schizophrenia presents with worsening negative symptoms, including avolition and anhedonia. He has been compliant with his medication. What is the most appropriate next step in management?

    a. Increase the dose of the current antipsychotic medication

    b. Switch to a different class of antipsychotic medication

    c. Refer for cognitive behavioral therapy (CBT)

    d. Start electroconvulsive therapy (ECT)

Seasonal Affective Disorder (SAD)

1. A 32-year-old woman presents with a history of feeling depressed during the fall and winter months for the past three years. She reports increased sleep, weight gain, and carbohydrate cravings during these periods. What is the most likely diagnosis?

   a. Major Depressive Disorder (MDD)

   b. Bipolar Disorder

   c. Seasonal Affective Disorder (SAD)

   d. Generalized Anxiety Disorder (GAD)

2. A 25-year-old man presents with feelings of sadness and loss of interest in activities during the winter months. He denies any other episodes of depression or manic symptoms. What is the most likely diagnosis?

   a. Major Depressive Disorder (MDD)

   b. Bipolar Disorder, Depressive Episode

   c. Adjustment Disorder with Depressed Mood

   d. Seasonal Affective Disorder (SAD)

3. A 40-year-old woman presents with symptoms of low energy, irritability, and difficulty concentrating starting in the fall and continuing through the winter. She reports improved mood and energy levels in the spring and summer. What is the most likely diagnosis?

   a. Bipolar Disorder, Depressive Episode

   b. Adjustment Disorder with Depressed Mood

   c. Major Depressive Disorder (MDD)

   d. Seasonal Affective Disorder (SAD)

4. A 30-year-old man presents with a pattern of depression symptoms that recur in late autumn and continue into the winter months. He reports that these symptoms have occurred for the past five years. What is the most appropriate initial treatment for this patient?

   a. Sertraline

   b. Cognitive Behavioral Therapy (CBT)

   c. Light therapy

   d. Fluoxetine

5. A 28-year-old woman presents with a pattern of depression symptoms that recur in the spring and continue into the summer months. She reports these symptoms for the past three years. What is the most likely diagnosis?

   a. Bipolar Disorder, Depressive Episode

   b. Major Depressive Disorder (MDD)

   c. Adjustment Disorder with Depressed Mood

   d. Seasonal Affective Disorder (SAD)

6. A 35-year-old man presents with recurrent episodes of depression that occur at the same time every year, starting in late October and lasting until early spring. He reports oversleeping, weight gain, and carbohydrate cravings during these episodes. What is the most likely diagnosis?

   a. Major Depressive Disorder (MDD), Recurrent

   b. Bipolar Disorder, Depressive Episode

   c. Seasonal Affective Disorder (SAD)

   d. Dysthymic Disorder

7. A 45-year-old woman presents with a history of depression that recurs in the fall and winter months. She reports feeling tired, oversleeping, and gaining weight during these periods. What is the most appropriate initial treatment for this patient?

    a. Bupropion

    b. Cognitive Behavioral Therapy (CBT)

    c. Fluoxetine

    d. Light therapy

8. A 50-year-old man with a history of Seasonal Affective Disorder (SAD) presents with worsening symptoms of depression during the fall. He is currently taking sertraline. What is the most appropriate next step in management?

    a. Increase sertraline dose

    b. Add bupropion to sertraline therapy

    c. Start cognitive behavioral therapy (CBT)

    d. Initiate light therapy

9. A 38-year-old woman presents with a history of depression symptoms that worsen in the winter months. She reports feeling tired, craving carbohydrates, and gaining weight during these periods. What is the most likely diagnosis?

    a. Bipolar Disorder, Depressive Episode

    b. Major Depressive Disorder (MDD), Recurrent

    c. Adjustment Disorder with Depressed Mood

    d. Seasonal Affective Disorder (SAD)

10. A 42-year-old woman presents with recurrent episodes of depression that begin in the late fall and remit in early spring. She reports oversleeping, weight gain, and carbohydrate cravings during these episodes. What is the most appropriate initial treatment for this patient?

    a. Cognitive Behavioral Therapy (CBT)

    b. Sertraline

    c. Fluoxetine

    d. Light therapy

11. A 37-year-old man presents with recurrent episodes of depression that coincide with the change of seasons. He reports low energy, oversleeping, and increased appetite during these periods. What is the most likely diagnosis?

    a. Bipolar Disorder, Depressive Episode

    b. Major Depressive Disorder (MDD)

    c. Adjustment Disorder with Depressed Mood

    d. Seasonal Affective Disorder (SAD)

12. A 33-year-old woman presents with a history of depression that worsens in the winter months. She reports feeling tired, irritable, and craving carbohydrates. What is the most appropriate initial treatment for this patient?

    a. Cognitive Behavioral Therapy (CBT)

    b. Fluoxetine

    c. Sertraline

    d. Light therapy

13. A 40-year-old man presents with recurrent episodes of depression that occur during the winter months. He reports low energy, increased sleep, and difficulty concentrating. What is the most likely diagnosis?

    a. Bipolar Disorder, Depressive Episode

    b. Major Depressive Disorder (MDD)

    c. Adjustment Disorder with Depressed Mood

    d. Seasonal Affective Disorder (SAD)

14. A 35-year-old woman presents with a history of depression symptoms that worsen in the fall and winter months. She reports feeling tired, sleeping more than usual, and gaining weight. What is the most likely diagnosis?

    a. Bipolar Disorder, Depressive Episode

    b. Major Depressive Disorder (MDD), Recurrent

    c. Adjustment Disorder with Depressed Mood

    d. Seasonal Affective Disorder (SAD)

15. A 30-year-old man presents with a history of depression that recurs during the winter months. He reports low energy, increased sleep, and difficulty concentrating. What is the most appropriate initial treatment for this patient?

    a. Cognitive Behavioral Therapy (CBT)

    b. Fluoxetine

    c. Sertraline

    d. Light therapy

Sickle Cell Disease

1. A 10-year-old boy presents with severe pain in his arms and legs. He is a known case of sickle cell disease. His temperature is 38.5°C (101.3°F). On examination, he has tenderness over his long bones. What is the most likely diagnosis?

    a. Vaso-occlusive crisis

    b. Acute chest syndrome

    c. Aplastic crisis

    d. Splenic sequestration crisis

2. A 25-year-old woman with sickle cell disease presents with sudden onset chest pain, cough, and dyspnea. She is tachypneic with oxygen saturation of 88% on room air. What is the most likely diagnosis?

    a. Vaso-occlusive crisis

    b. Acute chest syndrome

    c. Aplastic crisis

    d. Splenic sequestration crisis

3. A 15-year-old boy with sickle cell disease presents with fever, sore throat, and difficulty swallowing. On examination, he has swelling and tenderness of the neck. What is the most likely diagnosis?

    a. Vaso-occlusive crisis

    b. Acute chest syndrome

    c. Aplastic crisis

    d. Cervical lymphadenitis

4. A 30-year-old woman with sickle cell disease presents with pallor and fatigue. She reports feeling weak and dizzy for the past few days. On examination, she is tachycardic with a heart rate of 110 bpm. What is the most likely diagnosis?

   a. Vaso-occlusive crisis

   b. Acute chest syndrome

   c. Aplastic crisis

   d. Splenic sequestration crisis

5. A 20-year-old man with sickle cell disease presents with sudden onset severe abdominal pain and distension. He is hypotensive with a palpable spleen on examination. What is the most likely diagnosis?

   a. Vaso-occlusive crisis

   b. Acute chest syndrome

   c. Aplastic crisis

   d. Splenic sequestration crisis

6. A 35-year-old woman with sickle cell disease presents with pain and swelling in her right leg. On examination, there is calf tenderness and erythema. What is the most likely diagnosis?

   a. Deep vein thrombosis

   b. Cellulitis

   c. Vaso-occlusive crisis

   d. Osteomyelitis

7. A 40-year-old man with sickle cell disease presents with pain in his left eye and decreased vision. On examination, there is conjunctival injection and a cherry-red spot on the retina. What is the most likely diagnosis?

   a. Retinal detachment

   b. Central retinal artery occlusion

   c. Vaso-occlusive crisis

   d. Ocular infarction

8. A 45-year-old woman with sickle cell disease presents with sudden onset severe pain in her right upper abdomen. On examination, there is tenderness over the liver and jaundice. What is the most likely diagnosis?

    a. Cholecystitis

    b. Acute hepatic sequestration crisis

    c. Acute pancreatitis

    d. Acute fatty liver of pregnancy

9. A 25-year-old man with sickle cell disease presents with fever, cough, and pleuritic chest pain. On examination, there are decreased breath sounds and dullness to percussion over the right lung base. What is the most likely diagnosis?

    a. Vaso-occlusive crisis

    b. Acute chest syndrome

    c. Aplastic crisis

    d. Pleurisy

10. A 30-year-old woman with sickle cell disease presents with bone pain and tenderness. On examination, there is swelling and warmth over her right humerus. What is the most likely diagnosis?

    a. Osteomyelitis

    b. Vaso-occlusive crisis

    c. Septic arthritis

    d. Cellulitis

11. A 35-year-old woman with sickle cell disease presents with pain and swelling in her right calf. On examination, there is erythema and warmth over the calf. Doppler ultrasound shows deep vein thrombosis (DVT). What is the most likely diagnosis?

    a. Vaso-occlusive crisis

    b. DVT

    c. Cellulitis

    d. Osteomyelitis

12. A 40-year-old man with sickle cell disease presents with fever and oliguria. On examination, he is hypotensive and has pallor. Laboratory studies show hemoglobin of 6 g/dL. What is the most likely diagnosis?

    a. Vaso-occlusive crisis

    b. Acute chest syndrome

    c. Aplastic crisis

    d. Renal medullary carcinoma

13. A 25-year-old woman with sickle cell disease presents with sudden onset severe pain in her right upper abdomen. On examination, there is tenderness over the liver. Laboratory studies show a significant increase in bilirubin levels. What is the most likely diagnosis?

    a. Cholecystitis

    b. Acute hepatic sequestration crisis

    c. Acute pancreatitis

    d. Acute fatty liver of pregnancy

14. A 30-year-old man with sickle cell disease presents with acute onset of severe pain in his right leg. On examination, the leg is swollen, erythematous, and warm to touch. What is the most likely diagnosis?

    a. Vaso-occlusive crisis

    b. Deep vein thrombosis

    c. Osteomyelitis

    d. Cellulitis

15. A 35-year-old woman with sickle cell disease presents with fever, headache, and altered mental status. On examination, she has nuchal rigidity. What is the most likely diagnosis?

    a. Meningitis

    b. Stroke

    c. Vaso-occlusive crisis

    d. Acute chest syndrome

Sinusitis

1. A 35-year-old woman presents with facial pain and pressure over her cheeks and forehead, along with purulent nasal discharge. She has a low-grade fever. What is the most likely diagnosis?

    a. Allergic rhinitis

    b. Acute bacterial sinusitis

    c. Nasal polyps

    d. Chronic sinusitis

2. A 45-year-old man with a history of chronic rhinosinusitis presents with nasal congestion, facial pain, and postnasal drip persisting for more than 12 weeks. What is the most likely diagnosis?

    a. Acute bacterial sinusitis

    b. Allergic rhinitis

    c. Chronic sinusitis

    d. Nasal polyps

3. A 30-year-old woman presents with facial pain, fever, and purulent nasal discharge that has persisted for 10 days despite over-the-counter treatments. What is the most appropriate initial management?

    a. Nasal corticosteroid spray

    b. Antihistamines

    c. Antibiotics

    d. Oral decongestants

4. A 40-year-old man presents with fever, headache, and nasal congestion that worsened after an upper respiratory infection. He has tenderness over his frontal sinuses. What is the most likely diagnosis?

    a. Acute bacterial sinusitis

    b. Allergic rhinitis

    c. Chronic sinusitis

    d. Nasal polyps

5. A 55-year-old woman with a history of recurrent sinus infections presents with nasal congestion, facial pain, and fatigue. She reports thick nasal discharge that is yellow-green in color. What is the most likely diagnosis?

    a. Acute bacterial sinusitis

    b. Allergic rhinitis

    c. Chronic sinusitis

    d. Nasal polyps

6. A 35-year-old man presents with fever, nasal congestion, and purulent nasal discharge. He reports worsening of symptoms after several days of upper respiratory tract infection symptoms. Which sinus is most commonly affected in this condition?

    a. Sphenoid sinus

    b. Maxillary sinus

    c. Frontal sinus

    d. Ethmoid sinus

7. A 40-year-old woman presents with facial pain, headache, and nasal congestion. She reports having recurrent episodes of sinusitis and nasal polyps. What is the most likely diagnosis?

    a. Acute bacterial sinusitis

    b. Chronic sinusitis

    c. Allergic rhinitis

    d. Fungal sinusitis

8. A 30-year-old man presents with nasal congestion, facial pain, and a persistent cough. He reports having allergies to dust and pollen. What is the most likely diagnosis?

    a. Acute bacterial sinusitis

    b. Allergic rhinitis

    c. Chronic sinusitis

    d. Nasal polyps

9. A 45-year-old woman presents with headaches, facial pain, and nasal congestion. She has been using over-the-counter nasal decongestants with minimal relief. On physical exam, you notice polyps in her nasal cavity. What is the most likely diagnosis?

   a. Acute bacterial sinusitis

   b. Allergic rhinitis

   c. Chronic sinusitis with nasal polyps

   d. Fungal sinusitis

10. A 35-year-old man presents with severe headaches, fever, and periorbital swelling. He has difficulty looking up and complains of double vision. What is the most likely diagnosis?

    a. Acute bacterial sinusitis

    b. Allergic rhinitis

    c. Orbital cellulitis

    d. Chronic sinusitis

11. A 40-year-old woman with chronic sinusitis presents with a history of recurrent sinus infections. She reports facial pain, nasal congestion, and thick nasal discharge. What is the initial step in managing her condition?

    a. Oral decongestants

    b. Topical nasal corticosteroid spray

    c. Antibiotics

    d. Surgical consultation

12. A 45-year-old man with chronic sinusitis presents with headaches and facial pain. He reports a history of asthma and aspirin sensitivity. What condition should be considered in this patient?

    a. Nasal polyps

    b. Chronic fungal sinusitis

    c. Allergic rhinitis

    d. Aspirin-exacerbated respiratory disease (AERD)

13. A 30-year-old woman presents with severe nasal congestion, facial pain, and purulent nasal discharge. She has a history of multiple episodes of sinusitis. What imaging study is most appropriate to evaluate her condition?

    a. CT scan of the sinuses

    b. MRI of the sinuses

    c. X-ray of the sinuses

    d. Ultrasound of the sinuses

14. A 35-year-old man with acute bacterial sinusitis fails to improve after 10 days of amoxicillin-clavulanate. What is the next step in management?

    a. Change to a different class of antibiotics

    b. Extend the duration of antibiotic therapy

    c. Add a nasal corticosteroid spray

    d. Obtain a sinus culture

15. A 40-year-old woman with chronic sinusitis and nasal polyps is started on intranasal corticosteroids. How do corticosteroids improve symptoms in this patient?

    a. By reducing inflammation and shrinking polyps

    b. By directly killing bacteria in the sinuses

    c. By improving mucociliary clearance

    d. By reducing nasal congestion

Stroke

1. A 65-year-old man presents to the emergency room with sudden onset of right-sided weakness and slurred speech that started 30 minutes ago. What is the most likely diagnosis?

    a. Transient ischemic attack (TIA)

    b. Ischemic stroke

    c. Hemorrhagic stroke

    d. Migraine with aura

2. A 70-year-old woman with a history of hypertension and diabetes presents with sudden severe headache, nausea, and vomiting. What is the most likely type of stroke?

    a. Transient ischemic attack (TIA)

    b. Ischemic stroke

    c. Hemorrhagic stroke

    d. Lacunar stroke

3. A 60-year-old man presents with sudden loss of vision in the left eye and left-sided weakness. Symptoms resolve completely within 10 minutes. What is the most likely diagnosis?

    a. Migraine with aura

    b. Ischemic stroke

    c. Transient ischemic attack (TIA)

    d. Hemorrhagic stroke

4. A 75-year-old woman presents with sudden onset of left-sided weakness and difficulty speaking. Symptoms began 2 hours ago and have not resolved. What is the most appropriate initial management?

    a. IV thrombolysis with alteplase

    b. Emergent neurosurgical consultation

    c. Blood pressure management

    d. Symptomatic treatment only

5. A 68-year-old man is brought to the emergency room with sudden-onset severe headache, altered mental status, and right-sided hemiparesis. What is the most likely type of stroke?

    a. Ischemic stroke

    b. Hemorrhagic stroke

    c. Lacunar stroke

    d. Transient ischemic attack (TIA)

6. A 62-year-old woman with atrial fibrillation presents with sudden-onset right-sided weakness and facial droop. What is the most likely cause of the stroke?

    a. Atherosclerosis

    b. Cardiogenic embolism

    c. Small vessel disease

    d. Vasculitis

7. A 55-year-old man with a history of smoking and hypertension presents with sudden-onset right-sided weakness and slurred speech. What is the most appropriate imaging study to confirm the diagnosis?

    a. CT angiography

    b. MRI of the brain

    c. Non-contrast CT scan of the brain

    d. Carotid ultrasound

8. A 70-year-old woman with diabetes and hypertension presents with sudden-onset left-sided weakness and difficulty speaking. What is the most important factor to assess for the eligibility of thrombolytic therapy?

    a. Time of symptom onset

    b. Presence of diabetes

    c. Blood pressure

    d. Age of the patient

9. A 65-year-old man with a history of smoking presents with sudden-onset left-sided weakness and right gaze preference. What is the most likely location of the stroke?

    a. Left middle cerebral artery

    b. Right middle cerebral artery

    c. Posterior cerebral artery

    d. Anterior cerebral artery

10. A 58-year-old woman with a history of hypertension presents with sudden-onset severe headache, nausea, and vomiting. What is the most appropriate initial management?

    a. IV thrombolysis with alteplase

    b. Emergent neurosurgical consultation

    c. Blood pressure management

    d. Non-contrast CT scan of the brain

11. A 72-year-old man with known carotid artery stenosis presents with sudden-onset right-sided weakness and difficulty speaking. What is the most likely cause of the stroke?

    a. Atherosclerosis

    b. Cardiogenic embolism

    c. Small vessel disease

    d. Vasculitis

12. A 60-year-old woman with diabetes and hypertension presents with sudden-onset right-sided weakness and slurred speech. What is the most appropriate initial imaging study?

    a. CT angiography

    b. MRI of the brain

    c. Non-contrast CT scan of the brain

    d. Carotid ultrasound

13. A 55-year-old woman with a history of smoking and hyperlipidemia presents with sudden-onset left-sided weakness and facial droop. What is the most likely cause of the stroke?

    a. Large artery atherosclerosis

    b. Cardiogenic embolism

    c. Small vessel disease

    d. Vasculitis

14. A 68-year-old man with a history of atrial fibrillation presents with sudden-onset right-sided weakness and visual changes. What is the most appropriate management strategy?

    a. IV thrombolysis with alteplase

    b. Emergent neurosurgical consultation

    c. Anticoagulation therapy

    d. Carotid endarterectomy

15. A 62-year-old woman with diabetes presents with sudden-onset left-sided weakness and difficulty speaking. What is the most appropriate next step in management?

    a. IV thrombolysis with alteplase

    b. Emergent carotid endarterectomy

    c. Blood pressure management

    d. Non-contrast CT scan of the brain

Systemic Lupus Erythematosus (SLE)

1. A 28-year-old female presents with a butterfly-shaped rash over her cheeks and nose, fatigue, and joint pain. Laboratory tests reveal positive antinuclear antibodies (ANA) and anti-double-stranded DNA (anti-dsDNA) antibodies. What is the most likely diagnosis?

    a. Rheumatoid arthritis

    b. Systemic Lupus Erythematosus (SLE)

    c. Sjögren's syndrome

    d. Polymyositis

2. A 35-year-old female presents with oral ulcers, photosensitivity, and arthritis. Laboratory tests show positive ANA and anti-Smith (anti-Sm) antibodies. What is the most likely diagnosis?

    a. Rheumatoid arthritis

    b. Systemic Lupus Erythematosus (SLE)

    c. Sjögren's syndrome

    d. Polymyositis

3. A 25-year-old female presents with a rash on her face, chest, and back that worsens with sun exposure, joint pain, and hair loss. Laboratory tests show positive ANA and anti-Ro (SSA) antibodies. What is the most likely diagnosis?

    a. Rheumatoid arthritis

    b. Systemic Lupus Erythematosus (SLE)

    c. Sjögren's syndrome

    d. Dermatomyositis

4. A 30-year-old female presents with fever, weight loss, and a malar rash. Laboratory tests show low complement levels (C3 and C4), positive ANA, and anti-dsDNA antibodies. What is the most likely diagnosis?

   a. Rheumatoid arthritis

   b. Systemic Lupus Erythematosus (SLE)

   c. Sjögren's syndrome

   d. Polymyalgia rheumatica

5. A 22-year-old female presents with fatigue, hair loss, and a rash on her face that worsens with sun exposure. She has a history of oral ulcers and arthritis. Laboratory tests show positive ANA and anti-dsDNA antibodies. What is the most likely diagnosis?

   a. Rheumatoid arthritis

   b. Systemic Lupus Erythematosus (SLE)

   c. Sjögren's syndrome

   d. Polymyositis

6. A 40-year-old female presents with Raynaud phenomenon, joint pain, and dry eyes. She has a history of dry mouth and fatigue. Laboratory tests show positive ANA and anti-Ro (SSA) antibodies. What is the most likely diagnosis?

   a. Rheumatoid arthritis

   b. Systemic Lupus Erythematosus (SLE)

   c. Sjögren's syndrome

   d. Mixed connective tissue disease

7. A 30-year-old female presents with fatigue, joint pain, and a malar rash. She has a history of mouth ulcers and alopecia. Laboratory tests show low complement levels (C3 and C4), positive ANA, and anti-dsDNA antibodies. What is the most likely diagnosis?

    a. Rheumatoid arthritis

    b. Systemic Lupus Erythematosus (SLE)

    c. Sjögren's syndrome

    d. Polymyalgia rheumatica

8. A 25-year-old female presents with joint pain, fatigue, and a malar rash. She has a history of photosensitivity and hair loss. Laboratory tests show positive ANA and anti-Smith (anti-Sm) antibodies. What is the most likely diagnosis?

    a. Rheumatoid arthritis

    b. Systemic Lupus Erythematosus (SLE)

    c. Sjögren's syndrome

    d. Polymyositis

9. A 35-year-old female presents with chest pain, shortness of breath, and a malar rash. She has a history of oral ulcers and joint pain. Laboratory tests show positive ANA and anti-dsDNA antibodies. EKG shows pericarditis. What is the most likely diagnosis?

    a. Rheumatoid arthritis

    b. Systemic Lupus Erythematosus (SLE)

    c. Sjögren's syndrome

    d. Polymyositis

10. A 30-year-old female presents with fatigue, joint pain, and a malar rash. She has a history of oral ulcers and alopecia. Laboratory tests show low complement levels (C3 and C4), positive ANA, and anti-dsDNA antibodies. What is the most likely diagnosis?

    a. Rheumatoid arthritis

    b. Systemic Lupus Erythematosus (SLE)

    c. Sjögren's syndrome

    d. Mixed connective tissue disease

11. A 28-year-old female presents with fever, joint pain, and a malar rash. She has a history of oral ulcers and fatigue. Laboratory tests show positive ANA and anti-dsDNA antibodies. What is the most likely diagnosis?

    a. Rheumatoid arthritis

    b. Systemic Lupus Erythematosus (SLE)

    c. Sjögren's syndrome

    d. Polymyositis

12. A 35-year-old female presents with headache, visual disturbances, and joint pain. She has a history of fatigue and a malar rash. Laboratory tests show positive ANA and anti-dsDNA antibodies. What is the most likely diagnosis?

    a. Rheumatoid arthritis

    b. Systemic Lupus Erythematosus (SLE)

    c. Sjögren's syndrome

    d. Antiphospholipid syndrome

13. A 30-year-old female presents with fever, joint pain, and a malar rash. She has a history of oral ulcers and hair loss. Laboratory tests show low complement levels (C3 and C4), positive ANA, and anti-dsDNA antibodies. What is the most likely diagnosis?

    a. Rheumatoid arthritis

    b. Systemic Lupus Erythematosus (SLE)

    c. Sjögren's syndrome

    d. Polymyositis

14. A 25-year-old female presents with fatigue, joint pain, and a malar rash. She has a history of oral ulcers and photosensitivity. Laboratory tests show positive ANA and anti-Ro (SSA) antibodies. What is the most likely diagnosis?

    a. Rheumatoid arthritis

    b. Systemic Lupus Erythematosus (SLE)

    c. Sjögren's syndrome

    d. Polymyositis

15. A 32-year-old female presents with fever, joint pain, and a malar rash. She has a history of oral ulcers and hair loss. Laboratory tests show low complement levels (C3 and C4), positive ANA, and anti-dsDNA antibodies. What is the most likely diagnosis?

    a. Rheumatoid arthritis

    b. Systemic Lupus Erythematosus (SLE)

    c. Sjögren's syndrome

    d. Polymyositis

Testicular Cancer

1. A 28-year-old male presents with a painless, firm mass in his left testicle. On examination, the left testicle is enlarged and non-tender. What is the most likely diagnosis?

    a. Epididymitis

    b. Testicular torsion

    c. Testicular cancer

    d. Hydrocele

2. A 30-year-old male presents with a history of testicular swelling and dull ache for the past month. Physical examination reveals a firm, painless mass in the right testicle. What is the most appropriate initial investigation?

    a. Ultrasound of the scrotum

    b. CT scan of the abdomen and pelvis

    c. Serum alpha-fetoprotein (AFP), beta-human chorionic gonadotropin (β-hCG), and lactate dehydrogenase (LDH) levels

    d. MRI of the scrotum

3. A 25-year-old male presents with a painless, firm mass in his left testicle. On examination, the left testicle is enlarged and non-tender. Ultrasound confirms a solid intratesticular mass. Serum markers show elevated β-hCG and LDH levels, with normal AFP. What is the most likely diagnosis?

    a. Seminoma

    b. Non-seminomatous germ cell tumor (NSGCT)

    c. Leydig cell tumor

    d. Sertoli cell tumor

4. A 32-year-old male presents with a painless, firm mass in his right testicle. On examination, the right testicle is enlarged and non-tender. Ultrasound confirms a solid intratesticular mass. Serum markers show elevated AFP and β-hCG levels, with normal LDH. What is the most likely diagnosis?

    a. Seminoma

    b. Embryonal carcinoma

    c. Choriocarcinoma

    d. Teratoma

5. A 28-year-old male presents with a painless, firm mass in his left testicle. On examination, the left testicle is enlarged and non-tender. Ultrasound confirms a solid intratesticular mass. Serum markers show normal AFP, β-hCG, and LDH levels. What is the most likely diagnosis?

    a. Seminoma

    b. Embryonal carcinoma

    c. Leydig cell tumor

    d. Sertoli cell tumor

6. A 30-year-old male presents with a painless, firm mass in his right testicle. On examination, the right testicle is enlarged and non-tender. Ultrasound confirms a solid intratesticular mass. Serum markers show elevated AFP and β-hCG levels, with normal LDH. What is the most likely diagnosis?

    a. Yolk sac tumor

    b. Seminoma

    c. Leydig cell tumor

    d. Sertoli cell tumor

7. A 35-year-old male presents with a painless, firm mass in his left testicle. On examination, the left testicle is enlarged and non-tender. Ultrasound confirms a solid intratesticular mass. Serum markers show elevated β-hCG and LDH levels, with normal AFP. What is the most likely diagnosis?

    a. Seminoma

    b. Embryonal carcinoma

    c. Leydig cell tumor

    d. Sertoli cell tumor

8. A 32-year-old male presents with a painless, firm mass in his right testicle. On examination, the right testicle is enlarged and non-tender. Ultrasound confirms a solid intratesticular mass. Serum markers show elevated AFP and β-hCG levels, with normal LDH. What is the most likely diagnosis?

    a. Seminoma

    b. Yolk sac tumor

    c. Choriocarcinoma

    d. Teratoma

9. A 28-year-old male presents with a painless, firm mass in his left testicle. On examination, the left testicle is enlarged and non-tender. Ultrasound confirms a solid intratesticular mass. Serum markers show normal AFP, β-hCG, and LDH levels. What is the most likely diagnosis?

    a. Seminoma

    b. Leydig cell tumor

    c. Sertoli cell tumor

    d. Testicular lymphoma

10. A 30-year-old male presents with a painless, firm mass in his right testicle. On examination, the right testicle is enlarged and non-tender. Ultrasound confirms a solid intratesticular mass. Serum markers show elevated AFP and β-hCG levels, with normal LDH. What is the most likely diagnosis?

    a. Yolk sac tumor

    b. Seminoma

    c. Leydig cell tumor

    d. Sertoli cell tumor

11. A 35-year-old male presents with a painless, firm mass in his left testicle. On examination, the left testicle is enlarged and non-tender. Ultrasound confirms a solid intratesticular mass. Serum markers show elevated β-hCG and LDH levels, with normal AFP. What is the most likely diagnosis?

    a. Seminoma

    b. Embryonal carcinoma

    c. Leydig cell tumor

    d. Sertoli cell tumor

12. A 32-year-old male presents with a painless, firm mass in his right testicle. On examination, the right testicle is enlarged and non-tender. Ultrasound confirms a solid intratesticular mass. Serum markers show elevated AFP and β-hCG levels, with normal LDH. What is the most likely diagnosis?

    a. Seminoma

    b. Yolk sac tumor

    c. Choriocarcinoma

    d. Teratoma

13. A 28-year-old male presents with a painless, firm mass in his left testicle. On examination, the left testicle is enlarged and non-tender. Ultrasound confirms a solid intratesticular mass. Serum markers show normal AFP, β-hCG, and LDH levels. What is the most likely diagnosis?

    a. Seminoma

    b. Leydig cell tumor

    c. Sertoli cell tumor

    d. Testicular lymphoma

14. A 30-year-old male presents with a painless, firm mass in his right testicle. On examination, the right testicle is enlarged and non-tender. Ultrasound confirms a solid intratesticular mass. Serum markers show elevated AFP and β-hCG levels, with normal LDH. What is the most likely diagnosis?

    a. Yolk sac tumor

    b. Seminoma

    c. Leydig cell tumor

    d. Sertoli cell tumor

15. A 35-year-old male presents with a painless, firm mass in his left testicle. On examination, the left testicle is enlarged and non-tender. Ultrasound confirms a solid intratesticular mass. Serum markers show elevated β-hCG and LDH levels, with normal AFP. What is the most likely diagnosis?

    a. Seminoma

    b. Embryonal carcinoma

    c. Leydig cell tumor

    d. Sertoli cell tumor

Thyroid Cancer

1. A 45-year-old female presents with a palpable thyroid nodule. Fine-needle aspiration biopsy (FNAB) reveals papillary thyroid carcinoma. Which of the following is the next appropriate step in management?

    a. Total thyroidectomy

    b. Radioactive iodine (RAI) therapy

    c. Observation with repeat FNAB in 6 months

    d. Genetic testing for RET proto-oncogene mutation

2. A 35-year-old male is found to have a thyroid nodule incidentally on imaging. FNAB shows a follicular neoplasm. What is the next best step in management?

    a. Total thyroidectomy

    b. Radioactive iodine (RAI) therapy

    c. Repeat FNAB with molecular testing

    d. Observation with repeat imaging in 6 months

3. A 50-year-old female presents with hoarseness and neck pain. Physical examination reveals a fixed, hard thyroid nodule. FNAB shows anaplastic thyroid carcinoma. What is the most appropriate initial management?

    a. Total thyroidectomy

    b. Chemotherapy and radiation therapy

    c. Radioactive iodine (RAI) therapy

    d. Supportive care and hospice referral

4. A 40-year-old female presents with a thyroid nodule. FNAB reveals medullary thyroid carcinoma. What is the next appropriate step in management?

    a. Total thyroidectomy with central neck dissection

    b. Radioactive iodine (RAI) therapy

    c. Observation with repeat FNAB in 6 months

    d. Genetic testing for RET proto-oncogene mutation

5. A 55-year-old male presents with a rapidly growing neck mass. FNAB shows lymphoma involving the thyroid gland. What is the most appropriate next step in management?

    a. Total thyroidectomy

    b. Chemotherapy and radiation therapy

    c. Radioactive iodine (RAI) therapy

    d. Observation with repeat imaging in 6 months

6. A 30-year-old female with a history of familial adenomatous polyposis presents with a thyroid nodule. FNAB reveals a follicular variant of papillary thyroid carcinoma. What is the next best step in management?

    a. Total thyroidectomy

    b. Radioactive iodine (RAI) therapy

    c. Observation with repeat FNAB in 6 months

    d. Genetic testing for RET proto-oncogene mutation

7. A 25-year-old female presents with palpitations and weight loss. Physical examination reveals a diffuse goiter. Thyroid function tests are consistent with hyperthyroidism. Thyroid scan shows increased uptake. What is the most likely diagnosis?

    a. Papillary thyroid carcinoma

    b. Graves' disease

    c. Follicular thyroid carcinoma

    d. Anaplastic thyroid carcinoma

8. A 60-year-old male presents with a thyroid nodule. FNAB shows suspicious cytology, but the patient has significant comorbidities and is not a candidate for surgery. What is the next best step in management?

    a. Start levothyroxine therapy

    b. Repeat FNAB in 6 months

    c. Trial of radioactive iodine (RAI) therapy

    d. Observation with periodic imaging

9. A 45-year-old female presents with a thyroid nodule. FNAB shows Hurthle cell neoplasm. What is the next best step in management?

    a. Total thyroidectomy

    b. Radioactive iodine (RAI) therapy

    c. Observation with repeat FNAB in 6 months

    d. Genetic testing for RET proto-oncogene mutation

10. A 55-year-old male presents with a thyroid nodule. FNAB shows cytologic features suspicious for papillary thyroid carcinoma, and molecular testing confirms BRAF V600E mutation. What is the next best step in management?

    a. Total thyroidectomy

    b. Radioactive iodine (RAI) therapy

    c. Observation with repeat FNAB in 6 months

    d. Genetic testing for RET proto-oncogene mutation

11. A 50-year-old female presents with a thyroid nodule. FNAB shows cytologic features suspicious for follicular neoplasm. Molecular testing shows RAS mutation. What is the next best step in management?

    a. Total thyroidectomy

    b. Radioactive iodine (RAI) therapy

    c. Observation with repeat FNAB in 6 months

    d. Genetic testing for RET proto-oncogene mutation

12. A 40-year-old male presents with a thyroid nodule. FNAB shows features of follicular adenoma. What is the next best step in management?

    a. Total thyroidectomy

    b. Radioactive iodine (RAI) therapy

    c. Observation with repeat FNAB in 6 months

    d. Genetic testing for RET proto-oncogene mutation

13. A 35-year-old female presents with a thyroid nodule. FNAB shows benign cytology. What is the next best step in management?

    a. Total thyroidectomy

    b. Radioactive iodine (RAI) therapy

    c. Observation with periodic follow-up

    d. Genetic testing for RET proto-oncogene mutation

14. A 45-year-old male presents with a thyroid nodule. FNAB shows features suspicious for medullary thyroid carcinoma. What is the next best step in management?

    a. Total thyroidectomy with central neck dissection

    b. Radioactive iodine (RAI) therapy

    c. Observation with repeat FNAB in 6 months

    d. Genetic testing for RET proto-oncogene mutation

15. A 55-year-old female presents with a thyroid nodule. FNAB shows cytologic features suspicious for lymphoma. What is the most appropriate next step in management?

    a. Total thyroidectomy

    b. Chemotherapy and radiation therapy

    c. Radioactive iodine (RAI) therapy

    d. Observation with repeat imaging in 6 months

Ulcerative Colitis

1. A 25-year-old woman presents with a 6-month history of bloody diarrhea, abdominal cramps, and weight loss. She has no family history of gastrointestinal diseases.What is the most likely diagnosis?

    a. Crohn's disease

    b. Ulcerative colitis

    c. Infectious colitis

    d. Irritable bowel syndrome

2. A 35-year-old man presents with a history of intermittent bloody diarrhea and tenesmus over the past year. He also reports feeling fatigued and has lost weight unintentionally.Which of the following findings on colonoscopy is most consistent with ulcerative colitis?

    a. Skip lesions and transmural inflammation

    b. Cobblestone appearance and strictures

    c. Continuous colonic involvement with friable mucosa and pseudopolyps

    d. Rectal sparing with perianal fistulas

3. A 28-year-old woman with ulcerative colitis presents with fever, abdominal pain, and leukocytosis. Her abdomen is tender on examination.What is the most likely complication?

    a. Toxic megacolon

    b. Colonic perforation

    c. Diverticulitis

    d. Appendicitis

4. A 40-year-old man with a history of ulcerative colitis presents with new-onset arthritis in his knees and ankles. He also complains of eye pain and redness.What is the most likely diagnosis?

    a. Reactive arthritis (Reiter's syndrome)

    b. Ankylosing spondylitis

    c. Rheumatoid arthritis

    d. Psoriatic arthritis

5. A 30-year-old woman with ulcerative colitis is noted to have pyoderma gangrenosum-like lesions on her legs. What is the most appropriate management?

   a. Topical corticosteroids

   b. Oral antibiotics

   c. Systemic corticosteroids

   d. Surgical debridement

6. A 22-year-old man with ulcerative colitis presents with diarrhea and abdominal pain. His medications include mesalamine and azathioprine. What is the most likely cause of his symptoms?

   a. Mesalamine-induced nephrotoxicity

   b. Mesalamine-induced pancreatitis

   c. Azathioprine-induced myelosuppression

   d. Azathioprine-induced hepatitis

7. A 38-year-old woman with ulcerative colitis presents with worsening abdominal pain and fever. CT scan shows a collection of pus adjacent to the colon. What is the most likely diagnosis?

   a. Perianal fistula

   b. Colonic stricture

   c. Colonic perforation

   d. Diverticulitis

8. A 45-year-old man with ulcerative colitis presents with recurrent episodes of diarrhea, weight loss, and abdominal pain despite treatment with mesalamine and corticosteroids. What is the most appropriate next step in management?

   a. Increase corticosteroid dose

   b. Add azathioprine

   c. Perform colectomy

   d. Start infliximab

9. A 32-year-old woman with ulcerative colitis presents with bloody diarrhea and abdominal cramps. She is pregnant at 20 weeks gestation. What is the most appropriate management?

    a. Start oral corticosteroids

    b. Perform colonoscopy with biopsy

    c. Start mesalamine suppositories

    d. Refer for surgical consultation

10. A 50-year-old man with ulcerative colitis presents with chronic diarrhea and weight loss. Colonoscopy shows continuous colonic involvement with pseudopolyps. What is the most likely endoscopic finding?

    a. Aphthous ulcers

    b. Cobblestone appearance

    c. Continuous involvement with pseudopolyps

    d. Transmural inflammation

11. A 35-year-old man with ulcerative colitis presents with arthritis and uveitis. His colonoscopy shows continuous involvement with friable mucosa and pseudopolyps. What is the most likely extraintestinal manifestation of his disease?

    a. Erythema nodosum

    b. Pyoderma gangrenosum

    c. Ankylosing spondylitis

    d. Primary sclerosing cholangitis

12. A 40-year-old woman with ulcerative colitis presents with fever, severe abdominal pain, and distension. Abdominal X-ray shows colonic dilatation. What is the most likely diagnosis?

    a. Toxic megacolon

    b. Colonic perforation

    c. Diverticulitis

    d. Clostridium difficile infection

13. A 28-year-old man with ulcerative colitis presents with severe abdominal pain and bloody diarrhea. He has a temperature of 39°C (102.2°F) and tachycardia. What is the most appropriate initial management?

    a. Intravenous fluids and antibiotics

    b. Immediate colonoscopy

    c. Start corticosteroids

    d. Surgical consultation

14. A 45-year-old woman with ulcerative colitis presents with perianal pain and discharge. Examination reveals an abscess. What is the most appropriate initial management?

    a. Surgical drainage

    b. Antibiotic therapy

    c. Azathioprine therapy

    d. Colonoscopy

15. A 50-year-old man with ulcerative colitis presents with dyspnea and pleuritic chest pain. CT scan shows a large pleural effusion. What is the most likely diagnosis?

    a. Pulmonary embolism

    b. Pleuritis

    c. Pulmonary hypertension

    d. Lupus pneumonitis

Urinary Tract Infection (UTI)

1. A 25-year-old female presents with dysuria, urgency, and suprapubic pain. She has no significant medical history. Urinalysis shows pyuria and bacteriuria. What is the most appropriate initial management?

    a. Amoxicillin

    b. Ciprofloxacin

    c. Nitrofurantoin

    d. Trimethoprim/sulfamethoxazole (TMP/SMX)

2. A 30-year-old male presents with fever, flank pain, and dysuria. Urinalysis shows pyuria, bacteriuria, and hematuria. Which of the following is the most appropriate next step in management?

    a. Empirical treatment with TMP/SMX

    b. Obtain a urine culture and start antibiotics

    c. Refer for urology consultation

    d. Start intravenous ceftriaxone

3. A 65-year-old female resident of a nursing home presents with confusion and urinary incontinence. She has a history of dementia and urinary catheterization. Urinalysis shows pyuria and bacteriuria. What is the most appropriate initial management?

    a. Empirical treatment with TMP/SMX

    b. Ceftriaxone

    c. Nitrofurantoin

    d. Remove urinary catheter and start ciprofloxacin

4. A 40-year-old pregnant female presents with dysuria and frequency. Urinalysis shows pyuria and bacteriuria. What is the most appropriate initial management?

    a. Ciprofloxacin

    b. Amoxicillin-clavulanate

    c. Nitrofurantoin

    d. TMP/SMX

5. A 55-year-old male with diabetes presents with dysuria, frequency, and fever. Urinalysis shows pyuria and bacteriuria. What is the most appropriate initial management?

    a. Empirical treatment with TMP/SMX

    b. Obtain a urine culture and start antibiotics

    c. Refer to urology for imaging studies

    d. Start intravenous ceftriaxone

6. A 70-year-old male presents with dysuria, urinary frequency, and suprapubic pain. He has a history of benign prostatic hyperplasia. Urinalysis shows pyuria and bacteriuria. What is the most appropriate initial management?

    a. Empirical treatment with TMP/SMX

    b. Ciprofloxacin

    c. Nitrofurantoin

    d. Refer for transrectal ultrasound

7. A 25-year-old sexually active female presents with dysuria and urinary frequency. She denies fever or flank pain. Urinalysis shows pyuria and bacteriuria. What is the most appropriate initial management?

    a. Empirical treatment with TMP/SMX

    b. Obtain a urine culture and start antibiotics

    c. Refer for pelvic ultrasound

    d. Start ciprofloxacin

8. A 60-year-old female presents with fever, chills, and costovertebral angle tenderness. She has a history of recurrent UTIs and recent urinary catheterization. Urinalysis shows pyuria, bacteriuria, and hematuria. What is the most appropriate initial management?

    a. Empirical treatment with TMP/SMX

    b. Ceftriaxone

    c. Nitrofurantoin

    d. Start intravenous vancomycin

9. A 35-year-old female presents with recurrent episodes of dysuria, frequency, and urgency. She has no significant medical history. Urinalysis shows pyuria and bacteriuria. What is the most appropriate next step in management?

    a. Refer to urology for cystoscopy

    b. Obtain a urine culture and start antibiotics

    c. Trial of cranberry extract

    d. Start nitrofurantoin

10. A 45-year-old male with a history of renal transplantation presents with fever, dysuria, and graft tenderness. Urinalysis shows pyuria and bacteriuria. What is the most appropriate initial management?

    a. Empirical treatment with TMP/SMX

    b. Ceftriaxone

    c. Nitrofurantoin

    d. Start intravenous piperacillin-tazobactam

11. A 55-year-old male presents with fever, chills, and left flank pain radiating to the groin. Urinalysis shows pyuria and bacteriuria. What is the most appropriate initial management?

    a. Empirical treatment with TMP/SMX

    b. Obtain a urine culture and start antibiotics

    c. Refer for urology consultation

    d. Start intravenous ceftriaxone

12. A 70-year-old female presents with fever, dysuria, and confusion. Urinalysis shows pyuria and bacteriuria. What is the most appropriate initial management?

    a. Empirical treatment with TMP/SMX

    b. Ceftriaxone

    c. Nitrofurantoin

    d. Remove urinary catheter and start ciprofloxacin

13. A 30-year-old pregnant female presents with dysuria and frequency. Urinalysis shows pyuria and bacteriuria. What is the most appropriate initial management?

    a. Ciprofloxacin

    b. Amoxicillin-clavulanate

    c. Nitrofurantoin

    d. TMP/SMX

14. A 50-year-old male with diabetes presents with dysuria, frequency, and fever. Urinalysis shows pyuria and bacteriuria. What is the most appropriate initial management?

    a. Empirical treatment with TMP/SMX

    b. Obtain a urine culture and start antibiotics

    c. Refer to urology for imaging studies

    d. Start intravenous ceftriaxone

15. A 65-year-old male presents with dysuria, urinary frequency, and suprapubic pain. He has a history of benign prostatic hyperplasia. Urinalysis shows pyuria and bacteriuria. What is the most appropriate initial management?

    a. Empirical treatment with TMP/SMX

    b. Ciprofloxacin

    c. Nitrofurantoin

    d. Refer for transrectal ultrasound

Venous Thromboembolism (VTE)

1. A 65-year-old female presents with sudden onset of left leg swelling and pain. She has a history of hypertension and recent surgery. On physical examination, her left leg is warm, swollen, and tender. What is the most likely diagnosis?

    a. Deep vein thrombosis (DVT)

    b. Cellulitis

    c. Peripheral artery disease (PAD)

    d. Varicose veins

2. A 50-year-old male presents with sudden onset of shortness of breath and pleuritic chest pain. He is tachycardic and hypoxic. His Wells score is 5 points. What is the next step in management?

    a. Start anticoagulation therapy immediately

    b. Perform a D-dimer test

    c. Order a ventilation-perfusion (V/Q) scan

    d. Perform a CT pulmonary angiography (CTPA)

3. A 45-year-old female presents with swelling and pain in her right calf that started yesterday. She has a history of obesity and uses oral contraceptives. On examination, her right calf is swollen and tender. What is the most appropriate initial test?

    a. D-dimer test

    b. Compression ultrasonography of the right leg

    c. CTPA

    d. Echocardiogram

4. A 60-year-old male presents with sudden onset of dyspnea and chest pain. He has a history of atrial fibrillation and recent hip replacement surgery. On examination, he is tachypneic and hypotensive. What is the most likely diagnosis?

    a.   Acute myocardial infarction

    b.   Pulmonary embolism (PE)

    c.   Pneumonia

    d.   Aortic dissection

5. A 55-year-old female presents with sudden onset of shortness of breath and chest pain. She has a history of breast cancer and recent chemotherapy. On examination, she is tachycardic and hypoxic. What is the most appropriate initial test?

    a.   Echocardiography

    b.   D-dimer test

    c.   CTPA

    d.   V/Q scan

6. A 70-year-old male presents with sudden onset of pleuritic chest pain and hemoptysis. He has a history of chronic obstructive pulmonary disease (COPD) and recent surgery. What is the initial management strategy?

    a.   Start anticoagulation therapy immediately

    b.   Perform a D-dimer test

    c.   Order a V/Q scan

    d.   Perform a CTPA

7. A 65-year-old female presents with swelling and pain in her left leg that started this morning. She has a history of heart failure and diabetes mellitus. On examination, her left leg is swollen and tender. What is the initial test of choice?

    a. D-dimer test

    b. Compression ultrasonography of the left leg

    c. CTPA

    d. Echocardiogram

8. A 50-year-old male presents with sudden onset of dyspnea and pleuritic chest pain. He is tachypneic and hypoxic. His Wells score is 4 points. What is the next step in management?

    a. Start anticoagulation therapy immediately

    b. Perform a D-dimer test

    c. Order a V/Q scan

    d. Perform a CTPA

9. A 45-year-old female presents with swelling and pain in her right calf that started 2 days ago. She has a history of obesity and recent long-haul flight. On examination, her right calf is swollen and tender. What is the initial management strategy?

    a. Start anticoagulation therapy immediately

    b. Perform a D-dimer test

    c. Order a V/Q scan

    d. Perform a compression ultrasonography of the right leg

10. A 60-year-old male presents with sudden onset of dyspnea and chest pain. He has a history of atrial fibrillation and recent hip replacement surgery. On examination, he is tachypneic and hypotensive. What is the most appropriate initial test?

    a. Echocardiography

    b. D-dimer test

    c. CTPA

    d. V/Q scan

11. A 55-year-old female presents with sudden onset of shortness of breath and chest pain. She has a history of breast cancer and recent chemotherapy. On examination, she is tachycardic and hypoxic. What is the most appropriate initial test?

    a. Echocardiography

    b. D-dimer test

    c. CTPA

    d. V/Q scan

12. A 70-year-old male presents with sudden onset of pleuritic chest pain and hemoptysis. He has a history of chronic obstructive pulmonary disease (COPD) and recent surgery. What is the initial management strategy?

    a. Start anticoagulation therapy immediately

    b. Perform a D-dimer test

    c. Order a V/Q scan

    d. Perform a CTPA

13. A 65-year-old female presents with swelling and pain in her left leg that started this morning. She has a history of heart failure and diabetes mellitus. On examination, her left leg is swollen and tender. What is the initial test of choice?

    a. D-dimer test

    b. Compression ultrasonography of the left leg

    c. CTPA

    d. Echocardiogram

14. A 50-year-old male presents with sudden onset of dyspnea and pleuritic chest pain. He is tachypneic and hypoxic. His Wells score is 4 points. What is the next step in management?

    a. Start anticoagulation therapy immediately

    b. Perform a D-dimer test

    c. Order a V/Q scan

    d. Perform a CTPA

15. A 45-year-old female presents with swelling and pain in her right calf that started 2 days ago. She has a history of obesity and recent long-haul flight. On examination, her right calf is swollen and tender. What is the initial management strategy?

    a. Start anticoagulation therapy immediately

    b. Perform a D-dimer test

    c. Order a V/Q scan

    d. Perform a compression ultrasonography of the right leg

Vitiligo

1. A 25-year-old woman presents with depigmented patches on her face and hands that have been progressively increasing in size over the past year. She denies any preceding trauma or use of topical medications. What is the most likely diagnosis?

    1. Tinea versicolor

    2. Pityriasis alba

    3. Vitiligo

    4. Post-inflammatory hypopigmentation

2. A 35-year-old man presents with depigmented patches on his face, hands, and genitalia. He has a family history of similar skin changes in his father. What is the most likely underlying mechanism of this condition?

    1. Autoimmune destruction of melanocytes

    2. Decreased melanin production

    3. Excessive sun exposure

    4. Fungal infection

3. A 30-year-old woman presents with depigmented patches on her elbows and knees. She has no other medical history and is not taking any medications. What is the characteristic appearance of lesions in this condition?

    1. Raised, erythematous plaques

    2. Hypopigmented macules with irregular borders

    3. Hyperpigmented patches with scaling

    4. Ulcerated papules

4. A 28-year-old woman presents with a recent onset of depigmented patches on her face and neck. She reports a tingling sensation and pain in these areas.What is the most likely cause of the tingling sensation and pain reported by the patient?

    1. Superficial fungal infection

    2. Autoimmune inflammation affecting nerves

    3. Hypersensitivity reaction

    4. Excessive sun exposure

5. A 32-year-old man presents with depigmented patches on his face, neck, and back. On examination, there is a clear-cut depigmentation with no other lesions.What is the most appropriate initial diagnostic test for this patient?

    1. Wood's lamp examination

    2. Skin biopsy

    3. Fungal culture

    4. Complete blood count

6. A 40-year-old woman with a history of vitiligo presents with new depigmented patches on her shins and forearms. She is otherwise healthy and not taking any medications.What is the most appropriate next step in management for this patient?

    1. Initiate topical corticosteroid therapy

    2. Prescribe oral antifungal therapy

    3. Refer to a dermatologist for evaluation

    4. Monitor without intervention

7. A 45-year-old man presents with depigmented patches on his face, neck, and hands. He has a history of Hashimoto's thyroiditis and type 1 diabetes mellitus. What is the most likely association between his medical conditions and the skin findings?

    1. Endocrine dysfunction predisposing to melanocyte destruction

    2. Immune-mediated destruction of melanocytes

    3. Excessive sun exposure leading to melanocyte damage

    4. Genetic predisposition to melanin deficiency

8. A 50-year-old woman presents with depigmented patches on her face, hands, and feet. She reports that the patches have been stable in size and number for the past five years. What is the most appropriate management strategy for this patient?

    1. Initiate combination therapy with topical corticosteroids and calcineurin inhibitors

    2. Start oral corticosteroids

    3. Perform surgical grafting of normal skin onto depigmented areas

    4. Monitor without intervention

9. A 35-year-old man presents with depigmented patches on his face and trunk. He reports previous use of topical corticosteroids without improvement. What is the most appropriate next step in management for this patient?

    1. Initiate topical calcineurin inhibitors

    2. Refer for phototherapy

    3. Perform a skin biopsy

    4. Prescribe oral corticosteroids

10. A 40-year-old woman presents with depigmented patches on her face and hands. She reports a recent episode of stress due to family issues. What is the most likely trigger for the new lesions in this patient?

    1. Excessive sun exposure

    2. Psychological stress

    3. Fungal infection

    4. Allergic reaction to skincare products

11. A 30-year-old man presents with depigmented patches on his face, trunk, and extremities. On examination, there is a clear border between the depigmented and normal skin. What is the most appropriate initial treatment for this patient?

    1. Topical corticosteroids

    2. Phototherapy with narrow-band UVB

    3. Topical calcineurin inhibitors

    4. Surgical grafting of normal skin

12. A 25-year-old woman presents with depigmented patches on her face, hands, and feet. She reports a family history of similar skin changes in her mother. What is the most likely pattern of distribution of these depigmented patches?

    1. Diffuse and widespread

    2. Limited to sun-exposed areas

    3. Segmental or localized

    4. Acral and mucosal

13. A 35-year-old woman presents with depigmented patches on her face and extremities. She is concerned about the cosmetic appearance of these patches. What is the most appropriate initial approach to addressing her concerns?

    1. Initiate combination therapy with topical corticosteroids and calcineurin inhibitors

    2. Recommend camouflage makeup

    3. Perform surgical grafting of normal skin onto depigmented areas

    4. Refer for phototherapy

14. A 40-year-old man presents with depigmented patches on his face and trunk. He reports a tingling sensation and pain in the affected areas. What is the most likely cause of the tingling sensation and pain reported by the patient?

    1. Superficial fungal infection

    2. Autoimmune inflammation affecting nerves

    3. Hypersensitivity reaction

    4. Excessive sun exposure

15. A 45-year-old woman presents with depigmented patches on her face and hands. She reports that the patches have been stable in size and number for the past ten years. What is the most appropriate management strategy for this patient?

    1. Initiate combination therapy with topical corticosteroids and calcineurin inhibitors

    2. Start oral corticosteroids

    3. Perform surgical grafting of normal skin onto depigmented areas

    4. Monitor without intervention

Acne

1. Answer: B. Acne vulgaris

   Explanation: Acne vulgaris typically presents with comedones (blackheads and whiteheads) on the face, often in adolescents due to increased sebum production and follicular hyperkeratosis.

2. Answer: C. Isotretinoin (Accutane)

   Explanation: Severe nodulocystic acne requires systemic treatment with isotretinoin, which is highly effective in reducing sebum production and preventing scarring.

3. Answer: B. Oral contraceptives

   Explanation: Hormonal acne, characterized by lesions on the lower face and jawline, often responds well to oral contraceptives that can modulate hormone levels and reduce sebum production.

4. Answer: C. Cognitive behavioral therapy

   Explanation: Acne excoriée is a psychological disorder characterized by compulsive picking of acne lesions. Cognitive behavioral therapy is effective in managing this condition by addressing the underlying behavior.

5. Answer: C. Acne keloidalis nuchae

   Explanation: Acne keloidalis nuchae is characterized by firm, keloid-like lesions on the occipital scalp, often triggered by chronic irritation from shaving.

6. Answer: D. Observation without treatment

   Explanation: Pediatric acne often resolves spontaneously without treatment. Observation is recommended unless the acne becomes severe or causes significant distress.

7. Answer: C. Drug-induced acneiform eruption

   Explanation: Drug-induced acneiform eruptions can occur as a side effect of medications such as corticosteroids, anticonvulsants, and lithium.

8. Answer: B. Acne rosacea

   Explanation: Acne rosacea is characterized by persistent erythema, telangiectasias, and papulopustules on the central face, often affecting middle-aged adults.

9. Answer: D. Laser therapy

   Explanation: Laser therapy is effective for treating post-inflammatory hyperpigmentation in patients with darker skin types, minimizing the risk of further pigmentary changes.

10. Answer: C. Isotretinoin (Accutane)

    Explanation: Acne conglobata is a severe form of nodulocystic acne characterized by interconnected nodules with sinus tracts. Isotretinoin is the treatment of choice due to its effectiveness in reducing sebum production and preventing scarring.

11. Answer: A. Topical benzoyl peroxide

    Explanation: Topical benzoyl peroxide is considered safe during pregnancy and is a first-line treatment for mild to moderate acne in pregnant women.

12. Answer: B. Chemical peel

    Explanation: Chemical peels can improve the appearance of atrophic acne scars by promoting skin regeneration and collagen production.

13. Answer: C. Topical benzoyl peroxide wash

    Explanation: Topical benzoyl peroxide wash is effective in treating acne on the body, especially in athletes who wear tight-fitting clothing prone to friction and sweat accumulation.

14. Answer: A. Isotretinoin (Accutane)

Explanation: Isotretinoin is indicated for severe, recalcitrant acne that has not responded to other treatments. It effectively reduces sebum production and prevents scarring.

15. Answer: A. Hidradenitis suppurativa

Explanation: Hidradenitis suppurativa presents with painful nodules and abscesses in intertriginous areas, distinct from acne which primarily affects the face and upper trunk.

Allergic Rhinitis

1. Answer: B. Allergic rhinitis

   Explanation: Sarah's symptoms of seasonal sneezing, watery eyes, and worsening outdoors suggest allergic rhinitis, triggered by environmental allergens typically present during spring and fall.

2. Answer: A. Oral antihistamines

   Explanation: Oral antihistamines are recommended as first-line treatment for allergic rhinitis in children to alleviate symptoms of sneezing, itching, and rhinorrhea.

3. Answer: A. Fever

   Explanation: The presence of fever suggests a possible infectious etiology such as sinusitis rather than allergic rhinitis, which typically does not cause fever.

4. Answer: C. Nasal polyps

   Explanation: Chronic nasal congestion, pale boggy mucosa, and history of allergies are suggestive of nasal polyps, which can occur secondary to allergic rhinitis.

5. Answer: B. Dust mites

   Explanation: Symptoms worsened by exposure to carpet suggest sensitivity to dust mites, a common indoor allergen triggering allergic rhinitis symptoms.

6. Answer: C. Saline nasal irrigation

   Explanation: Saline nasal irrigation is a safe and effective non-pharmacological treatment option for allergic rhinitis during pregnancy.

7. Answer: C. Sinusitis

   Explanation: The presence of purulent discharge, fever, and facial pain suggests acute sinusitis rather than allergic rhinitis.

8. Answer: B. Add intranasal corticosteroids

   Explanation: Adding intranasal corticosteroids is recommended for patients with persistent symptoms of allergic rhinitis despite treatment with oral antihistamines.

9. Answer: B. Chronic sinusitis

   Explanation: Chronic sinusitis is commonly associated with the development of nasal polyps, which can occur secondary to persistent inflammation.

10. Answer: B. Perennial allergic rhinitis

    Explanation: Perennial allergic rhinitis refers to symptoms that persist throughout the year, often triggered by indoor allergens such as dust mites, pet dander, or mold.

11. Answer: C. Decongestants

    Explanation: Decongestants can exacerbate asthma symptoms and are generally avoided in patients with allergic rhinitis and asthma.

12. Answer: C. Occupational allergic rhinitis

    Explanation: Occupational allergic rhinitis occurs due to exposure to allergens in the workplace, in this case, likely triggered by flowers or pollen in the flower shop.

13. Answer: B. Recommend allergen avoidance measures

    Explanation: Initial management of allergic rhinitis includes recommending allergen avoidance measures to minimize exposure to triggering allergens.

14. Answer: A. Seasonal allergic rhinitis

    Explanation: Seasonal allergic rhinitis occurs in response to specific allergens present during certain seasons, such as pollen during spring or summer.

15. Answer: B. Perennial allergic rhinitis

    Explanation: Perennial allergic rhinitis refers to year-round symptoms triggered by indoor allergens such as dust mites, pet dander, or mold.

Alzheimer's Disease

1. Answer: D. Alzheimer's disease

    Explanation: The clinical presentation of progressive forgetfulness and impaired short-term memory, along with medial temporal lobe atrophy on MRI, is characteristic of Alzheimer's disease.

2. Answer: C. Order an MRI of the brain

    Explanation: Given the symptoms and history, an MRI of the brain would help to evaluate for structural changes such as atrophy or vascular lesions, which are important in the diagnosis of Alzheimer's disease.

3. Answer: B. Posterior cortical atrophy

    Explanation: Posterior cortical atrophy presents with visual symptoms, apraxia, and aphasia, distinct from the amnestic or language variants typically seen in Alzheimer's disease.

4. Answer: D. Lewy body dementia

    Explanation: Lewy body dementia is characterized by fluctuating cognition, visual hallucinations, REM sleep behavior disorder, and parkinsonism, which are not typical of Alzheimer's disease.

5. Answer: A. Semantic variant of primary progressive aphasia

    Explanation: Semantic variant of primary progressive aphasia presents with fluent but empty speech, anomia, and left posterior temporoparietal atrophy, which are distinct from typical Alzheimer's disease.

6. Answer: B. Normal pressure hydrocephalus

    Explanation: Normal pressure hydrocephalus presents with a triad of cognitive impairment, gait disturbance (positive Romberg sign), and urinary incontinence. It can mimic Alzheimer's disease clinically.

7. Answer: B. Order an MRI of the brain

    Explanation: An MRI of the brain is indicated to evaluate for structural changes that may suggest Alzheimer's disease or another cause of dementia.

8. Answer: A. Alzheimer's disease

    Explanation: Elevated tau protein levels in the cerebrospinal fluid are consistent with Alzheimer's disease pathology, characterized by neurofibrillary tangles containing tau protein.

9. Answer: B. Semantic variant of primary progressive aphasia

    Explanation: Semantic variant of primary progressive aphasia is characterized by fluent but empty speech, anomia, and left perisylvian atrophy on MRI, distinct from typical Alzheimer's disease.

10. Answer: B. Frontotemporal dementia

    Explanation: Frontotemporal dementia presents with behavioral changes, social withdrawal, and early signs of parkinsonism, which are distinct from Alzheimer's disease.

11. Answer: A. Alzheimer's disease

    Explanation: Alzheimer's disease commonly presents with progressive memory loss and impairment in complex tasks such as arithmetic, along with normal neurological examination initially.

12. Answer: B. Posterior cortical atrophy

    Explanation: Posterior cortical atrophy is characterized by visual symptoms, difficulty with spatial orientation, and bilateral posterior parietal and occipital lobe atrophy on imaging, distinguishing it from typical Alzheimer's disease.

13. Answer: B. Semantic variant of primary progressive aphasia

    Explanation: Semantic variant of primary progressive aphasia presents with progressive language impairment, anxiety, and asymmetric frontotemporal atrophy on MRI, distinguishing it from Alzheimer's disease.

14. Answer: A. Initiate treatment with donepezil

    Explanation: Given the symptoms and clinical suspicion of Alzheimer's disease, initiating treatment with a cholinesterase inhibitor like donepezil is appropriate as per current guidelines.

15. Answer: C. Frontotemporal dementia

    Explanation: Frontotemporal dementia presents with behavioral changes, language impairment, and frontal lobe atrophy, which are distinct from typical Alzheimer's disease.

Anemia

1. Answer: A. Iron deficiency anemia

    Explanation: The patient's symptoms, gender, and history of heavy menstrual bleeding are consistent with iron deficiency anemia, which is the most common type of anemia worldwide.

2. Answer: B. Vitamin B12 deficiency anemia

    Explanation: The symptoms described (tingling, difficulty walking, sore tongue) along with macrocytic red blood cells are characteristic of vitamin B12 deficiency anemia, often seen in vegetarians due to inadequate intake of vitamin B12.

3. Answer: D. Sickle cell anemia

    Explanation: The patient's symptoms, ethnic background, and the presence of sickle-shaped red blood cells confirm the diagnosis of sickle cell anemia, an inherited hemoglobinopathy common among individuals of African descent.

4. Answer: C. Anemia of chronic disease

    Explanation: The patient's history of chronic diseases (coronary artery disease and diabetes mellitus) and the laboratory findings (low hemoglobin with normal MCV) suggest anemia of chronic disease, which is characterized by chronic inflammation or underlying diseases.

5. Answer: A. Iron deficiency anemia

    Explanation: Iron deficiency anemia is common in pregnancy due to increased iron requirements for fetal growth and maternal blood volume expansion.

6. Answer: D. Alcohol-induced anemia

    Explanation: Chronic alcohol abuse can lead to vitamin deficiencies, particularly vitamin B12 and folate, causing macrocytic anemia.

7. Answer: A. Iron deficiency anemia

    Explanation: Irregular menstrual periods are a common cause of iron deficiency anemia in young women due to chronic blood loss.

8. Answer: C. Thalassemia

   Explanation: Thalassemia is common in individuals of Mediterranean, Southeast Asian, and African descent and is characterized by reduced synthesis of globin chains, leading to microcytic anemia.

9. Answer: D. Drug-induced thrombocytopenia

   Explanation: Regular aspirin use can lead to drug-induced thrombocytopenia, causing bleeding tendencies but not typically affecting the red blood cell indices.

10. Answer: D. Chronic kidney disease

    Explanation: Anemia of chronic kidney disease is normocytic and normochromic, commonly seen due to decreased production of erythropoietin.

11. Answer: C. Gastrointestinal bleeding

    Explanation: Gastrointestinal bleeding, often induced by NSAIDs and peptic ulcers, can lead to chronic blood loss and subsequent iron deficiency anemia.

12. Answer: B. Vitamin B12 deficiency anemia

    Explanation: A strict vegan diet can lead to vitamin B12 deficiency, causing macrocytic anemia and neurological symptoms.

13. Answer: D. Hemolytic anemia

    Explanation: The presence of jaundice, dark urine, elevated LDH, and fragmented red blood cells (schistocytes) indicates hemolytic anemia, which can be triggered by infections such as viral illnesses.

14. Answer: B. Folate deficiency anemia

    Explanation: Folate deficiency can occur during pregnancy due to increased requirements for fetal development, leading to megaloblastic anemia.

15. Answer: C. Hereditary spherocytosis

    Explanation: Hereditary spherocytosis is a congenital hemolytic anemia characterized by spherocytes on peripheral blood smear and a family history of similar symptoms.

Angina Pectoris

1. Answer: B) Stable angina

   Explanation: Stable angina is characterized by chest pain or discomfort that occurs predictably with exertion and is relieved by rest or nitroglycerin. The patient's history of hypertension and hyperlipidemia further supports this diagnosis.

2. Answer: A) Emotional stress

   Explanation: Emotional stress is a common trigger for stable angina due to its effect on increasing heart rate and blood pressure.

3. Answer: B) Unstable angina

   Explanation: Unstable angina is characterized by chest pain at rest or with minimal exertion that is prolonged (lasting more than 20 minutes) and associated with ECG changes like ST-segment depression or T-wave inversion.

4. Answer: C) Variant angina (Prinzmetal angina)

   Explanation: Variant angina is characterized by chest pain at rest due to coronary artery spasm, often seen in younger patients and frequently associated with smoking.

5. Answer: B) Nitroglycerin

   Explanation: Nitroglycerin is a cornerstone of therapy for both acute relief and chronic management of stable angina by promoting coronary vasodilation.

6. Answer: B) Bradycardia

   Explanation: Beta-blockers can cause bradycardia, which may exacerbate symptoms in patients with stable angina, especially if their heart rate is already low.

7. Answer: B) Chest pain relieved by exertion

   Explanation: In stable angina, chest pain typically occurs with exertion or stress and is relieved by rest or nitroglycerin.

8. Answer: A) Immediate angiography

Explanation: This presentation suggests progression to unstable angina. Immediate angiography is indicated to evaluate the extent of coronary artery disease and plan further management.

9. Answer: C) Nitroglycerin

Explanation: Nitroglycerin is used for acute relief of angina symptoms triggered by exertion or stress.

10. Answer: A) Diltiazem

Explanation: Diltiazem, a calcium channel blocker, can be used as an alternative or add-on therapy in patients with stable angina who have inadequate symptom control with beta-blockers and nitrates.

11. Answer: C) Variant angina

Explanation: Variant angina (Prinzmetal angina) is characterized by chest pain at rest due to coronary artery spasm, often associated with transient ST-segment elevation on ECG.

12. Answer: D) Young age (20-30 years)

Explanation: Stable angina is more commonly seen in older individuals and is typically associated with risk factors such as hypertension, diabetes mellitus, and dyslipidemia.

13. Answer: B) Unstable angina

Explanation: Unstable angina is characterized by chest pain at rest or with minimal exertion, lasting more than 20 minutes, and associated with ECG changes like ST-segment depression.

14. Answer: C) Add ranolazine

Explanation: Ranolazine is an antianginal medication that can be added to existing therapy in patients with stable angina who have inadequate symptom relief with other medications like nitroglycerin.

15. Answer: C) Pain relieved by nitroglycerin

Explanation: Stable angina is typically relieved by nitroglycerin or rest, whereas unstable angina often requires urgent medical attention due to worsening or persistent symptoms at rest.

Anxiety Disorders

1. Answer: C) Generalized Anxiety Disorder (GAD)

   Explanation: GAD is characterized by excessive worry and anxiety about a number of events or activities, lasting for at least 6 months and causing significant distress or impairment.

2. Answer: B) Panic Disorder

   Explanation: Panic disorder involves recurrent panic attacks and persistent worry about having additional attacks or their consequences.

3. Answer: C) Social Anxiety Disorder

   Explanation: Social anxiety disorder is characterized by intense fear of social situations where the individual fears being judged or scrutinized by others.

4. Answer: D) Obsessive-Compulsive Disorder (OCD)

   Explanation: OCD involves obsessions (intrusive thoughts) and compulsions (ritualistic behaviors performed to reduce anxiety).

5. Answer: B) Panic Disorder

   Explanation: Panic disorder is characterized by recurrent panic attacks and persistent worry about having additional attacks.

6. Answer: C) Generalized Anxiety Disorder (GAD)

   Explanation: GAD is characterized by excessive worry and anxiety about various aspects of life, lasting for at least 6 months.

7. Answer: D) Specific Phobia

   Explanation: Specific phobia involves intense fear of a specific object or situation, leading to avoidance behavior.

8. Answer: D) Obsessive-Compulsive Disorder (OCD)

   Explanation: OCD involves obsessions (unwanted, intrusive thoughts) and compulsions (ritualistic behaviors) aimed at reducing anxiety.

9. Answer: D) Obsessive-Compulsive Disorder (OCD)

   Explanation: OCD involves intrusive, unwanted thoughts (obsessions) and repetitive behaviors (compulsions) performed to reduce anxiety.

10. Answer: A) Panic Disorder

    Explanation: Panic disorder involves recurrent panic attacks and persistent worry about having additional attacks or their consequences.

11. Answer: D) Specific Phobia

    Explanation: Specific phobia involves intense fear of a specific object or situation, leading to avoidance behavior.

12. Answer: A) Hypochondriasis

    Explanation: Hypochondriasis (now known as Illness Anxiety Disorder) involves preoccupation with having or acquiring a serious illness, despite reassurances from medical professionals.

13. Answer: C) Social Anxiety Disorder

    Explanation: Social anxiety disorder involves intense fear of social situations where the individual fears being judged or embarrassed.

14. Answer: D) Specific Phobia

    Explanation: Specific phobia involves intense fear and avoidance of a specific object or situation.

15. Answer: C) Generalized Anxiety Disorder (GAD)

    Explanation: GAD is characterized by excessive worry and anxiety about a variety of events or activities, lasting for at least 6 months.

Asthma

1. Answer: C) Asthma exacerbation

   Explanation: The sudden onset of dyspnea, cough, wheezing, and a history of allergies with episodic wheezing suggests asthma exacerbation. Pneumonia typically presents with fever, productive cough, and focal chest signs. Pulmonary embolism presents with sudden onset dyspnea, pleuritic chest pain, and may have signs of deep vein thrombosis. COPD exacerbation would typically present with a history of smoking and chronic cough with increased sputum production.

2. Answer: A) Asthma

   Explanation: The persistent dry cough, worse at night and early morning, along with wheezing and absence of smoking history or allergies, are typical of asthma. Chronic bronchitis presents with a productive cough for at least 3 months in 2 consecutive years. Bronchiectasis presents with chronic productive cough and recurrent infections. Pulmonary fibrosis typically presents with progressive dyspnea on exertion and fine bibasilar inspiratory crackles.

3. Answer: B) Short-acting beta agonist (SABA)

   Explanation: In children with asthma exacerbations, the initial treatment of choice is a short-acting beta agonist (SABA) like albuterol. Oral corticosteroids are used for moderate to severe exacerbations not responding to SABA. LABAs are used as maintenance therapy in conjunction with ICS. ICS is used as first-line maintenance therapy for persistent asthma.

4. Answer: B) Pulmonary function tests (PFTs)

   Explanation: In a patient with chronic cough and dyspnea, PFTs would be the most appropriate initial test to assess for airflow limitation consistent with COPD. Chest X-ray may show hyperinflation but is less specific. Bronchoscopy may be considered if there is suspicion of another pathology. HRCT is more sensitive than a chest X-ray for detecting emphysema.

5. Answer: B) Asthma

   Explanation: The episodic nature of symptoms triggered by exercise and allergens, along with a history of hay fever and wheezing, is suggestive of asthma. Chronic bronchitis is characterized by chronic productive cough. Pulmonary embolism presents with sudden onset dyspnea and pleuritic chest pain. Pneumonia typically presents with fever, productive cough, and focal chest signs.

6. Answer: C) Inhaled corticosteroids (ICS)

   Explanation: In a patient with symptoms consistent with allergic asthma, ICS is the initial treatment of choice for maintenance therapy. Montelukast is an alternative but less preferred option. Oral corticosteroids are used for exacerbations not controlled by ICS. LAMA is typically used in COPD, not first-line for asthma.

7. Answer: D) COPD

   Explanation: The history of smoking, chronic cough, dyspnea on exertion, and airflow limitation that is not fully reversible with bronchodilators are characteristic of COPD. Asthma typically shows significant reversibility with bronchodilators on PFTs. Chronic bronchitis presents with a productive cough. Bronchiectasis presents with chronic productive cough and recurrent infections.

8. Answer: C) Bronchiectasis

   Explanation: The history of recurrent sinus infections, chronic productive cough with large amounts of purulent sputum, and worsening symptoms during respiratory infections are typical of bronchiectasis. Asthma typically presents with episodic symptoms and wheezing. Chronic bronchitis presents with chronic productive cough. Pneumonia presents with fever, productive cough, and focal chest signs.

9. Answer: C) Short-acting beta agonist (SABA)

   Explanation: In a patient with acute exacerbation of asthma, the initial treatment of choice is a SABA like albuterol. ICS are used for maintenance therapy. LABA are used as adjuncts to ICS in maintenance therapy. Oral corticosteroids are used for moderate to severe exacerbations not responding to SABA.

10. Answer: C) Pulmonary fibrosis

Explanation: The chronic non-productive cough, progressive dyspnea on exertion, absence of history of allergies or smoking, and fine bibasilar inspiratory crackles suggest pulmonary fibrosis. Asthma typically presents with episodic symptoms and wheezing. Chronic bronchitis presents with chronic productive cough. Bronchiectasis presents with chronic productive cough and recurrent infections.

11. Answer: C) Pulmonary function tests (PFTs)

Explanation: In a patient with suspected allergic asthma, PFTs would be the most appropriate initial test to assess for airflow limitation and reversibility. Chest X-ray may show hyperinflation but is less specific. HRCT is more sensitive than a chest X-ray for detecting structural lung abnormalities. Bronchoscopy is generally reserved for evaluating other lung diseases or complications.

12. Answer: D) COPD

Explanation: The history of smoking, chronic cough, dyspnea on exertion, and partial reversibility of airflow limitation with bronchodilators are characteristic of COPD. Asthma typically shows significant reversibility with bronchodilators on PFTs. Chronic bronchitis presents with a productive cough. Bronchiectasis presents with chronic productive cough and recurrent infections.

13. Answer: D) Inhaled corticosteroid (ICS)

Explanation: In a patient with symptoms consistent with allergic asthma, ICS is the initial treatment of choice for maintenance therapy. Oral corticosteroids are used for exacerbations not controlled by ICS. SABA are used for acute exacerbations. LABA are used as adjuncts to ICS in maintenance therapy.

14. Answer: D) COPD

Explanation: The history of smoking, chronic cough, dyspnea on exertion, and airflow limitation that is not fully reversible with bronchodilators are characteristic of COPD. Asthma typically shows significant reversibility with bronchodilators on PFTs. Chronic bronchitis presents with a productive cough. Bronchiectasis presents with chronic productive cough and recurrent infections.

15. Answer: A) Asthma

Explanation: The intermittent nature of symptoms worse at night and early morning, along with wheezing and absence of smoking history or allergies, are typical of asthma. Chronic bronchitis presents with a productive cough for at least 3 months in 2 consecutive years. Pulmonary embolism presents with sudden onset dyspnea and pleuritic chest pain. Pneumonia presents with fever, productive cough, and focal chest signs.

Atherosclerosis

1. Answer: C) Atherosclerosis of peripheral arteries

    Explanation: Intermittent claudication is a classic symptom of peripheral artery disease (PAD) caused by atherosclerosis in peripheral arteries, leading to reduced blood flow during exertion.

2. Answer: A) Myocardial infarction due to plaque rupture and thrombosis

    Explanation: ST-segment elevation myocardial infarction (STEMI) typically results from acute thrombotic occlusion of a coronary artery due to plaque rupture and subsequent thrombosis, a hallmark feature of advanced atherosclerosis.

3. Answer: C) Thrombotic stroke from atherosclerosis in the intracranial arteries

    Explanation: Atherosclerosis can lead to thrombosis and subsequent stroke in intracranial arteries, causing focal neurologic deficits such as those described.

4. Answer: C) Lifestyle modification and pharmacotherapy

    Explanation: Initial management of stable angina due to atherosclerosis involves lifestyle changes (e.g., diet, exercise) and pharmacotherapy (e.g., statins, antiplatelet agents) to reduce cardiovascular risk factors.

5. Answer: A) Atherosclerosis of the abdominal aorta

    Explanation: Atherosclerosis is a common cause of abdominal aortic aneurysms, particularly in older individuals with cardiovascular risk factors such as smoking and hypertension.

6. Answer: C) Atherosclerosis of pelvic arteries

    Explanation: Atherosclerosis affecting pelvic arteries can lead to reduced blood flow to the penis, contributing to erectile dysfunction, especially in patients with diabetes and hypertension.

7. Answer: C) Atherosclerosis of the aortic valve

    Explanation: Aortic stenosis in elderly patients is most commonly due to atherosclerosis and calcification of the aortic valve leaflets.

8. Answer: C) Popliteal artery

    Explanation: Rest pain in the legs is characteristic of advanced peripheral artery disease (PAD) affecting arteries such as the popliteal artery, often due to atherosclerosis.

9. Answer: B) Atherosclerosis of intracranial arteries

   Explanation: Atherosclerosis of intracranial arteries can cause TIAs or strokes due to thrombotic or embolic occlusion, leading to small infarcts seen on imaging.

10. Answer: C) Femoral artery

    Explanation: Exercise-induced leg pain (claudication) suggests peripheral artery disease (PAD) affecting arteries like the femoral artery, commonly due to atherosclerosis in smokers.

11. Answer: C) Atherosclerosis of peripheral arteries

    Explanation: Chronic non-healing ulcers on the feet are often due to poor perfusion caused by atherosclerosis in peripheral arteries, exacerbated by hypertension and diabetes.

12. Answer: A) Atherosclerotic plaque rupture

    Explanation: Atherosclerotic plaque rupture leading to thrombosis is a common cause of ischemic stroke, particularly in the middle cerebral artery territory.

13. Answer: A) Coronary artery spasm

    Explanation: Variant angina (Prinzmetal angina) presents with chest pain at rest due to transient coronary artery spasm, rather than atherosclerotic plaque rupture.

14. Answer: A) Atherosclerosis of the abdominal aorta

    Explanation: Atherosclerosis is a common cause of abdominal aortic aneurysms, which can rupture and present with sudden-onset severe abdominal pain.

15. Answer: C) Chronic ischemic heart disease

    Explanation: Chronic ischemic heart disease, often due to atherosclerosis in the coronary arteries, can lead to reduced left ventricular function and global hypokinesis.

Bipolar Disorder

1. Answer: B. Bipolar disorder

    Explanation: Bipolar disorder is characterized by episodes of mania or hypomania alternating with episodes of depression. The alternating nature of his symptoms over time is indicative of bipolar disorder rather than major depressive disorder, schizophrenia, or generalized anxiety disorder.

2. Answer: B. Olanzapine

    Explanation: Olanzapine is an antipsychotic commonly used for acute manic episodes in bipolar disorder. It helps control symptoms such as agitation, aggression, and psychotic features. Lithium is also a first-line treatment for bipolar disorder, but it is not the initial choice for acute mania.

3. Answer: A. Lithium toxicity

    Explanation: Symptoms such as diarrhea, tremor, and confusion are suggestive of lithium toxicity. Regular monitoring of lithium levels is necessary to prevent toxicity, which can occur due to factors such as dehydration, drug interactions, or impaired renal function.

4. Answer: D. Lamotrigine

    Explanation: Lamotrigine is considered safer than lithium, valproate, or carbamazepine during pregnancy due to lower risks of teratogenicity and developmental delays. It is often the preferred mood stabilizer for pregnant women with bipolar disorder.

5. Answer: A. Augment current medication with a second mood stabilizer

    Explanation: If a patient with bipolar disorder has not responded to monotherapy, augmenting with a second mood stabilizer or an antipsychotic is often the next step to achieve better symptom control.

6. Answer: A. Bipolar II disorder

    Explanation: Bipolar II disorder is characterized by recurrent episodes of depression and hypomania (less severe than full-blown mania). Unlike bipolar I disorder, manic episodes do not occur in bipolar II disorder.

7. Answer: A. Lithium-induced nephrogenic diabetes insipidus

   Explanation: Lithium can cause nephrogenic diabetes insipidus, characterized by symptoms such as excessive thirst, polyuria, and electrolyte imbalances. It is important to monitor renal function and electrolytes regularly in patients taking lithium.

8. Answer: D. Valproate

   Explanation: Valproate is commonly used in the treatment of rapid cycling bipolar disorder due to its effectiveness in stabilizing mood swings. It is particularly helpful in cases where other mood stabilizers may be less effective.

9. Answer: A. Olanzapine-induced metabolic syndrome

   Explanation: Olanzapine is associated with metabolic side effects such as weight gain, increased appetite, dyslipidemia, and insulin resistance, collectively known as metabolic syndrome. Regular monitoring of weight and metabolic parameters is essential.

10. Answer: B. Lithium

    Explanation: Lithium is effective for both acute mania and hypomania. It is often considered the initial treatment of choice for managing hypomanic episodes in bipolar disorder.

11. Answer: A. Add lithium or lamotrigine

    Explanation: For patients with bipolar depression who do not respond adequately to antidepressants alone, adding a mood stabilizer such as lithium or lamotrigine is recommended to stabilize mood and prevent switching into mania.

12. Answer: B. Every 3 months

    Explanation: Regular monitoring of lithium levels, renal function, and thyroid function is recommended every 3 months in stable patients to prevent toxicity and ensure therapeutic levels.

13. Answer: C. Carbamazepine-induced hyponatremia

    Explanation: Carbamazepine can cause hyponatremia, especially in elderly patients, leading to symptoms such as nausea, vomiting, confusion, and seizures. Monitoring of sodium levels is crucial during treatment with carbamazepine.

14. Answer: B. Bipolar disorder, mixed episode

Explanation: A mixed episode in bipolar disorder involves symptoms of both mania (or hypomania) and depression occurring nearly every day for at least one week. It is characterized by rapid mood swings, irritability, and impulsivity.

15. Answer: A. Intramuscular olanzapine

Explanation: Intramuscular antipsychotics such as olanzapine are often used in acute settings to rapidly control severe agitation and psychosis in patients with bipolar disorder who may not be adherent to oral medications.

Bronchitis

1. Answer: C. Pneumonia

    Explanation: The presence of fever, productive cough with purulent sputum, and crackles on lung auscultation suggests a lower respiratory tract infection such as pneumonia, rather than acute bronchitis, chronic bronchitis, or asthma.

2. Answer: B. Chronic bronchitis

    Explanation: Chronic bronchitis is characterized by a productive cough lasting at least 3 months for 2 consecutive years. The patient's smoking history, chronic productive cough, and dyspnea on exertion are consistent with this diagnosis.

3. Answer: C. Viral upper respiratory tract infection

    Explanation: Acute bronchitis typically presents with cough and possibly mild systemic symptoms, but usually lacks findings of lower respiratory involvement on physical examination, distinguishing it from pneumonia or chronic bronchitis.

4. Answer: D. COPD exacerbation

    Explanation: The patient's history of COPD, worsening dyspnea, increased sputum production, and auscultatory findings (wheezing and crackles) are consistent with an exacerbation of COPD rather than acute bronchitis, chronic bronchitis, or pneumonia.

5. Answer: D. Supportive care

    Explanation: This patient's symptoms are consistent with uncomplicated acute bronchitis, which is usually viral in origin and self-limiting. Supportive care, such as adequate hydration and symptomatic relief, is the mainstay of management.

6. Answer: B. Chronic bronchitis

    Explanation: Chronic bronchitis is defined by a productive cough on most days for at least 3 months in 2 consecutive years in a patient with a history of smoking. The patient's symptoms and history are consistent with this diagnosis.

7.   Answer: C. Pneumonia

Explanation: The presence of fever, dyspnea, and crackles on lung examination suggests a lower respiratory tract infection such as pneumonia rather than acute bronchitis, chronic bronchitis, or tuberculosis, given her clinical presentation.

8.   Answer: C. Asthma

Explanation: The presence of wheezing without fever or significant sputum production suggests asthma rather than acute bronchitis, chronic bronchitis, or pneumonia. Asthma is characterized by reversible airflow obstruction and bronchial hyperresponsiveness.

9.   Answer: B. Chronic bronchitis

Explanation: Chronic bronchitis is characterized by a chronic productive cough lasting at least 3 months for 2 consecutive years, typically in smokers. The patient's history and physical findings are consistent with this diagnosis.

10. Answer: C. Bronchiectasis

Explanation: Bronchiectasis is characterized by irreversible dilatation of bronchi due to chronic inflammation and infection. The patient's symptoms, recurrent infections, foul-smelling sputum, and radiographic findings support this diagnosis.

11. Answer: A. Acute bronchitis

Explanation: Acute bronchitis typically presents with cough and possibly mild systemic symptoms, but lung examination is usually normal. The absence of significant findings differentiates it from chronic bronchitis, pneumonia, or asthma.

12. Answer: C. Bronchiectasis

Explanation: The presence of cyanosis, digital clubbing, and chronic productive cough suggests bronchiectasis, which is characterized by irreversible bronchial dilatation and recurrent respiratory infections. This differentiates it from acute bronchitis, chronic bronchitis, or pneumonia.

13. Answer: A. Empirical antibiotics

Explanation: This patient's symptoms of productive cough, fever, and rhonchi suggest a lower respiratory tract infection, possibly bacterial pneumonia. Empirical antibiotics are indicated in this scenario, distinguishing it from acute bronchitis or chronic bronchitis.

14. Answer: D. Smoking cessation counseling

Explanation: Given the patient's history of chronic cough, sputum production, and smoking, the initial step in management should include addressing smoking cessation. This is crucial in the management of chronic bronchitis and its associated complications.

15. Answer: C. Asthma

Explanation: The patient's symptoms of episodic wheezing, chest tightness, and nocturnal exacerbation are typical of asthma. Asthma is characterized by reversible airflow obstruction and bronchial hyperresponsiveness, distinguishing it from acute bronchitis, chronic bronchitis, or pneumonia.

Cancer

1. Answer: C. Low-dose CT scan of the chest

    Explanation: Former smokers aged 55-80 years with a significant smoking history (30 pack-years) should undergo annual lung cancer screening with low-dose CT scan to detect early-stage lung cancer.

2. Answer: A. Order a mammogram and ultrasound

    Explanation: Imaging with mammogram and ultrasound is the initial step in evaluating breast masses. Biopsy is indicated based on imaging findings to confirm the diagnosis.

3. Answer: D. Shared decision-making regarding PSA testing

    Explanation: Prostate cancer screening guidelines recommend shared decision-making between the patient and provider regarding PSA testing in men aged 55-69 years.

4. Answer: B. Order a colonoscopy

    Explanation: Rectal bleeding and changes in bowel habits in a patient aged 50 years or older warrant further evaluation with colonoscopy to assess for colorectal cancer.

5. Answer: A. Perform a full-body skin examination

    Explanation: Patients with fair skin and a history of significant sun exposure should undergo regular full-body skin examinations to detect early signs of melanoma.

6. Answer: C. Pap smear and HPV testing annually

    Explanation: Cervical cancer screening guidelines recommend Pap smear and HPV testing every 5 years for women aged 30-65 years, or Pap smear alone every 3 years.

7. Answer: A. Transvaginal ultrasound

    Explanation: Persistent symptoms such as bloating, pelvic pain, and early satiety in a woman over 40 should prompt evaluation with transvaginal ultrasound to assess for ovarian cancer.

8. Answer: A. Order a scrotal ultrasound

    Explanation: A painless testicular mass in a young adult male should prompt evaluation with scrotal ultrasound to assess for testicular cancer.

9. Answer: C. CT scan of the abdomen and pelvis

   Explanation: Jaundice, weight loss, and clay-colored stools in a patient with a history of heavy alcohol use raise concern for pancreatic cancer. CT scan is the initial investigation of choice.

10. Answer: A. Upper endoscopy with biopsy

    Explanation: Progressive dysphagia in an older adult should prompt evaluation with upper endoscopy to assess for esophageal cancer, with biopsy for definitive diagnosis.

11. Answer: C. Perform a fine-needle aspiration (FNA) biopsy

    Explanation: A painless thyroid nodule in an adult should be evaluated with thyroid ultrasound and FNA biopsy to assess for thyroid cancer.

12. Answer: D. Cystoscopy with biopsy

    Explanation: Painless gross hematuria in an older adult with a history of smoking warrants evaluation with cystoscopy and biopsy to assess for bladder cancer.

13. Answer: B. Order a transrectal ultrasound (TRUS) and biopsy

    Explanation: Elevated PSA levels and a firm nodule on digital rectal examination indicate the need for further evaluation with transrectal ultrasound (TRUS) and biopsy to diagnose prostate cancer.

14. Answer: B. CT scan of the abdomen and pelvis

    Explanation: Flank pain, hematuria, unintentional weight loss, and fatigue raise concern for renal cell carcinoma. CT scan is the initial investigation of choice.

15. Answer: A. Fine-needle aspiration (FNA) biopsy of a lymph node

    Explanation: Painless lymphadenopathy, night sweats, and unintentional weight loss raise concern for lymphoma. Fine-needle aspiration biopsy of a lymph node is the initial investigation for diagnosis.

Candidiasis

1. Answer: C. Candidiasis

   Explanation: The symptoms of vaginal itching, thick white discharge resembling cottage cheese, and erythematous mucosa are classic for Candida vulvovaginitis.

2. Answer: B. Oral thrush

   Explanation: The presence of white plaques that can be scraped off, leaving erythematous mucosa, is characteristic of oral thrush (oral candidiasis).

3. Answer: B. Candida esophagitis

   Explanation: Whitish plaques on the esophageal mucosa in an immunocompromised patient with dysphagia and odynophagia suggest Candida esophagitis.

4. Answer: C. Candidal diaper dermatitis

   Explanation: Well-defined erythematous plaques with satellite lesions in the diaper area suggest candidal diaper dermatitis, often seen in infants.

5. Answer: B. Candidal intertrigo

   Explanation: Erythematous plaques with satellite papules and pustules in the inguinal folds are characteristic of candidal intertrigo, common in individuals with diabetes mellitus.

6. Answer: D. Candidal nail infection

   Explanation: Chronic paronychia with nail plate separation and yellow discoloration suggests a candidal nail infection, which can occur in immunocompromised individuals.

7. Answer: B. Candidal interdigital infection

   Explanation: White, macerated areas with a slightly pungent odor between the toes suggest a candidal interdigital infection, which may not respond to typical antifungal treatments.

8. Answer: C. Candidal intertrigo

   Explanation: Pruritic, red, scaly patches in skin folds exacerbated by heat and humidity suggest candidal intertrigo, common in moist environments.

9. Answer: D. Candidal vulvovaginitis

    Explanation: Erythematous plaques with satellite papules and pustules in the vulvar area are characteristic of candidal vulvovaginitis.

10. Answer: D. Autoimmune polyendocrinopathy-candidiasis-ectodermal dystrophy (APECED)

    Explanation: APECED is a genetic autoimmune syndrome associated with chronic mucocutaneous candidiasis due to defective T-cell function.

11. Answer: B. Candida esophagitis

    Explanation: Whitish plaques on the esophageal mucosa in an immunocompromised patient with dysphagia suggest Candida esophagitis, a common complication of chemotherapy and radiation therapy.

12. Answer: B. Candida colitis

    Explanation: Yellowish plaques adherent to the colonic mucosa in an HIV-positive patient with chronic diarrhea suggest Candida colitis.

13. Answer: D. Fungal sinusitis

    Explanation: Unilateral erythematous nasal mucosa with purulent discharge in a diabetic patient suggests fungal sinusitis, commonly caused by Candida species.

14. Answer: B. Candidal intertrigo

    Explanation: Well-defined erythematous plaques with satellite papules and pustules in the groin area suggest candidal intertrigo, which may not respond to typical antifungal treatments.

15. Answer: D. Candidal nail infection

    Explanation: Purulent discharge from the nail bed in a diabetic patient suggests a candidal nail infection, which can cause paronychia and other nail changes.

Celiac Disease

1. Answer: C. Celiac disease

    Explanation: Chronic diarrhea, bloating, weight loss, iron deficiency anemia, and positive tTG-IgA are characteristic of Celiac disease, an autoimmune disorder triggered by gluten consumption.

2. Answer: B. Celiac disease

    Explanation: Celiac disease can present with malabsorption, vitamin deficiencies, and steatorrhea due to damage to the small intestine mucosa caused by gluten ingestion.

3. Answer: C. Upper endoscopy with duodenal biopsy

    Explanation: Celiac disease diagnosis requires confirmation with upper endoscopy and biopsy showing characteristic histopathological changes (e.g., villous atrophy, crypt hyperplasia) in the small intestine.

4. Answer: C. Order serum anti-tTG antibodies

    Explanation: Serum anti-tTG antibodies are a sensitive and specific initial screening test for Celiac disease, especially in individuals with associated symptoms and family history.

5. Answer: C. Celiac disease

    Explanation: Positive anti-EMA antibodies and symptoms of malabsorption (diarrhea, fatigue) suggest Celiac disease, characterized by autoimmune-mediated damage to the small intestine mucosa upon gluten exposure.

6. Answer: B. Serum anti-tTG antibodies

    Explanation: Chronic anemia, especially refractory to iron supplementation, along with vitamin deficiencies and recurrent oral ulcers, should prompt testing for Celiac disease with serum anti-tTG antibodies.

7. Answer: D. Perform upper endoscopy with biopsy

    Explanation: Upper endoscopy with biopsy is essential to confirm the diagnosis of Celiac disease, particularly when clinical suspicion is high and other causes of malabsorption have been ruled out.

8. Answer: B. Perform upper endoscopy with biopsy

   Explanation: Despite positive serum anti-tTG antibodies, the diagnosis of Celiac disease should be confirmed with upper endoscopy and biopsy to assess for characteristic histological changes in the small intestine.

9. Answer: B. Celiac disease

   Explanation: Chronic diarrhea, nutrient deficiencies (e.g., vitamin D, calcium), and extraintestinal symptoms (headaches, muscle pain) suggest Celiac disease, an autoimmune disorder triggered by gluten ingestion.

10. Answer: D. Celiac disease

    Explanation: Positive serum anti-tTG antibodies, HLA-DQ2 genotype, and symptoms such as anemia, weight loss, and dermatitis herpetiformis are characteristic of Celiac disease.

11. Answer: A. Initiate gluten-free diet

    Explanation: Positive serum anti-tTG antibodies in the setting of symptoms and possible gluten sensitivity warrant initiation of a gluten-free diet, though confirmation with biopsy may still be necessary for diagnosis.

12. Answer: A. Celiac disease

    Explanation: Positive anti-EMA antibodies, malabsorption symptoms (diarrhea, weight loss), and vitamin deficiencies are indicative of Celiac disease, which requires confirmation with biopsy.

13. Answer: B. Perform upper endoscopy with biopsy

    Explanation: Despite positive serum anti-tTG antibodies, the diagnosis of Celiac disease should be confirmed with upper endoscopy and biopsy to assess for characteristic histological changes in the small intestine.

14. Answer: C. Celiac disease

    Explanation: Chronic diarrhea, iron deficiency anemia, positive serum anti-tTG antibodies, and a history of migraines and mouth ulcers suggest Celiac disease, which should be confirmed with biopsy.

15. Answer: B. Perform upper endoscopy with biopsy

   Explanation: Positive serum anti-tTG antibodies and symptoms of malabsorption (low calcium, vitamin D) indicate a need for upper endoscopy with biopsy to confirm the diagnosis of Celiac disease.

Chronic Kidney Disease

1. Answer: C. Stage 3

   Explanation: Stage 3 CKD is characterized by moderate kidney damage with eGFR of 30-59 mL/min/1.73 m². Symptoms such as fatigue and swelling typically appear at this stage.

2. Answer: B. Hyperkalemia

   Explanation: CKD can lead to impaired potassium excretion, causing hyperkalemia, which can manifest with nausea, vomiting, confusion, and potentially life-threatening cardiac arrhythmias.

3. Answer: B. Renal osteodystrophy

   Explanation: Renal osteodystrophy occurs due to mineral and bone disorder in CKD, characterized by abnormalities in calcium, phosphorus, and parathyroid hormone levels, leading to bone pain and fractures.

4. Answer: A. Volume overload

   Explanation: Volume overload is common in CKD patients on dialysis due to fluid retention, leading to symptoms such as dyspnea and pedal edema.

5. Answer: B. Hypocalcemia

   Explanation: Hypocalcemia can occur in CKD due to decreased activation of vitamin D and impaired calcium absorption, leading to symptoms such as muscle cramps and paresthesias.

6. Answer: B. Chronic kidney disease

   Explanation: Symptoms such as frequent urination, nocturia, swelling (due to fluid retention), and elevated serum creatinine are indicative of CKD, commonly seen in patients with diabetes and hypertension.

7. Answer: A. Uremia

   Explanation: Uremia refers to the accumulation of urea and other nitrogenous waste products in the blood due to impaired kidney function, leading to symptoms such as fatigue, nausea, and metallic taste.

8. Answer: D. Renal colic

   Explanation: Renal colic, often caused by kidney stones, can present with severe flank pain and oliguria in CKD patients, necessitating urgent evaluation and management.

9. Answer: B. Hyperkalemia

    Explanation: Hyperkalemia can lead to neurological symptoms such as confusion and seizures, especially in patients with advanced CKD where potassium excretion is impaired.

10. Answer: C. Arrhythmia

    Explanation: Hyperkalemia in CKD can lead to life-threatening cardiac arrhythmias, including bradycardia, atrioventricular block, and ventricular tachycardia.

11. Answer: D. Renal osteodystrophy

    Explanation: Renal osteodystrophy refers to bone changes in CKD due to abnormalities in calcium, phosphate, and parathyroid hormone levels, leading to bone pain and fractures.

12. Answer: A. Hyperphosphatemia

    Explanation: Hyperphosphatemia in CKD can lead to pruritus, often severe, due to deposition of calcium-phosphate complexes in the skin.

13. Answer: D. Renal anemia

    Explanation: Renal anemia is common in CKD due to decreased production of erythropoietin by the kidneys, leading to normocytic anemia.

14. Answer: B. Hypocalcemia

    Explanation: Hypocalcemia can occur in CKD due to impaired activation of vitamin D and calcium-phosphate imbalance, leading to symptoms such as muscle weakness and paresthesias.

15. Answer: A. Acute kidney injury

    Explanation: Symptoms such as confusion, peripheral edema, and decreased urine output suggest acute kidney injury on the background of CKD, often precipitated by factors such as dehydration or medication toxicity.

Chronic Obstructive Pulmonary Disease (COPD)

1. Answer: B. Pulmonary function tests (PFTs)

    Explanation: PFTs are essential for diagnosing COPD, showing a reduced FEV1/FVC ratio (<0.70) indicative of airflow obstruction.

2. Answer: B. Nebulized short-acting bronchodilators

    Explanation: Management of COPD exacerbation involves bronchodilators (short-acting beta-agonists and anticholinergics) as first-line therapy to relieve airflow obstruction.

3. Answer: B. PFTs before and after bronchodilator

    Explanation: PFTs showing reversible airflow limitation (increase in FEV1 ≥12% or ≥200 mL post-bronchodilator) suggest asthma, whereas persistent airflow limitation is indicative of COPD.

4. Answer: D. Combination of NRT and behavioral counseling

    Explanation: Combining NRT (patch, gum, lozenge) with behavioral counseling is more effective for smoking cessation in patients with COPD compared to monotherapy.

5. Answer: A. Home oxygen therapy

    Explanation: Long-term oxygen therapy (LTOT) is indicated in COPD patients with severe hypoxemia (PaO2 ≤55 mmHg) to improve survival and reduce complications.

6. Answer: A. Start empirical antibiotics

    Explanation: Suspected pneumonia in COPD exacerbation warrants empirical antibiotics covering typical pathogens (e.g., Streptococcus pneumoniae, Haemophilus influenzae).

7. Answer: C. Pulmonary rehabilitation

    Explanation: Pulmonary rehabilitation is beneficial for COPD patients to improve exercise tolerance, dyspnea, and quality of life through structured exercise training and education.

8. Answer: B. Switch to long-acting beta-agonist (LABA)

    Explanation: Step-up therapy in COPD includes adding a long-acting bronchodilator (LABA or LAMA) for persistent symptoms despite short-acting bronchodilator use.

9. Answer: B. Perform echocardiogram

    Explanation: Worsening dyspnea and new-onset atrial fibrillation in COPD suggest potential cardiac decompensation. Echocardiogram helps assess cardiac function and guide management.

10. Answer: A. Start selective serotonin reuptake inhibitor (SSRI)

    Explanation: Depression is common in COPD. Starting an SSRI is appropriate for managing depressive symptoms in this patient without suicidal ideation.

11. Answer: A. Oral nutritional supplements

    Explanation: Oral nutritional supplements are recommended for COPD patients with unintentional weight loss and decreased appetite to improve nutritional status.

12. Answer: A. Encourage use of air purifiers

    Explanation: Indoor air pollutants can exacerbate COPD symptoms. Using air purifiers with HEPA filters can help reduce exposure to indoor allergens and pollutants.

13. Answer: A. Long-term macrolide therapy

    Explanation: Long-term macrolide therapy (e.g., azithromycin) reduces COPD exacerbation frequency and improves quality of life in patients with frequent exacerbations.

14. Answer: B. Influenza vaccine

    Explanation: Annual influenza vaccination is recommended for all COPD patients to reduce the risk of influenza-related complications and exacerbations.

15. Answer: C. Improved exercise tolerance and quality of life

    Explanation: Pulmonary rehabilitation improves exercise capacity, dyspnea, and quality of life in COPD patients through exercise training and education.

Congestive Heart Failure (CHF)

1. Answer: B. Echocardiogram

    Explanation: Echocardiogram is essential for diagnosing CHF, assessing left ventricular function, and identifying structural heart abnormalities.

2. Answer: B. Non-invasive positive pressure ventilation (NIPPV)

    Explanation: Management of acute decompensated CHF with acute pulmonary edema includes NIPPV to improve oxygenation and reduce work of breathing.

3. Answer: C. Beta-blockers

    Explanation: Beta-blockers (e.g., carvedilol, metoprolol) are recommended in HFrEF to reduce mortality and hospitalizations by blocking the harmful effects of sympathetic activation.

4. Answer: A. Loop diuretics

    Explanation: Symptomatic relief in HFpEF focuses on volume management with diuretics (e.g., loop diuretics like furosemide) to reduce pulmonary congestion and symptoms.

5. Answer: B. IV potassium supplementation

    Explanation: Hypokalemia in CHF patients should be corrected cautiously with IV potassium to prevent arrhythmias and muscle weakness.

6. Answer: B. Cardiac resynchronization therapy (CRT)

    Explanation: CRT is indicated in selected CHF patients with reduced ejection fraction and ventricular dyssynchrony to improve symptoms and reduce hospitalizations.

7. Answer: A. Reduce diuretic dose

    Explanation: Worsening renal function in CHF patients may require reducing diuretic dose to optimize renal perfusion and prevent further deterioration.

8. Answer: A. Transthoracic echocardiogram

    Explanation: Transthoracic echocardiogram is essential for assessing valvular heart disease (e.g., mitral stenosis) and its contribution to CHF symptoms.

9. Answer: B. Simplify medication regimen

Explanation: Simplifying the medication regimen (e.g., once-daily dosing, reducing pill burden) improves adherence and reduces hospitalizations in CHF patients.

10. Answer: B. Initiate direct oral anticoagulant (DOAC)

Explanation: In CHF patients with atrial fibrillation and CHA2DS2-VASc score ≥2, DOACs (e.g., apixaban, dabigatran) are preferred for stroke prevention.

11. Answer: A. Increase loop diuretic dose

Explanation: Management of acute decompensated CHF with volume overload includes increasing loop diuretic dose to achieve euvolemia and relieve symptoms.

12. Answer: B. Cardiac rehabilitation program

Explanation: Cardiac rehabilitation improves exercise tolerance, quality of life, and functional status in CHF patients through structured exercise training and education.

13. Answer: C. Refer for iron supplementation

Explanation: Iron deficiency in CHF patients should be corrected with oral or IV iron supplementation to improve symptoms and quality of life.

14. Answer: A. Continuous positive airway pressure (CPAP)

Explanation: CPAP therapy is effective in treating obstructive sleep apnea in CHF patients, improving sleep quality and daytime symptoms.

15. Answer: B. Left ventricular assist device (LVAD)

Explanation: LVAD improves survival and quality of life in selected severe CHF patients who are candidates for advanced heart failure therapy.

Crohn's Disease

1. Answer: B) Crohn's disease

    Explanation: Chronic abdominal pain, diarrhea, weight loss, fever, and fatigue are typical symptoms of Crohn's disease. The presence of a palpable mass in the right lower quadrant suggests possible involvement of the terminal ileum, common in Crohn's disease. IBS typically presents with abdominal pain and altered bowel habits without systemic symptoms. Ulcerative colitis primarily affects the colon and presents with bloody diarrhea. Diverticulitis typically presents with localized left lower quadrant pain.

2. Answer: A) Colonoscopy with biopsy

    Explanation: In a patient with suspected Crohn's disease presenting with abdominal pain, diarrhea, and rectal bleeding, colonoscopy with biopsy is the most appropriate initial test to evaluate the extent and severity of intestinal inflammation and to obtain tissue samples for histopathological confirmation. Stool cultures are typically done to rule out infectious causes. Ultrasound and CT scans may be useful for assessing complications such as abscesses or fistulas but are not the initial diagnostic tests for Crohn's disease.

3. Answer: A) Crohn's disease

    Explanation: The presence of chronic diarrhea, abdominal pain, fatigue, oral ulcers, and perianal complications (abscesses and fistulas) are characteristic of Crohn's disease. Ulcerative colitis primarily involves the colon and presents with bloody diarrhea. Celiac disease typically presents with malabsorption symptoms and is associated with gluten intolerance. IBS presents with abdominal pain and altered bowel habits but does not typically cause perianal complications or oral ulcers.

4. Answer: A) Skip lesions in the small intestine

    Explanation: Crohn's disease often presents with skip lesions, which are characterized by areas of normal bowel interspersed with inflamed segments. This pattern is typically seen in the small intestine but can also occur in any part of the gastrointestinal tract affected by Crohn's disease. Continuous colonic involvement is more characteristic of ulcerative colitis. Diffuse rectal thickening can occur in proctitis but is not specific to Crohn's disease. Sigmoid colon strictures can occur in both Crohn's disease and ulcerative colitis but are not typically the initial finding on imaging.

5. Answer: B) Ulcerative colitis

    Explanation: Chronic diarrhea, weight loss, rectal bleeding, and autoimmune thyroiditis suggest ulcerative colitis, which primarily affects the colon. Crohn's disease can also cause similar symptoms but is more commonly associated with skip lesions and extraintestinal manifestations like perianal disease rather than autoimmune thyroiditis. Diverticulitis presents with localized left lower quadrant pain and fever. Infectious colitis may present with similar symptoms but would typically have an acute onset and history of recent infection exposure.

6. Answer: B) Corticosteroids

    Explanation: Corticosteroids are often used as the initial treatment for moderate to severe Crohn's disease to induce remission. Mesalamine is used primarily in ulcerative colitis and may have limited benefit in Crohn's disease. Methotrexate and infliximab are used for maintenance therapy and in refractory cases of Crohn's disease.

7. Answer: B) Cobblestone appearance of the mucosa

    Explanation: Crohn's disease is characterized by a cobblestone appearance of the mucosa on endoscopy, which results from the presence of deep ulcerations separated by areas of normal mucosa. Continuous involvement of the colon is more typical of ulcerative colitis. Pseudopolyps can occur in both diseases but are more common in ulcerative colitis. Diffuse rectal strictures can occur in Crohn's disease but are less specific to the initial colonoscopic findings.

8. Answer: B) CT scan of the abdomen and pelvis

    Explanation: In a patient with suspected Crohn's disease and signs of abdominal mass or complications such as abscesses, a CT scan of the abdomen and pelvis is the most appropriate initial imaging test. It can assess the extent and severity of inflammation, identify complications, and guide management decisions. Ultrasound may be used for initial evaluation but is less sensitive than CT scan for assessing bowel wall thickening and extraintestinal manifestations. MRI is useful for evaluating small bowel involvement and complications. Barium enema is not typically used as an initial imaging modality for Crohn's disease.

9. Answer: D) Adalimumab

    Explanation: Adalimumab, a TNF-alpha inhibitor, is often used as initial therapy for moderate to severe Crohn's disease, especially in patients with extraintestinal manifestations such as migratory arthritis and erythema nodosum. Mesalamine is used primarily in ulcerative colitis. Corticosteroids are used for induction of remission but are not typically considered initial therapy in this case. Azathioprine may be used for maintenance therapy but is less commonly used as initial treatment compared to TNF-alpha inhibitors.

10. Answer: A) Skip lesions in the small intestine

    Explanation: Crohn's disease often presents with skip lesions, which are characterized by areas of normal bowel interspersed with inflamed segments. This pattern is typically seen in the small intestine but can also occur in any part of the gastrointestinal tract affected by Crohn's disease. Continuous colonic involvement is more characteristic of ulcerative colitis. Diffuse rectal thickening can occur in proctitis but is not specific to Crohn's disease. Sigmoid colon strictures can occur in both Crohn's disease and ulcerative colitis but are not typically the initial finding on imaging.

11. Answer: B) Cobblestone appearance of the mucosa

Explanation: Crohn's disease is characterized by a cobblestone appearance of the mucosa on endoscopy, which results from the presence of deep ulcerations separated by areas of normal mucosa. Continuous involvement of the colon is more typical of ulcerative colitis. Pseudopolyps can occur in both diseases but are more common in ulcerative colitis. Diffuse rectal strictures can occur in Crohn's disease but are less specific to the initial colonoscopic findings.

12. Answer: B) CT scan of the abdomen and pelvis

Explanation: In a patient with suspected Crohn's disease and signs of abdominal mass or complications such as abscesses, a CT scan of the abdomen and pelvis is the most appropriate initial imaging test. It can assess the extent and severity of inflammation, identify complications, and guide management decisions. Ultrasound may be used for initial evaluation but is less sensitive than CT scan for assessing bowel wall thickening and extraintestinal manifestations. MRI is useful for evaluating small bowel involvement and complications. Barium enema is not typically used as an initial imaging modality for Crohn's disease.

13. Answer: D) Adalimumab

Explanation: Adalimumab, a TNF-alpha inhibitor, is often used as initial therapy for moderate to severe Crohn's disease, especially in patients with extraintestinal manifestations such as migratory arthritis and erythema nodosum. Mesalamine is used primarily in ulcerative colitis. Corticosteroids are used for induction of remission but are not typically considered initial therapy in this case. Azathioprine may be used for maintenance therapy but is less commonly used as initial treatment compared to TNF-alpha inhibitors.

14. Answer: A) Skip lesions in the small intestine

   Explanation: Crohn's disease often presents with skip lesions, which are characterized by areas of normal bowel interspersed with inflamed segments. This pattern is typically seen in the small intestine but can also occur in any part of the gastrointestinal tract affected by Crohn's disease. Continuous colonic involvement is more characteristic of ulcerative colitis. Diffuse rectal thickening can occur in proctitis but is not specific to Crohn's disease. Sigmoid colon strictures can occur in both Crohn's disease and ulcerative colitis but are not typically the initial finding on imaging.

15. Answer: B) Cobblestone appearance of the mucosa

   Explanation: Crohn's disease is characterized by a cobblestone appearance of the mucosa on endoscopy, which results from the presence of deep ulcerations separated by areas of normal mucosa. Continuous involvement of the colon is more typical of ulcerative colitis. Pseudopolyps can occur in both diseases but are more common in ulcerative colitis. Diffuse rectal strictures can occur in Crohn's disease but are less specific to the initial colonoscopic findings.

Deep Vein Thrombosis (DVT)

1. Answer: A) Doppler ultrasound

   Explanation: Doppler ultrasound is the initial diagnostic test of choice for suspected DVT due to its high sensitivity and specificity in detecting thrombi within deep veins.

2. Answer: B) Pulmonary embolism

   Explanation: This patient's presentation is suggestive of a pulmonary embolism, a common complication of DVT in patients with cancer, characterized by dyspnea, pleuritic chest pain, and hemodynamic instability.

3. Answer: C) Order bilateral lower extremity ultrasound

   Explanation: Given the clinical suspicion for DVT post-surgery, ultrasound imaging of the lower extremities is indicated to confirm the diagnosis before starting anticoagulation therapy.

4. Answer: B) Acute arterial occlusion

   Explanation: Acute arterial occlusion presents with sudden-onset severe limb pain, pallor, coldness, absent pulses, and decreased sensation, which are not typical of DVT.

5. Answer: D) Bilateral lower extremity ultrasound

   Explanation: Given the patient's risk factors (oral contraceptives increase the risk of DVT), bilateral lower extremity ultrasound is warranted to confirm the diagnosis before initiating treatment.

6. Answer: C) Deep vein thrombosis

   Explanation: Homans' sign (calf pain with dorsiflexion of the foot) can indicate DVT, although it is not highly specific. Confirmatory imaging such as ultrasound is required for diagnosis.

7. Answer: C) Perform bilateral lower extremity ultrasound

   Explanation: Given the recent prolonged flight (a risk factor for DVT), ultrasound imaging of the lower extremities is the next step to confirm or rule out DVT before starting treatment.

8. Answer: D) Bilateral lower extremity ultrasound

   Explanation: Given the new-onset unilateral leg symptoms and risk factors (congestive heart failure), ultrasound imaging is necessary to confirm the presence of DVT before considering treatment options.

9. Answer: D) CT pulmonary angiography

   Explanation: This patient's presentation is concerning for pulmonary embolism, a complication of DVT. CT pulmonary angiography is the initial test of choice to confirm or rule out pulmonary embolism.

10. Answer: C) Perform bilateral lower extremity ultrasound

    Explanation: Post-operative DVT is a common complication after hip replacement surgery. Ultrasound imaging is needed to confirm the diagnosis before initiating treatment.

11. Answer: A) Chronic venous insufficiency

    Explanation: Chronic venous insufficiency can develop as a sequela of previous DVT, leading to persistent leg swelling and discoloration due to impaired venous return.

12. Answer: A) Warmth and erythema of the calf

    Explanation: Warmth and erythema of the calf are signs of inflammation associated with DVT. Physical examination findings can aid in the clinical suspicion of DVT.

13. Answer: C) Pulmonary embolism

    Explanation: Hemoptysis (coughing up blood) is a concerning sign of pulmonary embolism, a complication of DVT. This patient requires prompt evaluation for pulmonary embolism.

14. Answer: D) Bilateral lower extremity ultrasound

    Explanation: Factor V Leiden mutation is a thrombophilic disorder that increases the risk of DVT. Given the acute presentation, ultrasound is necessary to confirm DVT before treatment.

15. Answer: C) Perform CT pulmonary angiography

    Explanation: This patient's presentation is concerning for pulmonary embolism. CT pulmonary angiography is indicated to confirm or rule out pulmonary embolism before starting anticoagulation therapy.

Depression

1. Answer: A. Major depressive disorder

   Explanation: Emily's symptoms are characteristic of major depressive disorder (MDD), as they involve persistent sadness, anhedonia, and other depressive symptoms lasting at least two weeks. The absence of manic episodes differentiates it from bipolar disorder.

2. Answer: B. Sertraline

   Explanation: Sertraline, an SSRI (Selective Serotonin Reuptake Inhibitor), is a first-line medication for treating major depressive disorder. It helps alleviate symptoms of depression by increasing serotonin levels in the brain.

3. Answer: A. Switch to venlafaxine

   Explanation: If a patient does not respond to an SSRI such as fluoxetine after an adequate trial period, switching to another class of antidepressant such as venlafaxine (a serotonin-norepinephrine reuptake inhibitor) is a reasonable next step.

4. Answer: D. Duloxetine

   Explanation: Duloxetine is an SNRI (Serotonin-Norepinephrine Reuptake Inhibitor) that is effective in treating both depression and chronic pain conditions like fibromyalgia and diabetic peripheral neuropathy.

5. Answer: D. Risk of suicidal ideation

   Explanation: Patients with severe depression are at increased risk of suicidal ideation and behavior. Close monitoring and appropriate management, including hospitalization if necessary, are crucial to ensure patient safety.

6. Answer: B. Referral to a substance abuse program

   Explanation: Addressing the alcohol dependence is crucial before initiating antidepressant therapy, as substance use disorders can complicate the treatment of depression and may require specialized treatment.

7. Answer: A. Sertraline

    Explanation: Sertraline is often considered safer than other SSRIs during pregnancy due to lower risks of teratogenicity and adverse pregnancy outcomes. However, all decisions should be made in consultation with a healthcare provider.

8. Answer: A. Augment current medication with lithium

    Explanation: Augmenting the current antidepressant with lithium or another augmenting agent (such as an atypical antipsychotic) is often considered in cases of treatment-resistant depression.

9. Answer: A. Risk of teratogenicity with antidepressants

    Explanation: The risk of teratogenicity and other adverse effects of antidepressants during pregnancy should be discussed with Olivia, weighing the potential benefits and risks of treatment.

10. Answer: B. Bupropion

    Explanation: Bupropion is less likely to cause sexual dysfunction compared to SSRIs like fluoxetine, sertraline, and paroxetine, making it a suitable choice for patients concerned about this side effect.

11. Answer: A. Persistent depressive disorder (dysthymia)

    Explanation: Persistent depressive disorder (dysthymia) is characterized by chronic depressive symptoms lasting for at least two years, with periods of milder symptoms that do not meet the criteria for major depressive disorder.

12. Answer: A. MAOIs (Monoamine oxidase inhibitors)

    Explanation: MAOIs, such as phenelzine and tranylcypromine, are often effective for atypical depression characterized by symptoms like hypersomnia, weight gain, and mood reactivity.

13. Answer: C. Mirtazapine

    Explanation: Mirtazapine is often chosen for patients with depression who have insomnia and significant fatigue due to its sedating effects and potential to improve sleep quality.

14. Answer: A. SSRI-induced weight gain

    Explanation: Weight gain and excessive sleepiness can be side effects of SSRIs such as fluoxetine or sertraline. Monitoring for these side effects is important to manage and potentially switch medications if necessary.

15. Answer: A. Immediate psychiatric hospitalization

    Explanation: Hannah's presentation with suicidal ideation and feelings of worthlessness warrants immediate psychiatric evaluation and, if necessary, hospitalization to ensure her safety and provide intensive treatment.

Diabetes Mellitus (Type 1 and Type 2)

1. Answer: A. Type 1 diabetes mellitus

    Explanation: The classic symptoms of polyuria, polydipsia, weight loss, and hyperglycemia with ketonuria point towards Type 1 diabetes mellitus, which often presents acutely due to insulin deficiency.

2. Answer: B. Type 2 diabetes mellitus

    Explanation: This patient's obesity, insulin resistance (evidenced by acanthosis nigricans), and elevated HbA1c are typical of Type 2 diabetes mellitus, which is common in middle-aged and older adults.

3. Answer: C. Gestational diabetes mellitus

    Explanation: Gestational diabetes mellitus typically manifests during pregnancy and increases the risk of complications for both the mother and the fetus. It usually resolves after delivery.

4. Answer: B. Type 2 diabetes mellitus

    Explanation: This patient's symptoms, including obesity, hypertension, and signs of insulin resistance (central obesity, buffalo hump), along with elevated blood glucose, suggest Type 2 diabetes mellitus.

5. Answer: D. Reactive hypoglycemia

    Explanation: Reactive hypoglycemia typically occurs after meals and is more common in individuals who have undergone gastric bypass surgery or have other gastrointestinal disorders. It is characterized by episodes of low blood glucose levels.

6. Answer: A. Diabetic retinopathy

    Explanation: The presence of hemorrhages, cotton wool spots, and new-onset visual symptoms in a patient with Type 2 diabetes mellitus suggests diabetic retinopathy, a common microvascular complication.

7. Answer: B. Type 2 diabetes mellitus

    Explanation: This patient's symptoms of hyperglycemia, neuropathy (tingling in hands and feet), recurrent infections, and elevated HbA1c are consistent with Type 2 diabetes mellitus.

8. Answer: A. Diabetic ketoacidosis (DKA)

    Explanation: This patient's severe hyperglycemia, metabolic acidosis (low bicarbonate and pH), and

    dehydration are characteristic of diabetic ketoacidosis, which is more common in Type 1 diabetes mellitus

    but can occur in Type 2 diabetes mellitus as well.

9. Answer: A. Diabetic ketoacidosis (DKA)

    Explanation: This patient's severe hyperglycemia, metabolic acidosis (low bicarbonate and pH), and history

    of missed insulin injections are consistent with diabetic ketoacidosis, a severe complication of Type 1

    diabetes mellitus.

10. Answer: B. Hyperosmolar hyperglycemic state (HHS)

    Explanation: This patient's extremely high serum glucose, hyperosmolality, severe dehydration, and

    absence of significant ketosis are typical of hyperosmolar hyperglycemic state, a serious complication seen

    more commonly in Type 2 diabetes mellitus.

11. Answer: D. Insulin lispro

    Explanation: Insulin lispro is a rapid-acting insulin analogue used to cover meals and correct hyperglycemia

    in patients with Type 1 and Type 2 diabetes mellitus.

12. Answer: C. Increasing bedtime snack carbohydrate intake

    Explanation: Increasing bedtime snack carbohydrate intake can help prevent nocturnal hypoglycemia by

    providing a sustained source of glucose during the night, especially in patients at risk, such as those on

    basal insulin therapy.

13. Answer: C. Lactic acidosis

    Explanation: Lactic acidosis is a rare but serious adverse effect of metformin, especially in patients with

    renal impairment or other predisposing factors. It is characterized by elevated lactate levels and metabolic

    acidosis.

14. Answer: A. Start angiotensin-converting enzyme (ACE) inhibitor or angiotensin receptor blocker (ARB)

    Explanation: Treatment of microalbuminuria in patients with diabetes mellitus involves starting an ACE

    inhibitor or ARB to delay progression to macroalbuminuria and reduce the risk of diabetic nephropathy.

15. Answer: C. Peripheral neuropathy

    Explanation: This patient's symptoms of neuropathic pain, diminished sensation, and positive monofilament testing are characteristic of diabetic peripheral neuropathy, a common complication of diabetes mellitus.

Diabetic Neuropathy

1. Answer: A. Distal symmetric polyneuropathy

   Explanation: Distal symmetric polyneuropathy is the most common type of diabetic neuropathy, characterized by symmetric sensory loss in a stocking-glove distribution.

2. Answer: C. Monofilament testing

   Explanation: Monofilament testing (10-gram Semmes-Weinstein monofilament) is a simple and effective screening tool for detecting loss of protective sensation in diabetic neuropathy.

3. Answer: B. Autonomic neuropathy

   Explanation: Autonomic neuropathy in diabetes affects cardiovascular, gastrointestinal, and genitourinary systems, leading to symptoms such as orthostatic hypotension and gastroparesis.

4. Answer: A. Gabapentin

   Explanation: Gabapentin and pregabalin are first-line medications for managing neuropathic pain, including painful diabetic neuropathy, due to their efficacy and safety profile.

5. Answer: C. Offload pressure with a total contact cast

   Explanation: Offloading pressure with a total contact cast is crucial for managing diabetic foot ulcers, preventing further complications in patients with neuropathy.

6. Answer: A. Carpal tunnel syndrome

   Explanation: Carpal tunnel syndrome is a common mononeuropathy in diabetes, characterized by median nerve compression at the wrist, causing pain and sensory deficits.

7. Answer: B. Autonomic neuropathy

   Explanation: Autonomic neuropathy in diabetes can affect erectile function (diabetic autonomic neuropathy), leading to erectile dysfunction due to impaired neurovascular responses.

8. Answer: B. Autonomic neuropathy

   Explanation: Autonomic neuropathy can affect gastrointestinal motility (gastroparesis) in diabetes, causing symptoms such as early satiety, bloating, and nausea.

9. Answer: B. Autonomic neuropathy

    Explanation: Autonomic neuropathy in diabetes can affect bladder function (diabetic cystopathy), leading to urinary symptoms such as urgency, frequency, and incomplete emptying.

10. Answer: B. Charcot foot

    Explanation: Charcot foot is a complication of diabetic neuropathy characterized by progressive bone and joint destruction, leading to deformity and increased risk of foot ulcers.

11. Answer: B. Switch to pregabalin

    Explanation: Pregabalin is another first-line medication for neuropathic pain, including painful diabetic neuropathy, and can be considered if gabapentin is ineffective or not tolerated.

12. Answer: A. Inspect feet daily for cuts and blisters

    Explanation: Daily foot inspection is crucial for early detection of minor injuries in diabetic patients with neuropathy, reducing the risk of foot ulcers and infections.

13. Answer: B. Annually

    Explanation: Annual screening for diabetic neuropathy, including sensory testing with monofilament, is recommended to detect early nerve damage in asymptomatic patients.

14. Answer: B. Debridement and culture-directed antibiotics

    Explanation: Early aggressive management of infected foot ulcers with debridement and appropriate antibiotics reduces the risk of amputation in diabetic patients with neuropathy.

15. Answer: C. Regularly check blood glucose before driving

    Explanation: Patients with diabetic neuropathy should regularly monitor blood glucose levels and ensure they are within safe limits before driving to maintain driving safety.

Diabetic Retinopathy

1. Answer: A. Non-proliferative diabetic retinopathy (NPDR)

   Explanation: Microaneurysms and dot-blot hemorrhages are characteristic findings of NPDR, an early stage of diabetic retinopathy.

2. Answer: C. Diabetic macular edema (DME)

   Explanation: Yellow exudates and macular edema are characteristic findings of DME, a complication of diabetic retinopathy involving the macula.

3. Answer: B. Proliferative diabetic retinopathy (PDR)

   Explanation: Neovascularization, vitreous hemorrhage, and fibrous proliferation are characteristic findings of PDR, an advanced stage of diabetic retinopathy.

4. Answer: A. Non-proliferative diabetic retinopathy (NPDR)

   Explanation: Cotton wool spots and intraretinal hemorrhages are characteristic findings of NPDR, indicating early changes in diabetic retinopathy.

5. Answer: C. Diabetic macular edema (DME)

   Explanation: Yellowish deposits at the macula and cystoid spaces on OCT are characteristic findings of DME, which can lead to vision loss in diabetic patients.

6. Answer: B. Proliferative diabetic retinopathy (PDR)

   Explanation: Retinal hemorrhages, dilated retinal veins, cotton wool spots, and neovascularization are characteristic of PDR, a severe complication of diabetic retinopathy.

7. Answer: A. Non-proliferative diabetic retinopathy (NPDR)

   Explanation: Pale optic disc, narrowed arterioles, and scattered intraretinal hemorrhages are characteristic of NPDR, indicating early changes in diabetic retinopathy.

8. Answer: C. Diabetic macular edema (DME)

   Explanation: Lipid exudates and cystoid macular edema are characteristic findings of DME, a common complication in diabetic retinopathy.

9. Answer: C. Central retinal artery occlusion (CRAO)

    Explanation: Cherry-red spot, retinal edema, and segmented blood column in a retinal artery are characteristic findings of CRAO, a rare but serious condition.

10. Answer: A. Non-proliferative diabetic retinopathy (NPDR)

    Explanation: Scattered cotton wool spots and hard exudates are characteristic findings of NPDR, indicating early changes in diabetic retinopathy.

11. Answer: B. Proliferative diabetic retinopathy (PDR)

    Explanation: Vitreous hemorrhage and fibrovascular proliferation are characteristic findings of PDR, indicating advanced diabetic retinopathy.

12. Answer: C. Diabetic macular edema (DME)

    Explanation: Yellowish deposits at the macula and cystoid macular edema are characteristic findings of DME, a common complication in diabetic retinopathy.

13. Answer: B. Proliferative diabetic retinopathy (PDR)

    Explanation: Neovascularization, vitreous hemorrhage, and fibrous proliferation are characteristic findings of PDR, indicating advanced diabetic retinopathy.

14. Answer: A. Non-proliferative diabetic retinopathy (NPDR)

    Explanation: Microaneurysms, intraretinal hemorrhages, and cotton wool spots are characteristic findings of NPDR, indicating early changes in diabetic retinopathy.

15. Answer: C. Diabetic macular edema (DME)

    Explanation: Lipid exudates and cystoid macular edema are characteristic findings of DME, a common complication in diabetic retinopathy.

Dyslipidemia

1. Answer: D. Recommend lifestyle modifications and recheck lipid levels in 3 months

    Explanation: In a patient without known cardiovascular disease but with elevated LDL cholesterol, initial management involves lifestyle modifications including diet and exercise. Lipid-lowering drug therapy is considered if lifestyle changes do not achieve target levels after 3 months.

2. Answer: A. Start high-intensity statin therapy

    Explanation: Patients with diabetes aged 40-75 years should be on a moderate- to high-intensity statin regardless of baseline lipid levels. This patient's LDL cholesterol level warrants high-intensity statin therapy.

3. Answer: B. Initiate fibrate therapy

    Explanation: In severe hypertriglyceridemia (triglycerides >500 mg/dL) with acute pancreatitis, fibrates are preferred to reduce triglyceride levels and prevent further episodes of pancreatitis.

4. Answer: A. Initiate moderate-intensity statin therapy

    Explanation: Patients with a family history of premature coronary artery disease and LDL cholesterol levels ≥ 130 mg/dL should be started on moderate-intensity statin therapy to reduce cardiovascular risk.

5. Answer: B. Add ezetimibe to his current therapy

    Explanation: This patient has suboptimal HDL cholesterol levels despite statin therapy. Adding ezetimibe can further lower LDL cholesterol levels and improve overall lipid management.

6. Answer: A. Start high-intensity statin therapy

    Explanation: Patients with diabetes aged 40-75 years should be on a moderate- to high-intensity statin regardless of baseline lipid levels. This patient's LDL cholesterol level warrants high-intensity statin therapy.

7. Answer: A. Familial hypercholesterolemia (FH)

    Explanation: Xanthomas and severe elevations in LDL cholesterol (LDL >190 mg/dL) suggest familial hypercholesterolemia, a genetic disorder predisposing to premature cardiovascular disease.

8. Answer: D. Evaluate for familial chylomicronemia syndrome

   Explanation: Recurrent abdominal pain after meals and severe hypertriglyceridemia (>1000 mg/dL) suggest familial chylomicronemia syndrome, which requires specific management.

9. Answer: A. Start moderate-intensity statin therapy

   Explanation: Patients with rheumatoid arthritis are at increased risk of cardiovascular disease. This patient's LDL cholesterol level warrants initiation of moderate-intensity statin therapy.

10. Answer: A. Initiate high-intensity statin therapy

    Explanation: Patients with clinical atherosclerotic cardiovascular disease (ASCVD) and LDL cholesterol ≥ 190 mg/dL should be on high-intensity statin therapy to reduce cardiovascular risk.

11. Answer: A. Start high-intensity statin therapy

    Explanation: Patients with peripheral arterial disease (PAD) should be on high-intensity statin therapy to reduce cardiovascular risk, regardless of baseline lipid levels.

12. Answer: A. Start moderate-intensity statin therapy

    Explanation: Patients with diabetes aged 40-75 years should be on a moderate- to high-intensity statin regardless of baseline lipid levels. This patient's LDL cholesterol level warrants moderate-intensity statin therapy.

13. Answer: A. Familial hypercholesterolemia (FH)

    Explanation: Xanthomas and severe elevations in LDL cholesterol (LDL >190 mg/dL) suggest familial hypercholesterolemia, a genetic disorder predisposing to premature cardiovascular disease.

14. Answer: D. Recommend lifestyle modifications and recheck lipid levels in 6 months

    Explanation: In patients with metabolic syndrome and without established cardiovascular disease, lifestyle modifications are the first-line approach. Pharmacotherapy is considered if lifestyle changes are inadequate.

15. Answer: B. Add ezetimibe to his current therapy

    Explanation: This patient has suboptimal HDL cholesterol levels despite statin therapy. Adding ezetimibe can further lower LDL cholesterol levels and improve overall lipid management.

Eczema

1. Answer: C. Atopic dermatitis

   Explanation: Atopic dermatitis (eczema) typically presents in infancy with pruritic, erythematous patches on the face and extensor surfaces, often associated with a personal or family history of allergies.

2. Answer: B. Fragrances

   Explanation: Fragrances are common triggers for exacerbating eczema symptoms in susceptible individuals, causing irritation and allergic reactions.

3. Answer: B. Psoriasis

   Explanation: Psoriasis presents with well-defined, erythematous plaques with silvery scales, commonly affecting extensor surfaces and scalp, in contrast to the flexural distribution seen in atopic dermatitis.

4. Answer: A. Topical corticosteroids

   Explanation: Topical corticosteroids are first-line for managing acute exacerbations of atopic dermatitis due to their anti-inflammatory and immunosuppressive effects.

5. Answer: B. Topical calcineurin inhibitors

   Explanation: Topical calcineurin inhibitors (e.g., tacrolimus, pimecrolimus) are recommended for managing chronic atopic dermatitis in adults, providing anti-inflammatory effects without the side effects of long-term corticosteroid use.

6. Answer: A. Superinfection with Staphylococcus aureus

   Explanation: Eczema in flexural areas is prone to bacterial superinfection, often with Staphylococcus aureus, due to skin barrier dysfunction and scratching.

7. Answer: A. Apply emollients immediately after bathing

   Explanation: Applying emollients immediately after bathing helps lock in moisture and improves skin barrier function in atopic dermatitis, preventing dryness and itchiness.

8. Answer: C. Elimination diet guided by allergy testing

   Explanation: Some individuals with atopic dermatitis may benefit from an elimination diet guided by allergy testing to identify and avoid specific food triggers that exacerbate their symptoms.

9. Answer: B. Cognitive behavioral therapy (CBT)

   Explanation: Cognitive behavioral therapy (CBT) can help patients with chronic eczema manage psychological distress, improve coping strategies, and enhance quality of life.

10. Answer: D. Moisturize hands with emollients regularly

    Explanation: Regular use of emollients helps maintain skin barrier function and prevents occupational dermatitis in individuals prone to eczema, such as healthcare workers.

11. Answer: B. Topical calcineurin inhibitors

    Explanation: Topical calcineurin inhibitors are effective in managing eczema-related pruritus by reducing inflammation and itch, especially when topical corticosteroids alone are insufficient.

12. Answer: C. Shower immediately after exercise

    Explanation: Showering immediately after exercise helps remove sweat and allergens from the skin, reducing the risk of exacerbating eczema symptoms in individuals prone to sweat-induced flare-ups.

13. Answer: B. Dust mites

    Explanation: Dust mites are common environmental allergens that can exacerbate eczema symptoms, emphasizing the importance of allergen avoidance strategies such as using hypoallergenic bedding and regular cleaning.

14. Answer: A. Avoid sun exposure to prevent flare-ups

    Explanation: Sun exposure can exacerbate eczema symptoms in some individuals by triggering inflammation and increasing skin dryness, warranting sun protection measures to prevent flare-ups.

15. Answer: B. Topical calcineurin inhibitors

    Explanation: Topical calcineurin inhibitors (e.g., tacrolimus, pimecrolimus) are considered safer options for managing eczema during pregnancy due to their minimal systemic absorption and lower risk of adverse effects compared to topical corticosteroids.

Epilepsy

1. Answer: C) Order brain MRI

   Explanation: A new-onset seizure in an adult warrants investigation for an underlying cause such as structural brain abnormalities. Therefore, the next step should be brain MRI to evaluate for any intracranial pathology.

2. Answer: A) Phenytoin toxicity

   Explanation: Symptoms of nystagmus, ataxia, and double vision are consistent with phenytoin toxicity. This should be suspected in patients on phenytoin therapy presenting with neurological symptoms.

3. Answer: C) Stress

   Explanation: Stress is a recognized trigger for seizures in patients with epilepsy. Other triggers can include sleep deprivation, alcohol, and missed doses of antiepileptic medications.

4. Answer: C) Add another antiepileptic drug

   Explanation: When seizures continue despite optimal dosing of one antiepileptic drug, adding another AED is often the next step to achieve better seizure control.

5. Answer: C) Valproate

   Explanation: Valproate is associated with a higher risk of neural tube defects and other developmental abnormalities in the fetus compared to other antiepileptic drugs. It should be avoided if possible in women of childbearing age.

6. Answer: D) Complex partial seizure

   Explanation: Complex partial seizures often present with altered awareness and automatisms such as chewing or lip smacking. They may arise from the temporal lobe.

7. Answer: B) Discontinue lamotrigine and switch to levetiracetam

   Explanation: Rash is a common side effect of lamotrigine and can indicate a potentially serious hypersensitivity reaction. Discontinuation of lamotrigine and consideration of an alternative AED such as levetiracetam is appropriate.

8. Answer: C) Antiepileptic drug withdrawal

    Explanation: Non-compliance with antiepileptic medications can lead to withdrawal symptoms, including confusion, agitation, and potential breakthrough seizures.

9. Answer: C) Valproate

    Explanation: Valproate is considered first-line for the treatment of absence seizures. It has broad-spectrum activity against various seizure types, including absence seizures.

10. Answer: D) Tonic-clonic seizure

    Explanation: Tonic-clonic seizures are characterized by sudden loss of consciousness, tonic (stiffening) phase, followed by clonic (jerking) movements of the limbs.

11. Answer: D) Discuss potential risks and benefits with a healthcare provider.

    Explanation: It is important to discuss the potential risks and benefits of antiepileptic medications during pregnancy with a healthcare provider. Carbamazepine is generally preferred over valproate due to its lower teratogenic risk.

12. Answer: A) EEG

    Explanation: EEG is the most appropriate initial diagnostic test for evaluating suspected seizures and determining the seizure type.

13. Answer: A) Brain MRI

    Explanation: Brain MRI should be considered in patients with epilepsy who continue to have breakthrough seizures despite adherence to antiepileptic medications, to evaluate for structural abnormalities or other potential causes.

14. Answer: C) Topiramate side effects

    Explanation: Cognitive side effects such as difficulty concentrating and word-finding difficulties are common with topiramate therapy and should be monitored closely.

15. Answer: B) Hypersensitivity syndrome

Explanation: Rash and fever shortly after starting a new antiepileptic drug can indicate a hypersensitivity reaction, which can progress to a more serious condition known as drug reaction with eosinophilia and systemic symptoms (DRESS syndrome).

Erectile Dysfunction

1. Answer: C. Medication side effects

    Explanation: Antihypertensive medications can often lead to erectile dysfunction as a side effect.

2. Answer: B. Psychological factors

    Explanation: Stress and emotional issues such as anxiety and depression can lead to psychological erectile dysfunction.

3. Answer: A. Neuropathy

    Explanation: Diabetic neuropathy, due to poorly controlled diabetes, is a common cause of erectile dysfunction in diabetic patients.

4. Answer: C. Start testosterone replacement therapy

    Explanation: In cases of hypogonadism (low testosterone levels), testosterone replacement therapy is indicated.

5. Answer: C. Quit smoking

    Explanation: Smoking is a major risk factor for erectile dysfunction due to its impact on blood vessels and circulation.

6. Answer: C. Alcohol consumption

    Explanation: Excessive alcohol consumption can lead to temporary or long-term erectile dysfunction.

7. Answer: A. Hypogonadism

    Explanation: Decreased libido and muscle mass, along with erectile dysfunction, suggest low testosterone levels.

8. Answer: C. Exercise stress test

    Explanation: Chest pain on exertion in a patient with a family history of cardiovascular disease warrants evaluation for coronary artery disease.

9. Answer: C. Radiation therapy

    Explanation: Treatment for prostate cancer, including radiation therapy, can damage the structures necessary for an erection.

10. Answer: B. Drug use

   Explanation: Cocaine and other recreational drugs can impair erectile function.

11. Answer: A. Peyronie's disease

   Explanation: Peyronie's disease is characterized by the presence of fibrous plaques causing penile curvature and erectile dysfunction.

12. Answer: D. Tadalafil

   Explanation: Tadalafil is used to treat both BPH and erectile dysfunction due to its dual mechanism of action.

13. Answer: B. Vascular injury

   Explanation: Pelvic trauma can cause vascular injury, leading to erectile dysfunction.

14. Answer: B. Oral PDE-5 inhibitors

   Explanation: PDE-5 inhibitors are the first-line treatment for erectile dysfunction in the presence of comorbid conditions like hypertension and hyperlipidemia.

15. Answer: A. Psychological factors

   Explanation: The presence of morning erections suggests that the physical mechanisms are intact, pointing towards a psychological cause.

Fibromyalgia

1. Answer: C. Fibromyalgia

    Explanation: Fibromyalgia is characterized by widespread musculoskeletal pain, fatigue, and sleep disturbances. The presence of tenderness in multiple soft tissue areas (tender points) is also a key feature. The history of depression and anxiety is common in patients with fibromyalgia.

2. Answer: D. None of the above

    Explanation: Fibromyalgia does not typically cause elevations in inflammatory markers such as ESR or CRP, nor does it cause positive ANA. Diagnosis is clinical and based on symptoms and physical examination.

3. Answer: C. Regular low-impact aerobic exercise

    Explanation: Regular low-impact aerobic exercise, such as walking or swimming, is recommended for managing fibromyalgia symptoms. It helps reduce pain and improve overall function and well-being.

4. Answer: B. Amitriptyline

    Explanation: Amitriptyline, a tricyclic antidepressant, is commonly used to help improve sleep and reduce pain in patients with fibromyalgia. It has sedative properties that can aid in sleep.

5. Answer: C. Cognitive-behavioral therapy (CBT)

    Explanation: Cognitive-behavioral therapy (CBT) is effective in managing the cognitive difficulties and fatigue associated with fibromyalgia. It helps patients develop coping strategies and improve their overall quality of life.

6. Answer: B. Elimination of gluten and processed foods

    Explanation: Some patients with fibromyalgia may benefit from dietary modifications, such as eliminating gluten and processed foods, which can reduce inflammation and improve symptoms. However, dietary needs can vary among individuals.

7. Answer: A. Transcutaneous electrical nerve stimulation (TENS)

    Explanation: Transcutaneous electrical nerve stimulation (TENS) is a non-pharmacological therapy that can help reduce pain in fibromyalgia patients by delivering electrical impulses to nerve fibers.

8. Answer: B. Yoga and mindfulness meditation

Explanation: Yoga and mindfulness meditation are effective stress management techniques that can help reduce symptoms of fibromyalgia. They promote relaxation and improve overall mental and physical well-being.

9. Answer: B. Ergonomic workstation adjustments

Explanation: Ergonomic workstation adjustments can help reduce pain and improve comfort for patients with fibromyalgia. This includes proper chair support, desk height adjustments, and regular breaks.

10. Answer: B. Acupuncture

Explanation: Acupuncture has shown some evidence of benefit in reducing pain and improving function in patients with fibromyalgia. It is thought to work by stimulating the body's natural pain-relieving mechanisms.

11. Answer: A. Duloxetine

Explanation: Duloxetine is a serotonin-norepinephrine reuptake inhibitor (SNRI) that is effective in treating both fibromyalgia symptoms and depression. It helps reduce pain and improve mood.

12. Answer: B. Gentle stretching exercises before getting out of bed

Explanation: Gentle stretching exercises before getting out of bed can help reduce morning stiffness in patients with fibromyalgia by increasing blood flow and flexibility in muscles and joints.

13. Answer: B. Irritable bowel syndrome (IBS)

Explanation: Irritable bowel syndrome (IBS) is a common comorbid condition in patients with fibromyalgia and can cause gastrointestinal symptoms such as abdominal pain, bloating, and altered bowel habits.

14. Answer: B. Magnesium

Explanation: Magnesium supplements have shown some evidence of benefit in reducing pain and improving symptoms in patients with fibromyalgia. Magnesium plays a role in muscle function and energy production.

15. Answer: A. Tension-type headaches

Explanation: Tension-type headaches are commonly associated with fibromyalgia and are characterized by a constant, dull pain around the head. They can be triggered by muscle tension and stress.

Gastritis

1. Answer: C) NSAID-induced gastritis

    Explanation: NSAIDs are a common cause of gastritis, leading to mucosal damage and symptoms of epigastric pain that worsen after meals and improve with antacids.

2. Answer: C) Alcohol-induced gastritis

    Explanation: Heavy alcohol use can irritate the gastric mucosa, leading to gastritis characterized by nausea, vomiting, and epigastric pain that is relieved by eating.

3. Answer: B) Autoimmune gastritis

    Explanation: Pernicious anemia is associated with autoimmune gastritis, where autoantibodies attack parietal cells in the stomach, leading to reduced acid secretion and symptoms like epigastric pain, bloating, and early satiety.

4. Answer: D) Gastric erosions due to medication

    Explanation: Chronic renal failure patients on medications like NSAIDs or corticosteroids are at risk for medication-induced gastritis and gastric erosions, presenting with symptoms such as epigastric pain and gastrointestinal bleeding.

5. Answer: A) Start proton pump inhibitor (PPI) therapy

    Explanation: Given the history of aspirin use, NSAID-induced gastritis is likely. Starting PPI therapy can help alleviate symptoms and protect the gastric mucosa.

6. Answer: C) Urea breath test

    Explanation: Urea breath test is a non-invasive and accurate diagnostic test for detecting Helicobacter pylori infection in patients with symptoms of gastritis.

7. Answer: C) Reflux esophagitis

    Explanation: Symptoms worsened at night and relieved by eating are suggestive of reflux esophagitis, where gastric acid reflux into the esophagus causes symptoms similar to gastritis.

8. Answer: D) Alcoholic gastritis

    Explanation: Chronic alcohol use can lead to mucosal damage in the stomach, causing alcoholic gastritis with symptoms such as epigastric pain and gastrointestinal bleeding (hematemesis).

9. Answer: A) Helicobacter pylori infection

    Explanation: Epigastric pain aggravated by spicy foods is characteristic of H. pylori-induced gastritis. Testing for H. pylori infection is appropriate in this patient.

10. Answer: C) NSAID-induced gastritis

    Explanation: Chronic NSAID use can cause mucosal damage and symptoms such as epigastric pain, nausea, and weight loss due to NSAID-induced gastritis.

11. Answer: C) B12 deficiency gastritis

    Explanation: Strict vegetarians are at risk for vitamin B12 deficiency, which can lead to gastritis and symptoms such as epigastric pain and nausea.

12. Answer: B) Gastric erosions due to NSAIDs

    Explanation: Chronic NSAID use can lead to gastric erosions and symptoms such as epigastric pain and coffee-ground emesis (indicative of upper gastrointestinal bleeding).

13. Answer: B) Chronic stress gastritis

    Explanation: Epigastric pain worsened by stress is characteristic of chronic stress gastritis, which may not require specific treatment other than stress management.

14. Answer: C) Gastric erosions due to NSAIDs

    Explanation: Chronic NSAID use can cause gastric erosions and gastrointestinal bleeding, presenting with symptoms such as epigastric pain and black, tarry stools.

15. Answer: B) Autoimmune gastritis

    Explanation: Autoimmune gastritis can be associated with other autoimmune conditions such as thyroid disease, presenting with symptoms like epigastric pain, bloating, and early satiety.

Gastroesophageal Reflux Disease (GERD)

1. Answer: B. Gastroesophageal reflux disease (GERD)

   Explanation: John's symptoms of burning chest pain (heartburn), worsened by lying down or after meals, and regurgitation of acidic fluid are characteristic of GERD.

2. Answer: C. Gastroesophageal reflux disease (GERD)

   Explanation: Emily's symptoms, including chronic cough, hoarseness, throat clearing, and globus sensation, are often associated with GERD due to reflux of gastric contents into the esophagus and upper airway.

3. Answer: C. Lifestyle modifications

   Explanation: Initial management of mild GERD includes lifestyle modifications such as elevating the head of the bed, avoiding large meals, weight loss if overweight, and avoiding trigger foods and beverages.

4. Answer: C. Prescribe proton pump inhibitors (PPIs)

   Explanation: PPIs are the most effective medications for treating moderate to severe GERD symptoms by reducing gastric acid production, offering relief and promoting healing of esophageal mucosa.

5. Answer: D. Refer for pH monitoring

   Explanation: pH monitoring helps assess the extent and severity of acid reflux in patients with persistent symptoms despite PPI therapy, guiding further management such as surgical intervention.

6. Answer: B. Gastroesophageal reflux causing bronchospasm

   Explanation: GERD can exacerbate asthma symptoms by triggering bronchospasm due to aspiration of gastric contents into the airways, leading to reflux-induced asthma.

7. Answer: A. Eosinophilic esophagitis

   Explanation: Anna's symptoms of dysphagia (difficulty swallowing), weight loss, and occasional chest pain warrant consideration of eosinophilic esophagitis, an inflammatory condition of the esophagus.

8. Answer: A. Osteoporosis

   Explanation: Chronic PPI use has been associated with an increased risk of osteoporosis and fractures due to impaired calcium absorption, making regular bone density monitoring advisable.

9. Answer: D. Elevating the head of the bed

    Explanation: Elevating the head of the bed by 6 to 8 inches can help prevent nocturnal reflux by using gravity to keep gastric contents from moving into the esophagus while lying down.

10. Answer: A. Barrett's esophagus

    Explanation: Barrett's esophagus is a premalignant condition where normal squamous epithelium of the lower esophagus is replaced by metaplastic columnar epithelium due to chronic acid reflux.

11. Answer: A. Upper endoscopy

    Explanation: Upper endoscopy allows direct visualization of the esophagus to assess for erosive esophagitis, Barrett's esophagus, and other structural abnormalities in patients with refractory GERD symptoms.

12. Answer: D. Surveillance endoscopy every 3 years

    Explanation: Patients with Barrett's esophagus and a family history of esophageal cancer should undergo surveillance endoscopy every 3 years to monitor for dysplasia or progression to adenocarcinoma.

13. Answer: D. NSAID-induced esophagitis

    Explanation: NSAID-induced esophagitis can cause erosions and inflammation of the esophageal mucosa, leading to symptoms of chest pain, dysphagia, and heartburn.

14. Answer: D. Upper endoscopy with biopsy

    Explanation: Upper endoscopy with biopsy is recommended to evaluate dysphagia and assess for eosinophilic esophagitis, characterized by eosinophilic infiltration of the esophageal mucosa.

15. Answer: A. Nissen fundoplication

    Explanation: Nissen fundoplication is a surgical procedure where the upper part of the stomach is wrapped around the lower esophagus to strengthen the sphincter, preventing acid reflux.

Glaucoma

1. Answer: A. Primary open-angle glaucoma

    Explanation: Primary open-angle glaucoma is characterized by a gradual, asymptomatic loss of peripheral vision, elevated IOP, open anterior chamber angles, and normal optic disc appearance initially.

2. Answer: B. Acute angle-closure glaucoma

    Explanation: Acute angle-closure glaucoma presents with sudden onset of symptoms due to a sudden increase in IOP from angle closure. It is characterized by severe eye pain, redness, cloudy cornea, mid-dilated pupil, and elevated IOP.

3. Answer: A. Primary open-angle glaucoma

    Explanation: This patient has elevated IOP and characteristic optic disc changes (increased cup-to-disc ratio, notching, thinning of neuroretinal rim), consistent with primary open-angle glaucoma, which is often asymptomatic until late stages.

4. Answer: C. Normal-tension glaucoma

    Explanation: Normal-tension glaucoma presents with characteristic optic disc cupping and visual field loss despite normal IOP (<21 mmHg). It is often associated with vascular dysregulation and systemic conditions like hypertension.

5. Answer: D. Secondary glaucoma

    Explanation: Secondary glaucoma can occur secondary to other ocular or systemic conditions like diabetes mellitus. Elevated IOP and optic disc changes suggest glaucomatous damage due to secondary causes.

6. Answer: A. Primary open-angle glaucoma

    Explanation: Primary open-angle glaucoma can present with symptoms such as difficulty seeing in dim lighting (due to loss of peripheral vision) and halos around lights. IOP may be within normal limits initially.

7. Answer: D. Secondary glaucoma

    Explanation: Secondary glaucoma can occur following trauma, leading to structural changes in the eye like vertical elongation and optic disc cupping, with subsequent elevation in IOP and visual field loss.

8. Answer: B. Order visual field testing

   Explanation: Given the symptoms and normal IOP, the next step should be to confirm visual field defects with visual field testing to assess for possible glaucomatous damage despite normal IOP.

9. Answer: B. Perform immediate laser iridotomy

   Explanation: This patient presents with signs and symptoms consistent with acute angle-closure glaucoma. Immediate laser iridotomy is the preferred initial treatment to relieve pupillary block and lower IOP.

10. Answer: C. Perform visual field testing

    Explanation: Elevated IOP with a normal optic disc appearance warrants further evaluation with visual field testing to assess for early glaucomatous damage before initiating treatment.

11. Answer: A. Primary open-angle glaucoma

    Explanation: This patient presents with elevated IOP, characteristic optic disc cupping, and progressive visual field loss, consistent with primary open-angle glaucoma.

12. Answer: B. Repeat IOP measurement in 6 months

    Explanation: Normal IOP and optic disc appearance do not indicate glaucoma. It is appropriate to repeat IOP measurement in 6 months as part of routine eye care.

13. Answer: A. Primary open-angle glaucoma

    Explanation: Despite normal IOP, the presence of optic disc cupping and characteristic symptoms suggests primary open-angle glaucoma, which can occur even with IOP within normal limits.

14. Answer: C. Normal-tension glaucoma

    Explanation: This patient has characteristic optic disc changes and visual field loss despite normal IOP, consistent with normal-tension glaucoma.

15. Answer: D. Refer to an ophthalmologist

    Explanation: This patient presents with signs and symptoms suggestive of acute angle-closure glaucoma, requiring immediate evaluation and treatment by an ophthalmologist.

Gout

1. Answer: D. Gout

   Explanation: The classic presentation of gout includes sudden onset severe pain and swelling, commonly affecting the big toe. It is associated with hyperuricemia, and thiazide diuretics are a known risk factor.

2. Answer: A. Aspiration of the joint

   Explanation: In patients with chronic kidney disease, gout can present differently and joint aspiration is the most appropriate initial step to confirm the diagnosis and provide symptomatic relief.

3. Answer: B. IV corticosteroids

   Explanation: IV corticosteroids are indicated for the acute management of gout flare in patients who cannot tolerate NSAIDs or colchicine.

4. Answer: D. Initiate pegloticase

   Explanation: Pegloticase is indicated for patients with gout who have not achieved target uric acid levels with other urate-lowering therapies.

5. Answer: D. Long-term urate-lowering therapy

   Explanation: Patients with chronic tophaceous gout require long-term urate-lowering therapy to decrease the frequency of acute flares and to promote resolution of tophi.

6. Answer: C. Non-compliance with allopurinol

   Explanation: Non-compliance with allopurinol can lead to acute gout flares despite having normal uric acid levels.

7. Answer: B. Probenecid

   Explanation: Probenecid should be avoided in patients with a history of kidney stones or renal insufficiency, which is common in patients with gout.

8. Answer: D. Check for compliance with allopurinol

   Explanation: Before switching to another urate-lowering therapy, it is important to confirm patient compliance with the current regimen.

9. Answer: B. Oral colchicine

    Explanation: Colchicine is an appropriate initial treatment for acute gout flares, especially in patients who cannot take NSAIDs or corticosteroids.

10. Answer: A. Initiate allopurinol

    Explanation: Tophaceous gout requires long-term urate-lowering therapy to reduce tophi formation and prevent acute gouty attacks.

11. Answer: D. NSAIDs

    Explanation: NSAIDs are contraindicated in patients with chronic kidney disease due to the risk of renal impairment.

12. Answer: D. Corticosteroids

    Explanation: Corticosteroids are preferred in patients with peptic ulcer disease or gastrointestinal intolerance to NSAIDs.

13. Answer: C. Long-term allopurinol therapy

    Explanation: Long-term allopurinol therapy is indicated in patients with chronic tophaceous gout to reduce uric acid levels and prevent further tophi formation.

14. Answer: C. NSAIDs

    Explanation: NSAIDs are contraindicated in patients with chronic kidney disease due to the risk of renal impairment.

15. Answer: C. Non-compliance with allopurinol

    Explanation: Non-compliance with allopurinol can lead to acute gout flares despite having normal uric acid levels.

Graves' Disease

1. Answer: C. Graves' disease

   Explanation: Graves' disease is an autoimmune disorder characterized by hyperthyroidism, diffuse goiter, and often exophthalmos (proptosis).

2. Answer: A. Beta-blockers

   Explanation: Beta-blockers are used initially to manage symptoms such as tachycardia and tremors in patients with hyperthyroidism.

3. Answer: C. Graves' disease

   Explanation: Graves' disease is the most common cause of hyperthyroidism and is characterized by diffuse goiter, ophthalmopathy, and dermopathy.

4. Answer: A. Start methimazole

   Explanation: Methimazole or propylthiouracil are the initial treatments for Graves' disease to block thyroid hormone synthesis.

5. Answer: C. Graves' disease

   Explanation: Graves' disease is characterized by hyperthyroidism due to autoimmune stimulation of the thyroid gland.

6. Answer: B. Methimazole

   Explanation: Methimazole is an anti-thyroid drug used to inhibit thyroid hormone production in Graves' disease.

7. Answer: C. Radioactive iodine

   Explanation: Radioactive iodine should be avoided initially in younger patients or those with mild hyperthyroidism due to the risk of permanent hypothyroidism.

8. Answer: B. Thyroid stimulating immunoglobulin (TSI)

   Explanation: TSI is highly specific for Graves' disease and can be used to confirm the diagnosis.

9. Answer: C. Hypothyroidism

   Explanation: Hypothyroidism can occur after treatment for hyperthyroidism, particularly with radioactive iodine or surgery.

10. Answer: A. Methimazole

   Explanation: Methimazole is used initially to block thyroid hormone synthesis in patients with Graves' disease.

11. Answer: D. Start methimazole

   Explanation: Methimazole is the initial treatment of choice for Graves' disease to block thyroid hormone synthesis.

12. Answer: C. Graves' disease

   Explanation: Graves' disease is characterized by hyperthyroidism due to autoimmune stimulation of the thyroid gland.

13. Answer: B. Methimazole

   Explanation: Methimazole is an anti-thyroid drug used to inhibit thyroid hormone production in Graves' disease.

14. Answer: C. Radioactive iodine

   Explanation: Radioactive iodine should be avoided initially in younger patients or those with mild hyperthyroidism due to the risk of permanent hypothyroidism.

15. Answer: B. Thyroid stimulating immunoglobulin (TSI)

   Explanation: TSI is highly specific for Graves' disease and can be used to confirm the diagnosis.

Heart Attack (Myocardial Infarction)

1. Answer: C. ST-segment elevation myocardial infarction (STEMI)

    Explanation: The clinical presentation and ECG findings (ST-segment elevation) are characteristic of STEMI.

2. Answer: B. Non-ST-segment elevation myocardial infarction (NSTEMI)

    Explanation: The clinical presentation with troponin elevation and ECG findings of ST-segment depression and T-wave inversion suggest NSTEMI.

3. Answer: B. Immediate coronary angiography

    Explanation: Immediate coronary angiography with possible percutaneous coronary intervention (PCI) is indicated in STEMI.

4. Answer: A. Administer fibrinolytic therapy

    Explanation: In the presence of new-onset LBBB and symptoms suggestive of myocardial infarction, fibrinolytic therapy is indicated if PCI cannot be performed immediately.

5. Answer: D. Heparin

    Explanation: Heparin should be used cautiously in patients with chronic kidney disease due to the risk of bleeding and accumulation.

6. Answer: A. Fibrinolytic therapy

    Explanation: In the absence of contraindications, fibrinolytic therapy is indicated in STEMI, even in patients with aspirin allergy.

7. Answer: D. Intracranial hemorrhage within the past year

    Explanation: Intracranial hemorrhage within the past year is a contraindication to fibrinolytic therapy due to the risk of bleeding.

8. Answer: B. Immediate coronary angiography

    Explanation: Immediate coronary angiography with possible PCI is the preferred treatment for STEMI.

9. Answer: A. Administer fibrinolytic therapy

Explanation: Fibrinolytic therapy is indicated in the management of STEMI if PCI cannot be performed within 120 minutes of first medical contact.

10. Answer: B. Ventricular tachycardia

Explanation: Ventricular tachycardia is a common arrhythmic complication associated with STEMI.

11. Answer: B. Immediate coronary angiography

Explanation: Immediate coronary angiography with possible PCI is the preferred treatment for STEMI.

12. Answer: A. Administer fibrinolytic therapy

Explanation: Fibrinolytic therapy is indicated in the management of STEMI if PCI cannot be performed within 120 minutes of first medical contact.

13. Answer: B. Immediate coronary angiography

Explanation: Immediate coronary angiography with possible PCI is the preferred treatment for STEMI.

14. Answer: D. Heparin

Explanation: Heparin should be used cautiously in patients with chronic kidney disease due to the risk of bleeding and accumulation.

15. Answer: D. Intracranial hemorrhage within the past year

Explanation: Intracranial hemorrhage within the past year is a contraindication to fibrinolytic therapy due to the risk of bleeding.

Hemophilia

1. Answer: C. Prolonged aPTT (activated partial thromboplastin time)

    Explanation: The clinical presentation and family history are suggestive of hemophilia, which is characterized by a deficiency in clotting factors VIII or IX. The most common initial laboratory finding in hemophilia is a prolonged aPTT.

2. Answer: C. Factor VIII

    Explanation: Hemophilia A is caused by a deficiency of factor VIII. Patients typically present with bleeding episodes after minor trauma, which can include deep muscle hematomas.

3. Answer: C. Prolonged aPTT

    Explanation: Recurrent bleeding episodes after minor trauma, such as nosebleeds and prolonged bleeding after dental procedures, are suggestive of a clotting factor deficiency. Hemophilia would result in a prolonged aPTT.

4. Answer: C. Factor VIII

    Explanation: Hemophilia A (factor VIII deficiency) typically presents with spontaneous or trauma-induced joint bleeding. This patient's presentation is consistent with a joint bleed, which is common in hemophilia.

5. Answer: B. aPTT

    Explanation: Excessive bleeding from minor trauma, such as circumcision, suggests a bleeding disorder. Hemophilia should be suspected, and the most appropriate initial test is aPTT.

6. Answer: C. Factor VIII deficiency (Hemophilia A)

    Explanation: Hemophilia A (factor VIII deficiency) presents with recurrent episodes of spontaneous bleeding, often affecting muscles and joints. The onset is usually in childhood.

7. Answer: C. Factor VIII

    Explanation: Hemarthrosis (bleeding into the joint space) is a common manifestation of hemophilia, specifically hemophilia A, which is caused by a deficiency in factor VIII.

8. Answer: A. Factor VIII assay

    Explanation: This patient's symptoms are suggestive of von Willebrand disease rather than hemophilia. The best initial test to diagnose von Willebrand disease is a factor VIII assay.

9. Answer: A. Brain MRI

    Explanation: Severe headache and dizziness in a patient with hemophilia may suggest intracranial bleeding. A brain MRI is essential to evaluate for the presence of intracranial hemorrhage.

10. Answer: B. aPTT

    Explanation: Extensive bruising and prolonged bleeding after minor injuries are suggestive of a clotting factor deficiency. The initial test to evaluate for a clotting factor deficiency is aPTT.

11. Answer: B. aPTT

    Explanation: Bleeding from the gums and excessive bruising suggest a clotting disorder. The initial test to evaluate for a clotting factor deficiency is aPTT.

12. Answer: D. Recombinant factor VIII concentrate

    Explanation: The treatment of choice for acute joint bleeds in hemophilia A is recombinant factor VIII concentrate to replace the deficient clotting factor.

13. Answer: B. aPTT

    Explanation: Heavy menstrual bleeding and epistaxis suggest a clotting disorder. The initial test to evaluate for a clotting factor deficiency is aPTT.

14. Answer: D. Recombinant factor VIII concentrate

    Explanation: The treatment of choice for acute joint bleeds in hemophilia A is recombinant factor VIII concentrate.

15. Answer: B. aPTT

    Explanation: Recurrent gum bleeding after minor trauma suggests a clotting disorder. The initial test to evaluate for a clotting factor deficiency is aPTT.

Hepatitis (A, B, C)

1. Answer: C. HAV IgM

   Explanation: The clinical presentation of jaundice, dark urine, and clay-colored stools is suggestive of acute viral hepatitis. Hepatitis A virus (HAV) infection is associated with a positive IgM antibody to HAV.

2. Answer: C. HBsAg and HBeAg

   Explanation: Acute hepatitis B infection is characterized by the presence of HBsAg and HBeAg in the serum.

3. Answer: B. HCV RNA

   Explanation: Hepatitis C virus (HCV) infection is diagnosed by detecting HCV RNA in the blood. The history of blood transfusion before 1992 increases the risk of HCV infection.

4. Answer: B. Administer hepatitis A vaccine

   Explanation: The clinical presentation and exposure history are consistent with hepatitis A. The most appropriate next step is to administer hepatitis A vaccine to prevent further transmission.

5. Answer: A. HBsAg positive, HBeAg positive

   Explanation: Chronic hepatitis B infection is characterized by the persistence of HBsAg and the presence of HBeAg in the serum.

6. Answer: B. HCV RNA positive

   Explanation: Chronic hepatitis C infection is confirmed by detecting HCV RNA in the blood.

7. Answer: D. Improve personal hygiene practices

   Explanation: Hepatitis A virus (HAV) is transmitted via the fecal-oral route. Improving personal hygiene practices, such as handwashing, is crucial in preventing transmission.

8. Answer: A. HBsAg positive, HBcAb IgM positive

   Explanation: Acute hepatitis B infection is characterized by the presence of HBsAg and IgM antibody to hepatitis B core antigen (HBcAb IgM).

9. Answer: D. HCV RNA

    Explanation: The patient's history of multiple blood transfusions puts him at risk for hepatitis C virus (HCV) infection. Diagnosis is confirmed by detecting HCV RNA in the blood.

10. Answer: B. Improve personal hygiene practices

    Explanation: Hepatitis A virus (HAV) is transmitted via the fecal-oral route. Improving personal hygiene practices, such as handwashing, is crucial in preventing transmission, especially in healthcare settings.

11. Answer: C. HBsAg positive, HBeAg negative

    Explanation: Chronic hepatitis B infection is characterized by the persistence of HBsAg and the absence of HBeAg, with the presence of HBeAb.

12. Answer: D. HCV RNA

    Explanation: The patient's history of tattoos and blood transfusion increases the risk of hepatitis C virus (HCV) infection. Diagnosis is confirmed by detecting HCV RNA in the blood.

13. Answer: B. Improve personal hygiene practices

    Explanation: Hepatitis A virus (HAV) is transmitted via the fecal-oral route. Improving personal hygiene practices, such as handwashing, is crucial in preventing transmission, especially in food handlers.

14. Answer: B. HBsAg positive, HBcAb IgM positive

    Explanation: Acute hepatitis B infection is characterized by the presence of HBsAg and IgM antibody to hepatitis B core antigen (HBcAb IgM).

15. Answer: D. HCV RNA

    Explanation: The patient's history of blood transfusion increases the risk of hepatitis C virus (HCV) infection. Diagnosis is confirmed by detecting HCV RNA in the blood.

Herpes Simplex Virus (HSV)

1. Answer: B. Herpes simplex virus type 2 (HSV-2)

    Explanation: HSV-2 is the most common cause of genital herpes, typically presenting with painful vesicular lesions.

2. Answer: A. Herpes simplex virus type 1 (HSV-1)

    Explanation: HSV-1 commonly causes oral herpes, characterized by recurrent oral ulcers.

3. Answer: B. Cesarean section

    Explanation: Cesarean section is recommended for pregnant women with active genital herpes lesions to reduce the risk of neonatal herpes transmission.

4. Answer: C. Herpes simplex virus (HSV) infection

    Explanation: Disseminated HSV infection can occur in immunocompromised individuals, presenting with severe and widespread symptoms.

5. Answer: A. Herpes simplex keratitis

    Explanation: Herpes simplex keratitis presents with vesicular lesions on the forehead and eye, often associated with pain and vision changes.

6. Answer: B. Herpes simplex virus type 2 (HSV-2)

    Explanation: Recurrent painful genital ulcers in a sexually active individual are most likely due to HSV-2 infection.

7. Answer: D. Chronic ulceration

    Explanation: Individuals with HIV and recurrent genital herpes may experience chronic ulceration due to impaired immune response.

8. Answer: A. Acyclovir

    Explanation: Acyclovir is the first-line antiviral medication for the treatment of genital herpes.

9. Answer: A. Herpes simplex encephalitis

    Explanation: Herpes simplex encephalitis presents with fever, altered mental status, and characteristic CSF findings.

10. Answer: C. Varicella-zoster virus (VZV) infection

   Explanation: Varicella-zoster virus (VZV) infection presents with a vesicular rash typically affecting one side of the face or body, known as herpes zoster or shingles.

11. Answer: A. Herpes simplex virus type 1 (HSV-1)

   Explanation: Recurrent painful vesicular lesions on the lips are characteristic of HSV-1 infection, commonly known as cold sores.

12. Answer: A. Cesarean section

   Explanation: Cesarean section is recommended for pregnant women with active genital herpes lesions to prevent neonatal transmission.

13. Answer: A. Acyclovir resistance

   Explanation: Acyclovir resistance should be suspected in patients with persistent genital herpes lesions despite antiviral therapy, especially in immunocompromised individuals.

14. Answer: B. Herpes zoster (shingles)

   Explanation: Herpes zoster presents with a painful rash in a dermatomal distribution, typically in older adults or immunocompromised individuals who had chickenpox.

15. Answer: B. Herpes simplex virus type 2 (HSV-2)

   Explanation: Recurrent painful vesicular lesions on the labia are characteristic of HSV-2 infection.

Hypertension (High Blood Pressure)

1. Answer: D. Recommend lifestyle modifications

    Explanation: Lifestyle modifications including dietary changes, weight loss, exercise, and reduced sodium intake are the initial management steps in hypertension.

2. Answer: C. Check serum electrolytes

    Explanation: Hydrochlorothiazide can cause electrolyte imbalances, including hypokalemia, which can lead to muscle cramps. Checking serum electrolytes is necessary before making any changes to the medication regimen.

3. Answer: D. Lisinopril

    Explanation: Lisinopril is an ACE inhibitor that provides renal protective effects, particularly beneficial in patients with chronic kidney disease and diabetes.

4. Answer: A. Hydrochlorothiazide

    Explanation: Thiazide diuretics like hydrochlorothiazide are recommended as first-line treatment for hypertension in patients without compelling indications.

5. Answer: B. Start lifestyle modifications

    Explanation: Lifestyle modifications are the initial treatment for patients with elevated blood pressure and no comorbidities.

6. Answer: D. Terazosin

    Explanation: Terazosin is an alpha-blocker that is effective in treating hypertension and can also help with symptoms of BPH.

7. Answer: D. Propranolol

    Explanation: Propranolol is contraindicated in patients with asthma, severe bradycardia, and certain types of migraine headaches.

8. Answer: C. Hydrochlorothiazide

    Explanation: Thiazide diuretics like hydrochlorothiazide can increase serum uric acid levels and exacerbate gout.

9. Answer: A. Amlodipine

Explanation: Amlodipine is a calcium channel blocker that does not affect lung function and is safe to use in patients with COPD.

10. Answer: B. Amlodipine

Explanation: Amlodipine is a calcium channel blocker that is effective in treating hypertension and is often used in patients with coronary artery disease.

11. Answer: C. Lisinopril

Explanation: Lisinopril is an ACE inhibitor that is beneficial in patients with heart failure with reduced ejection fraction (HFrEF).

12. Answer: B. Methyldopa

Explanation: Methyldopa is a centrally acting alpha-2 agonist and is commonly used for hypertension in pregnancy.

13. Answer: A. Lisinopril

Explanation: Lisinopril is an ACE inhibitor that can increase potassium levels and should be avoided in patients with hyperkalemia.

14. Answer: D. Verapamil

Explanation: Verapamil is a calcium channel blocker that is effective in treating hypertension and is safe to use in patients with BPH.

15. Answer: B. Amlodipine

Explanation: Amlodipine is a calcium channel blocker that does not affect bone mineral density and is safe to use in patients with osteoporosis.

Hyperthyroidism

1. Answer: B. Graves' disease

   Explanation: Graves' disease is the most common cause of hyperthyroidism and is characterized by diffuse thyroid enlargement (goiter), ophthalmopathy, and dermatopathy. Positive thyroid peroxidase antibodies suggest an autoimmune etiology.

2. Answer: B. Toxic multinodular goiter

   Explanation: Toxic multinodular goiter is characterized by multiple hyperfunctioning thyroid nodules, leading to excess thyroid hormone production. These patients typically have a long-standing goiter and may present with symptoms of hyperthyroidism.

3. Answer: C. Hashimoto's thyroiditis

   Explanation: Although Hashimoto's thyroiditis is typically associated with hypothyroidism, patients can present with transient hyperthyroidism due to release of preformed thyroid hormone in the setting of inflammation.

4. Answer: B. Graves' disease

   Explanation: Graves' disease is an autoimmune disorder that results in hyperthyroidism, diffuse goiter, and thyroid eye disease. It is associated with smoking and a family history of autoimmune diseases.

5. Answer: C. Papillary thyroid carcinoma

   Explanation: Papillary thyroid carcinoma can present with signs and symptoms of hyperthyroidism due to the production of thyroid hormones by the tumor. Microcalcifications and a rapidly growing neck mass are concerning for malignancy.

6. Answer: A. Graves' disease

   Explanation: Graves' disease is characterized by diffuse goiter and radioactive iodine uptake. It is the most common cause of hyperthyroidism.

7. Answer: A. Graves' disease

   Explanation: Graves' disease is an autoimmune disorder associated with other autoimmune conditions. Diffuse thyroid enlargement and a hypoechoic pattern on ultrasound are consistent with Graves' disease.

8. Answer: A. Toxic multinodular goiter

    Explanation: Chronic iodine deficiency can lead to the development of toxic multinodular goiter, which presents with hyperthyroidism and diffuse thyroid enlargement with multiple nodules.

9. Answer: D. Iodine-induced hyperthyroidism

    Explanation: Chronic lithium therapy can induce iodine-induced hyperthyroidism due to increased iodine uptake by the thyroid gland.

10. Answer: C. Radiation-induced thyroiditis

    Explanation: Radiation therapy to the neck can lead to the development of radiation-induced thyroiditis and subsequent hyperthyroidism.

11. Answer: B. Postpartum thyroiditis

    Explanation: Postpartum thyroiditis can present with transient hyperthyroidism due to release of preformed thyroid hormone. Positive thyroid peroxidase antibodies are supportive of autoimmune thyroiditis.

12. Answer: C. Radiation-induced thyroiditis

    Explanation: Radioactive iodine therapy for Hodgkin lymphoma can lead to radiation-induced thyroiditis and subsequent hyperthyroidism.

13. Answer: B. Subacute thyroiditis

    Explanation: Subacute thyroiditis is a self-limited inflammatory condition of the thyroid gland that can present with transient hyperthyroidism. Tender thyroid enlargement and a recent upper respiratory tract infection are typical features.

14. Answer: B. Amiodarone-induced thyrotoxicosis

    Explanation: Amiodarone-induced thyrotoxicosis can present with signs and symptoms of hyperthyroidism in patients taking amiodarone, typically due to iodine-induced hyperthyroidism.

15. Answer: B. Subacute thyroiditis

Explanation: Subacute thyroiditis is a self-limited inflammatory condition of the thyroid gland that can present with transient hyperthyroidism. Tender thyroid enlargement and a recent upper respiratory tract infection are typical features.

Hypothyroidism

1. Answer: B. Hypothyroidism

    Explanation: The patient's symptoms (fatigue, weight gain, constipation), physical exam findings (dry skin, coarse hair, bradycardia), and laboratory results (elevated TSH, decreased free T4) are all consistent with hypothyroidism.

2. Answer: B. Hypothyroidism

    Explanation: The patient's symptoms (memory loss, depression, lethargy), physical exam findings (puffy face, dry skin, slow reflexes), and laboratory results (elevated TSH, decreased free T4) are consistent with hypothyroidism.

3. Answer: A. Hyperthyroidism

    Explanation: The patient's symptoms (weight loss, anxiety, palpitations), physical exam findings (diffusely enlarged thyroid gland), and laboratory results (low TSH, elevated free T4) are consistent with hyperthyroidism.

4. Answer: A. Primary hypothyroidism

    Explanation: Primary hypothyroidism is characterized by elevated TSH and decreased free T4 levels. The patient's symptoms (fatigue, cold intolerance, weight gain), and physical exam findings (dry skin, brittle hair, slow movements) are consistent with this diagnosis.

5. Answer: A. Primary hypothyroidism

    Explanation: The patient's symptoms (fatigue, constipation, muscle cramps), physical exam findings (puffy face, dry skin), and elevated TSH with normal free T4 suggest primary hypothyroidism.

6. Answer: C. Hashimoto's thyroiditis

    Explanation: Hashimoto's thyroiditis is characterized by elevated TSH, positive anti-thyroid peroxidase antibodies, and symptoms of hypothyroidism (fatigue, hair loss, weight gain, dry skin, brittle hair).

7.   Answer: B. Secondary hypothyroidism

Explanation: Secondary hypothyroidism occurs due to pituitary or hypothalamic dysfunction, leading to decreased TSH secretion. This patient's history of pituitary surgery and low TSH despite low free T4 are indicative of secondary hypothyroidism.

8.   Answer: D. Subacute thyroiditis

Explanation: Subacute thyroiditis is characterized by a tender thyroid gland, often preceded by an upper respiratory tract infection, elevated TSH, and low free T4 levels due to transient thyroid hormone release.

9.   Answer: C. Thyroid cancer

Explanation: Thyroid cancer can present with a painless thyroid nodule, low TSH levels, and normal free T4. This patient's presentation is consistent with thyroid cancer.

10. Answer: C. Thyroid cancer

Explanation: Thyroid cancer can present with a hard, fixed thyroid nodule, hoarseness, and difficulty swallowing. This patient's presentation is consistent with thyroid cancer.

11. Answer: D. Graves' disease

Explanation: Graves' disease is characterized by hyperthyroidism, exophthalmos, diffusely enlarged thyroid gland, low TSH, and elevated free T4 levels.

12. Answer: C. Thyroid cancer

Explanation: Thyroid cancer can present with a large, fixed thyroid mass, difficulty breathing, low TSH levels, and normal free T4.

13. Answer: B. Secondary hypothyroidism

Explanation: Secondary hypothyroidism occurs due to pituitary or hypothalamic dysfunction, leading to decreased TSH secretion. This patient's history of pituitary adenoma treated with surgery and low TSH despite normal free T4 are indicative of secondary hypothyroidism.

14. Answer: A. Primary hypothyroidism

    Explanation: Primary hypothyroidism is characterized by elevated TSH and decreased free T4 levels. The patient's symptoms (fatigue, weight gain, constipation), and physical exam findings (dry skin, coarse hair, bradycardia) are consistent with this diagnosis.

15. Answer: A. Primary hypothyroidism

    Explanation: The patient's symptoms (memory loss, depression, lethargy), physical exam findings (puffy face, dry skin, slow reflexes), and laboratory results (elevated TSH, decreased free T4) are consistent with primary hypothyroidism.

Insomnia

1. Answer :C. Primary Insomnia. This patient's symptoms are typical of primary insomnia, characterized by difficulty initiating or maintaining sleep, or non-restorative sleep, leading to impairment of daytime functioning.

2. Answer :C. Cognitive Behavioral Therapy for Insomnia (CBT-I). CBT-I is the first-line treatment for chronic insomnia. It addresses maladaptive behaviors and cognitions that contribute to insomnia.

3. Answer :e.Start CBT-I. This patient's insomnia is chronic, and CBT-I should be considered, as it addresses underlying behavioral and cognitive factors contributing to insomnia.

4. Answer :B. Nocturia. Nocturia, or waking up at night to urinate, is a common cause of insomnia, especially in older adults.

5. Answer :C. Primary Insomnia. This patient's symptoms are typical of primary insomnia, which is characterized by difficulty maintaining sleep and non-restorative sleep.

6. Answer :e.Shift Work Sleep Disorder. This patient's difficulty falling asleep is likely due to her rotating shift work schedule.

7. Answer :C. Obstructive Sleep Apnea. This patient's symptoms of loud snoring, gasping for air, and excessive daytime sleepiness are suggestive of obstructive sleep apnea.

8. Answer :d.Restless Legs Syndrome. This patient's symptoms of an overwhelming urge to move her legs, which worsens at night and improves with movement, are characteristic of restless legs syndrome.

9. Answer :C. Chronic pain. Chronic pain can disrupt sleep and is a common cause of insomnia.

10. Answer :C. Delayed Sleep Phase Disorder. This patient's difficulty falling asleep at a socially acceptable time and her preference for later bedtimes suggest delayed sleep phase disorder.

11. Answer :a,Insomnia Disorder. This patient's difficulty staying asleep and waking up early are characteristic of insomnia disorder.

12. Answer :e.Cognitive Behavioral Therapy for Insomnia (CBT-I). This patient's insomnia is likely related to stress and poor sleep hygiene, making CBT-I the most appropriate initial management.

13. Answer :B. Narcolepsy. This patient's symptoms of excessive daytime sleepiness, vivid dreams, and sudden loss of muscle tone during emotional situations are characteristic of narcolepsy.

14. Answer :a.Insomnia Disorder. This patient's difficulty falling asleep and light, easily disrupted sleep suggest insomnia disorder, possibly with a familial component.

15. Answer :C. Cognitive Behavioral Therapy for Insomnia (CBT-I). This patient's insomnia is likely related to stress and anxiety, making CBT-I the most appropriate initial management.

Irritable Bowel Syndrome (IBS)

1. Answer: B. Irritable Bowel Syndrome (IBS)

   Explanation: The patient's symptoms of abdominal pain and bloating, which improve after defecation, along with alternating constipation and diarrhea, are characteristic of IBS.

2. Answer: D. Rome IV criteria questionnaire

   Explanation: The Rome IV criteria questionnaire is used to diagnose IBS based on symptom patterns. It includes criteria related to abdominal pain, stool consistency, and defecation frequency.

3. Answer: A. High-fiber diet

   Explanation: A high-fiber diet is recommended as initial management for IBS symptoms, particularly for patients with diarrhea-predominant IBS.

4. Answer: D. Trial of a low-FODMAP diet

   Explanation: A low-FODMAP diet has been shown to reduce symptoms in patients with IBS, particularly those with constipation-predominant symptoms.

5. Answer: C. Irritable Bowel Syndrome (IBS)

   Explanation: The patient's symptoms of bloating, abdominal pain, and alternating diarrhea and constipation, exacerbated by stress, are typical of IBS.

6. Answer: C. Irritable Bowel Syndrome (IBS)

   Explanation: The negative stool studies and absence of significant findings on examination support the diagnosis of IBS, which is characterized by chronic abdominal pain and altered bowel habits in the absence of organic disease.

7. Answer: B. Trial of antispasmodic medication

   Explanation: Antispasmodic medications, such as hyoscyamine or dicyclomine, are often used to relieve abdominal pain and cramping in patients with IBS.

8. Answer: A. Trial of lubiprostone (Amitiza)

   Explanation: Lubiprostone is indicated for the treatment of constipation-predominant IBS (IBS-C) in adults and is an appropriate initial management option for this patient.

A PLUS EXAM REVIEW

9. Answer: A. Trial of a low-FODMAP diet

   Explanation: A low-FODMAP diet restricts fermentable carbohydrates and can be beneficial for patients with IBS who have symptoms triggered by certain foods, including dairy products.

10. Answer: D. Cognitive-behavioral therapy (CBT)

    Explanation: Cognitive-behavioral therapy, which includes stress management techniques, is recommended as a first-line treatment for patients with IBS.

11. Answer: A. Trial of a low-FODMAP diet

    Explanation: A low-FODMAP diet is effective for reducing symptoms in patients with IBS triggered by fermentable carbohydrates found in foods like onions and garlic.

12. Answer: D. Cognitive-behavioral therapy (CBT)

    Explanation: CBT, which includes techniques to manage stress and improve coping strategies, is recommended as initial management for patients with IBS.

13. Answer: B. Trial of rifaximin (Xifaxan)

    Explanation: Rifaximin is an antibiotic that has been shown to be effective in treating diarrhea-predominant IBS (IBS-D) by altering the gut microbiota.

14. Answer: C. Start a tricyclic antidepressant

    Explanation: Tricyclic antidepressants, such as amitriptyline, can help reduce abdominal pain in patients with IBS, particularly those with pain-predominant symptoms.

15. Answer: A. Trial of a low-FODMAP diet

    Explanation: A low-FODMAP diet can be effective for reducing symptoms triggered by certain foods, including dairy products, in patients with IBS.

Malaria

1. Answer: C. Atovaquone-proguanil

   Explanation: Atovaquone-proguanil is the treatment of choice for uncomplicated P. vivax malaria in non-pregnant patients.

2. Answer: A. Quinine plus doxycycline

   Explanation: Quinine plus doxycycline is the initial treatment for uncomplicated P. falciparum malaria in non-pregnant patients.

3. Answer: A. Quinine plus clindamycin

   Explanation: Quinine plus clindamycin is the treatment of choice for uncomplicated P. falciparum malaria in pregnant patients.

4. Answer: A. Chloroquine

   Explanation: Chloroquine is the treatment of choice for uncomplicated P. malariae malaria.

5. Answer: B. Intravenous quinine

   Explanation: Intravenous quinine is the initial treatment for severe P. falciparum malaria.

6. Answer: D. Artesunate plus clindamycin

   Explanation: Artesunate plus clindamycin is the treatment of choice for severe P. falciparum malaria with evidence of organ dysfunction.

7. Answer: B. Quinine plus doxycycline

   Explanation: Quinine plus doxycycline is the treatment of choice for Plasmodium knowlesi malaria.

8. Answer: A. Chloroquine

   Explanation: Chloroquine is the treatment of choice for uncomplicated P. vivax malaria in patients with G6PD deficiency.

9. Answer: D. Primaquine

   Explanation: Primaquine is used to eradicate liver hypnozoites in the treatment of P. ovale malaria.

10. Answer: B. Atovaquone-proguanil

    Explanation: Atovaquone-proguanil is effective for prophylaxis against chloroquine-resistant P. falciparum.

11. Answer: B. Chloroquine

    Explanation: Chloroquine is the treatment of choice for uncomplicated P. malariae malaria.

12. Answer: A. Artemether-lumefantrine

    Explanation: Artemether-lumefantrine is used for the treatment of uncomplicated P. falciparum malaria in non-pregnant, stable patients.

13. Answer: A. Quinine plus clindamycin

    Explanation: Quinine plus clindamycin is the treatment of choice for uncomplicated P. vivax malaria in pregnant patients.

14. Answer: B. Artemether-lumefantrine

    Explanation: Artemether-lumefantrine is used for the treatment of uncomplicated P. falciparum malaria in non-pregnant, stable patients.

15. Answer: B. Intravenous quinine

    Explanation: Intravenous quinine is the initial treatment for severe P. falciparum malaria.

Menopause

1. Answer: C) Menopause

   Explanation: Menopause is diagnosed after 12 consecutive months of amenorrhea in the absence of other causes. Symptoms such as hot flashes, night sweats, and mood swings are common.

2. Answer: C) Menopause

   Explanation: Menopausal symptoms such as vaginal dryness, painful intercourse, and urinary urgency can occur even while menstrual cycles are still regular.

3. Answer: D) Increased risk of both osteoporosis and heart disease

   Explanation: Menopause is associated with decreased estrogen levels, increasing the risk of osteoporosis and cardiovascular disease.

4. Answer: D) Lifestyle modifications (e.g., regular exercise)

   Explanation: Lifestyle modifications are recommended as first-line management for menopausal symptoms, including regular exercise to help reduce hot flashes and improve sleep.

5. Answer: C) Avoid HRT due to the history of breast cancer

   Explanation: Women with a history of breast cancer should generally avoid HRT due to the potential risk of recurrence.

6. Answer: D) Increased risk of metabolic syndrome

   Explanation: Menopause is associated with an increased risk of metabolic syndrome, including increased abdominal fat and changes in lipid profile.

7. Answer: B) Menopause-related changes

   Explanation: Menopause can cause symptoms such as dry skin, joint pain, and stiffness due to estrogen deficiency.

8. Answer: B) Vaginal estrogen cream

   Explanation: Vaginal estrogen cream is effective for treating vaginal atrophy and dyspareunia in postmenopausal women.

9. Answer: D) All of the above

   Explanation: Clonidine and gabapentin are effective non-hormonal therapies for managing hot flashes and night sweats in menopausal women.

10. Answer: B) Venlafaxine

    Explanation: Venlafaxine is an effective therapy for hot flashes in women who cannot or prefer not to use hormone therapy, such as those with a history of migraines.

11. Answer: A) Dual-energy X-ray absorptiometry (DXA) scan

    Explanation: DXA scan is the gold standard for diagnosing osteoporosis and assessing bone mineral density in menopausal women.

12. Answer: C) Dyslipidemia

    Explanation: Dyslipidemia, particularly elevated LDL cholesterol and decreased HDL cholesterol, is a significant cardiovascular risk factor in menopausal women.

13. Answer: C) Hormonal fluctuations

    Explanation: Hormonal fluctuations, particularly decreased estrogen levels, can cause palpitations in menopausal women.

14. Answer: B) No change in risk compared to premenopausal women

    Explanation: The risk of breast cancer in menopausal women does not change compared to premenopausal women, but other factors such as family history still influence risk.

15. Answer: B) Vaginal lubricants

    Explanation: Vaginal lubricants are a non-hormonal therapy option for managing vaginal dryness and discomfort in menopausal women.

Migraine Headaches

1. Answer:B) Migraine headache

    Explanation: Migraine headaches are typically severe, throbbing headaches associated with nausea,

    sensitivity to light (photophobia), and sometimes sensitivity to sound (phonophobia).

2. Answer:B) Migraine with aura

    Explanation: The zigzag lines and unilateral throbbing headache are characteristic of migraine with aura.

    Aura refers to transient neurological symptoms that precede or accompany the headache.

3. Answer:C)Cluster headache

    Explanation: Cluster headaches are characterized by severe unilateral pain around the eye, with ipsilateral

    lacrimation (tearing) and nasal congestion (rhinorrhea).

4. Answer:C)Subarachnoid hemorrhage

    Explanation: Sudden onset severe headache, often described as the worst headache of life, along with

    neck stiffness and photophobia, are characteristic of subarachnoid hemorrhage.

5. Answer:d)Language

    Explanation: Difficulty speaking during the aura phase suggests a language (or speech) aura, which is a

    type of sensory-motor aura.

6. Answer:C) Menstrual migraine

    Explanation: Migraines that occur around the menstrual cycle are termed menstrual migraines.

7. Answer:C) Cluster headache

    Explanation: Cluster headaches are characterized by recurrent, brief, severe headaches that occur in

    clusters or groups, typically over weeks to months.

8. Answer:a)Tension-type headache

    Explanation: Tension-type headaches are typically bilateral, pressing or tightening in quality, and not

    associated with nausea or vomiting.

9. Answer:C) Cluster headache

   Explanation: Headaches that occur after alcohol consumption and are unilateral with severe pain suggest cluster headaches.

10. Answer:B) Migraine headache

    Explanation: Migraines are characterized by unilateral pulsating headaches associated with nausea, photophobia, and sometimes aura, with a possible family history.

11. Answer:C) Chronic migraine

    Explanation: Chronic migraine is defined as headaches occurring on ≥15 days per month for >3 months, with features of migraine.

12. Answer:C) Cluster headache

    Explanation: The characteristic features of excruciating unilateral headaches, red eye, and drooping eyelid suggest cluster headaches.

13. Answer:B) Migraine headache

    Explanation: The presence of aura, visual disturbances, and sensory symptoms, followed by a throbbing headache with nausea and photophobia, are characteristic of migraine with aura.

14. Answer:d)Sinus headache

    Explanation: Headache associated with facial pain, worsened by bending over, and accompanied by nasal congestion and discharge suggests sinus headache.

15. Answer:B) Migraine headache

    Explanation: Recurrent headaches occurring during the menstrual cycle, severe and throbbing in nature, and associated with nausea, vomiting, and family history, are characteristic of menstrual migraines.

Multiple Sclerosis (MS)

1. Answer: C. Multiple Sclerosis (MS)

   Explanation: MS is characterized by demyelination in the central nervous system (CNS), leading to various neurological symptoms, including optic neuritis and motor deficits.

2. Answer: C. Multiple Sclerosis (MS)

   Explanation: MS often presents with relapsing-remitting neurological symptoms that worsen with heat exposure, due to impaired nerve conduction in demyelinated areas.

3. Answer: C. Multiple Sclerosis (MS)

   Explanation: MS typically presents with relapsing-remitting episodes of neurological symptoms, which can include optic neuritis, ataxia, and diplopia.

4. Answer: A. High-dose corticosteroids

   Explanation: Acute exacerbations of MS are typically treated with high-dose corticosteroids to reduce inflammation and accelerate recovery.

5. Answer: B. Discontinue DMT before conception

   Explanation: Many DMTs used in MS are contraindicated during pregnancy. It's recommended to discontinue DMTs before conception, if possible.

6. Answer: C. Multiple Sclerosis (MS)

   Explanation: MS can present with various neurological symptoms, including facial weakness, double vision, and sensory deficits, due to demyelination in the CNS.

7. Answer: B. Cerebellum

   Explanation: Lesions in the cerebellum can cause ataxia, intention tremor, and scanning speech, which are common in MS.

8. Answer: C. Neurogenic bladder

   Explanation: MS can cause neurogenic bladder due to dysfunction in the control of bladder emptying, leading to urgency, frequency, and incontinence.

9. Answer: A. Decreases pro-inflammatory cytokine production

    Explanation: Interferon beta-1a is thought to reduce the inflammatory response associated with MS, thereby decreasing relapses.

10. Answer: C. Add corticosteroids

    Explanation: Acute exacerbations in MS are typically treated with corticosteroids to reduce inflammation and severity of symptoms.

11. Answer: B. Baclofen

    Explanation: Baclofen is a centrally acting muscle relaxant commonly used to treat spasticity in MS.

12. Answer: C. Frontal lobes

    Explanation: Cognitive impairment and emotional lability in MS are often associated with lesions in the frontal lobes.

13. Answer: D. Dysesthesia

    Explanation: Dysesthesia refers to abnormal sensations such as burning, itching, or tingling, which are common in MS.

14. Answer: A. Start high-dose vitamin D supplementation

    Explanation: Vitamin D deficiency is common in MS and supplementation may have beneficial effects on disease progression.

15. Answer: B. Disease activity tends to improve during pregnancy

    Explanation: Pregnancy is associated with a reduced risk of relapse in MS, particularly during the third trimester.

Narcotic Addiction

1. Answer: A. Naloxone administration

   Explanation: Naloxone is an opioid antagonist used to reverse opioid overdose, including heroin. It should be administered immediately to reverse respiratory depression and other opioid effects.

2. Answer: A. Buprenorphine

   Explanation: Buprenorphine is a partial opioid agonist that helps manage opioid withdrawal and cravings, making it the first-line treatment for opioid use disorder.

3. Answer: D. Naltrexone

   Explanation: Naltrexone is an opioid antagonist that blocks the effects of opioids and is used for relapse prevention in individuals who have already detoxed from opioids.

4. Answer: B. Buprenorphine

   Explanation: Buprenorphine is effective in managing opioid withdrawal symptoms due to its partial agonist activity at the opioid receptors.

5. Answer: D. Buprenorphine

   Explanation: Buprenorphine is recommended for pregnant women with opioid use disorder due to its safety profile and effectiveness in reducing withdrawal symptoms.

6. Answer: B. Reduction in cravings and withdrawal symptoms

   Explanation: Methadone is a long-acting opioid agonist that reduces cravings and withdrawal symptoms, allowing individuals to function without euphoria or sedation.

7. Answer: D. Naltrexone

   Explanation: Naltrexone is an opioid antagonist that blocks the effects of opioids and reduces the risk of relapse in individuals who have completed detoxification.

8. Answer: A. Buprenorphine

   Explanation: Buprenorphine is recommended for patients with hepatitis C due to its lower risk of hepatotoxicity compared to methadone.

9. Answer: B. Lower risk of respiratory depression

   Explanation: Buprenorphine has a lower risk of respiratory depression compared to full opioid agonists like methadone.

10. Answer: C. Methadone

    Explanation: Methadone maintenance therapy is associated with higher retention rates in treatment programs compared to other medications for opioid use disorder.

11. Answer: B. Buprenorphine

    Explanation: Buprenorphine can be prescribed in an office-based setting by trained physicians, making it accessible for treatment of opioid use disorder.

12. Answer: C. Reduction in opioid cravings and withdrawal symptoms

    Explanation: Buprenorphine maintenance therapy aims to reduce opioid cravings and withdrawal symptoms, supporting long-term recovery.

13. Answer: D. Naltrexone

    Explanation: Naltrexone, an opioid antagonist, may exacerbate depression and is generally not recommended for patients with severe depression.

14. Answer: D. Naltrexone

    Explanation: Naltrexone is an opioid antagonist that is non-addictive and helps prevent relapse by blocking the effects of opioids.

15. Answer: A. Daily visits to the clinic for administration

    Explanation: Methadone is usually administered daily in a clinic under supervision to ensure compliance and safety.

Narcolepsy

1. Answer: B. Narcolepsy

   Explanation: Narcolepsy is characterized by excessive daytime sleepiness, cataplexy (sudden loss of muscle tone triggered by emotions), hypnagogic hallucinations (vivid dreams upon falling asleep), and sleep paralysis.

2. Answer: D. Refer for polysomnography

   Explanation: Polysomnography (overnight sleep study) followed by a multiple sleep latency test (MSLT) is the diagnostic gold standard for narcolepsy.

3. Answer: B. Sodium oxybate

   Explanation: Sodium oxybate (gamma-hydroxybutyrate) is the first-line treatment for cataplexy associated with narcolepsy.

4. Answer: D. Switch to armodafinil

   Explanation: Armodafinil is a longer-acting formulation of modafinil and can be considered when the effect of modafinil is insufficient.

5. Answer: D. Consider sodium oxybate

   Explanation: Sodium oxybate has been shown to improve both daytime sleepiness and nighttime sleep disturbances in patients with narcolepsy.

6. Answer: D. Consider pitolisant

   Explanation: Pitolisant is a histamine H3 receptor antagonist/inverse agonist that is approved for treatment of excessive daytime sleepiness in adults with narcolepsy.

7. Answer: C. Prescribe sodium oxybate

   Explanation: Sodium oxybate is the treatment of choice for cataplexy in patients with narcolepsy.

8. Answer: D. Sodium oxybate

   Explanation: Sodium oxybate should be used cautiously in patients with hypertension due to its potential to increase blood pressure.

9. Answer: D. Sodium oxybate

   Explanation: Sodium oxybate is contraindicated in patients with CKD due to its potential to worsen renal function.

10. Answer: D. Sodium oxybate

    Explanation: Sodium oxybate is contraindicated in patients with significant hepatic impairment due to its potential for exacerbating liver disease.

11. Answer: A. Modafinil

    Explanation: Modafinil is effective in treating excessive daytime sleepiness and is generally well-tolerated in patients with anxiety disorders.

12. Answer: A. Modafinil

    Explanation: Modafinil is effective in treating excessive daytime sleepiness and is generally well-tolerated in patients with depression.

13. Answer: C. Methylphenidate

    Explanation: Methylphenidate can be used cautiously in patients with bipolar disorder and narcolepsy to improve excessive daytime sleepiness.

14. Answer: A. Modafinil

    Explanation: Modafinil has lower abuse potential compared to other stimulants and is preferred in patients with substance use disorder.

15. Answer: C. Methylphenidate

    Explanation: Methylphenidate can increase intraocular pressure and is contraindicated in patients with glaucoma.

Nephrotic Syndrome

1. Answer: B. Nephrotic syndrome

   Explanation: Nephrotic syndrome is characterized by proteinuria (>3.5 g/day), hypoalbuminemia, hyperlipidemia, and edema.

2. Answer: A. Minimal change disease

   Explanation: Minimal change disease is the most common cause of nephrotic syndrome in children and young adults, often preceded by an upper respiratory tract infection.

3. Answer: A. Minimal change disease

   Explanation: Minimal change disease is characterized by diffuse effacement of podocyte foot processes on renal biopsy.

4. Answer: C. Membranous nephropathy

   Explanation: Membranous nephropathy is characterized by immune complex deposits along the basement membrane on renal biopsy.

5. Answer: B. Focal segmental glomerulosclerosis (FSGS)

   Explanation: Focal segmental glomerulosclerosis is characterized by segmental sclerosis and hyalinosis of glomeruli on renal biopsy.

6. Answer: D. IgA nephropathy

   Explanation: IgA nephropathy is characterized by mesangial hypercellularity and IgA deposits on renal biopsy.

7. Answer: C. Membranous nephropathy

   Explanation: Membranous nephropathy can be associated with hepatitis B and is characterized by immune complex deposition in a diffuse granular pattern on renal biopsy.

8. Answer: C. Membranous nephropathy

   Explanation: Membranous nephropathy can be secondary to malignancies and is characterized by thickening of the glomerular basement membrane on renal biopsy.

9. Answer: D. Secondary amyloidosis

   Explanation: Secondary amyloidosis can cause nephrotic syndrome and is characterized by apple-green birefringence under polarized light on renal biopsy.

10. Answer: D. Secondary amyloidosis

    Explanation: Secondary amyloidosis can be associated with rheumatoid arthritis and is characterized by deposition of amyloid fibrils on renal biopsy.

11. Answer: D. Light chain cast nephropathy

    Explanation: Light chain cast nephropathy (myeloma kidney) can cause nephrotic syndrome and is characterized by deposition of monoclonal immunoglobulin light chains on renal biopsy.

12. Answer: D. Diabetic nephropathy

    Explanation: Diabetic nephropathy is characterized by nodular mesangial expansion (Kimmelstiel-Wilson nodules) and thickened glomerular basement membrane on renal biopsy.

13. Answer: D. Hepatitis C-associated glomerulonephritis

    Explanation: Hepatitis C-associated glomerulonephritis can cause nephrotic syndrome and is characterized by an MPGN pattern on renal biopsy.

14. Answer: D. Lupus nephritis

    Explanation: Lupus nephritis can cause nephrotic syndrome and is characterized by a diffuse proliferative pattern with wire-loop lesions on renal biopsy.

15. Answer: D. Amyloidosis

    Explanation: Amyloidosis can cause nephrotic syndrome and is characterized by deposition of Congo red-positive material on renal biopsy.

Obsessive-Compulsive Disorder (OCD)

1. Answer: C. Obsessive-compulsive disorder (OCD)

   Explanation: The patient's symptoms of intrusive thoughts and compulsive behaviors (hand washing) are characteristic of OCD.

2. Answer: C. Obsessive-compulsive disorder (OCD)

   Explanation: The patient's obsessions about harm and avoidance behaviors are typical of OCD, particularly the harm-related subtype.

3. Answer: A. Obsessive-compulsive disorder (OCD)

   Explanation: The patient's preoccupation with symmetry and orderliness, along with time-consuming behaviors, are characteristic of OCD.

4. Answer: B. Obsessive-compulsive disorder (OCD)

   Explanation: The patient's fear of contamination and compulsive hand washing are typical symptoms of OCD.

5. Answer: A. Obsessive-compulsive disorder (OCD)

   Explanation: The patient's intrusive thoughts and compulsive checking behavior are characteristic of OCD.

6. Answer: A. Obsessive-compulsive disorder (OCD)

   Explanation: The patient's compulsive counting and belief that something bad will happen if he doesn't perform the ritual are typical of OCD.

7. Answer: A. Obsessive-compulsive disorder (OCD)

   Explanation: The patient's intrusive thoughts and compulsive behaviors (ritual tapping) are characteristic of OCD.

8. Answer: B. Obsessive-compulsive disorder (OCD)

   Explanation: The patient's obsessive doubts and repeated checking behavior are typical symptoms of OCD.

9. Answer: B. Obsessive-compulsive disorder (OCD)

   Explanation: The patient's fear of contamination, compulsive cleaning, and distress when the routine is interrupted are characteristic of OCD.

10. Answer: A. Obsessive-compulsive disorder (OCD)

    Explanation: The patient's obsessions about contamination and compulsive hand washing are typical symptoms of OCD.

11. Answer: A. Obsessive-compulsive disorder (OCD)

    Explanation: The patient's fear of harming others and performing rituals to prevent harm are characteristic of OCD, particularly the harm-related subtype.

12. Answer: A. Obsessive-compulsive disorder (OCD)

    Explanation: The patient's intrusive thoughts, compulsive washing, and anxiety about resisting the urge are characteristic of OCD.

13. Answer: A. Obsessive-compulsive disorder (OCD)

    Explanation: The patient's mental rituals (repeating words until they feel right) and time-consuming behaviors are characteristic of OCD.

14. Answer: A. Obsessive-compulsive disorder (OCD)

    Explanation: The patient's intrusive thoughts and compulsive checking behavior (locks) are typical symptoms of OCD.

15. Answer: B. Obsessive-compulsive disorder (OCD)

    Explanation: The patient's obsessions about contamination and compulsive hand washing are characteristic of OCD.

Osteoarthritis

1. Answer 1:B. Osteoarthritis. This patient's symptoms of chronic pain and stiffness, worse in the morning but improving throughout the day, along with Heberden's nodes (enlarged finger joints), are characteristic of osteoarthritis.

2. Answer 2:B. Osteoarthritis. This patient's symptoms of knee pain worsening with activity, improving with rest, crepitus, and tenderness over the knee joint are typical of osteoarthritis.

3. Answer 3:B. Osteoarthritis. This patient's symptoms of pain and swelling in the base of the thumb, aggravated by grasping objects and without trauma history, are characteristic of osteoarthritis.

4. Answer 4:C. Ankylosing spondylitis. This patient's symptoms of chronic low back pain and stiffness, worse in the mornings and improving with activity, along with no radiation of pain into the legs, are characteristic of ankylosing spondylitis rather than osteoarthritis.

5. Answer 5:B. Osteoarthritis. This patient's symptoms of knee pain worse with activity, stiffness after prolonged sitting (which improves with movement), and absence of systemic symptoms are typical of osteoarthritis.

6. Answer 6:B. Osteoarthritis. This patient's symptoms of chronic hip pain worse with weight-bearing and improved with rest, along with limited range of motion and crepitus, are characteristic of osteoarthritis.

7. Answer 7:Rheumatoid arthritis. This patient's symptoms of pain and swelling in multiple joints, morning stiffness lasting more than an hour, symmetric joint involvement, and presence of rheumatoid nodules are characteristic of rheumatoid arthritis.

8. Answer 8:B. Osteoarthritis. This patient's symptoms of pain and stiffness in the fingers, worse in the mornings and improving throughout the day, along with Heberden's nodes, are characteristic of osteoarthritis.

9. Answer 9:B. Osteoarthritis. This patient's symptoms of chronic pain and stiffness in hands and knees, worse with activity and improved with rest, along with Heberden's and Bouchard's nodes, are characteristic of osteoarthritis.

10. Answer 10:B. Osteoarthritis. This patient's symptoms of chronic knee pain worse with activity (climbing stairs, prolonged walking), crepitus, and tenderness over the knee joints are characteristic of osteoarthritis.

11. Answer 11:C. Gout. This patient's symptoms of sudden intense pain and swelling in the big toe are characteristic of acute gouty arthritis, not osteoarthritis.

12. Answer 12:C. Ankylosing spondylitis. This patient's symptoms of chronic low back pain and stiffness, worse in the mornings and improving with activity, are characteristic of ankylosing spondylitis, not osteoarthritis.

13. Answer 13:Rheumatoid arthritis. This patient's symptoms of pain and swelling in multiple joints, morning stiffness lasting more than an hour, symmetric joint involvement, and presence of rheumatoid nodules are characteristic of rheumatoid arthritis.

14. Answer 14:B. Osteoarthritis. This patient's symptoms of pain and stiffness in the fingers, worse in the mornings and improving throughout the day, along with Heberden's nodes, are characteristic of osteoarthritis.

15. Answer 15:B. Osteoarthritis. This patient's symptoms of chronic pain and stiffness in hands and knees, worse with activity and improved with rest, along with Heberden's and Bouchard's nodes, are characteristic of osteoarthritis.

Osteoporosis

1. Answer 1: C. Osteoporosis

    Explanation: Osteoporosis is characterized by low bone mass and microarchitectural deterioration of bone tissue, leading to increased bone fragility and susceptibility to fractures, particularly in postmenopausal women.

2. Answer 2: B. Vertebral compression fracture

    Explanation: Vertebral compression fractures are a common complication of osteoporosis, particularly in individuals with chronic steroid use. They present with acute back pain, often precipitated by minimal trauma.

3. Answer 3: B. Osteoporosis

    Explanation: Osteoporosis can lead to vertebral compression fractures, causing height loss and a stooped posture (kyphosis).

4. Answer 4: D. Order a hip X-ray

    Explanation: The patient's presentation is concerning for a hip fracture, which is a severe complication of osteoporosis. An X-ray is needed to confirm the diagnosis.

5. Answer 5: B. Dual-energy X-ray absorptiometry (DXA) scan

    Explanation: DXA scan is the gold standard for diagnosing osteoporosis by measuring bone mineral density (BMD) at the hip and spine.

6. Answer 6: B. Alendronate

    Explanation: Alendronate is a bisphosphonate that helps to increase bone density and reduce the risk of fractures in osteoporosis.

7. Answer 7: B. Vertebral compression fractures

    Explanation: Vertebral compression fractures are common in osteoporosis and present with height loss and back pain.

8. Answer 8: D. Order a hip X-ray

   Explanation: The patient's presentation is concerning for a hip fracture, a severe complication of osteoporosis. An X-ray is needed to confirm the diagnosis.

9. Answer 9: D. Teriparatide

   Explanation: Teriparatide is a recombinant form of parathyroid hormone that is used to stimulate bone formation in patients with severe osteoporosis.

10. Answer 10: B. Thyroid function tests

    Explanation: Thyroid function tests are appropriate for evaluating secondary causes of osteoporosis, as thyroid dysfunction can contribute to bone loss.

11. Answer 11: A. Vertebral compression fracture

    Explanation: Vertebral compression fractures are a common complication of osteoporosis, especially in individuals with chronic steroid use, and present with acute back pain.

12. Answer 12: D. Order a hip X-ray

    Explanation: The patient's presentation is concerning for a hip fracture, a severe complication of osteoporosis. An X-ray is needed to confirm the diagnosis.

13. Answer 13: B. Forward flexion of the spine

    Explanation: Height loss and stooped posture (kyphosis) are characteristic physical findings in patients with vertebral compression fractures due to osteoporosis.

14. Answer 14: B. Dual-energy X-ray absorptiometry (DXA) scan

    Explanation: DXA scan is the gold standard for diagnosing osteoporosis by measuring bone mineral density (BMD) at the hip and spine.

15. Answer 15: B. Alendronate

    Explanation: Alendronate is a bisphosphonate that helps to increase bone density and reduce the risk of fractures in osteoporosis.

Panic Disorder

1. Answer 1: B. Panic disorder

    Explanation: Panic disorder is characterized by recurrent unexpected panic attacks, which are abrupt surges of intense fear or discomfort that peak within minutes.

2. Answer 2: A. Panic disorder

    Explanation: Panic disorder is characterized by recurrent unexpected panic attacks, which are abrupt surges of intense fear or discomfort that peak within minutes.

3. Answer 3: A. Panic disorder

    Explanation: Panic disorder is characterized by recurrent unexpected panic attacks, which are abrupt surges of intense fear or discomfort that peak within minutes.

4. Answer 4: B. Cognitive-behavioral therapy (CBT)

    Explanation: Cognitive-behavioral therapy (CBT) is a first-line treatment for panic disorder and has been shown to be effective in reducing the frequency and severity of panic attacks.

5. Answer 5: A. Panic disorder

    Explanation: Panic disorder is characterized by recurrent unexpected panic attacks, which are abrupt surges of intense fear or discomfort that peak within minutes.

6. Answer 6: A. Panic disorder

    Explanation: Panic disorder is characterized by recurrent unexpected panic attacks, which are abrupt surges of intense fear or discomfort that peak within minutes.

7. Answer 7: A. Panic disorder

    Explanation: Panic disorder is characterized by recurrent unexpected panic attacks, which are abrupt surges of intense fear or discomfort that peak within minutes.

8. Answer 8: B. Cognitive-behavioral therapy (CBT)

    Explanation: Cognitive-behavioral therapy (CBT) is a first-line treatment for panic disorder and has been shown to be effective in reducing the frequency and severity of panic attacks.

9. Answer 9: A. Panic disorder

    Explanation: Panic disorder is characterized by recurrent unexpected panic attacks, which are abrupt

    surges of intense fear or discomfort that peak within minutes.

10. Answer 10: A. Panic disorder

    Explanation: Panic disorder is characterized by recurrent unexpected panic attacks, which are abrupt

    surges of intense fear or discomfort that peak within minutes.

11. Answer 11: A. Panic disorder

    Explanation: Panic disorder is characterized by recurrent unexpected panic attacks, which are abrupt

    surges of intense fear or discomfort that peak within minutes.

12. Answer 12: B. Cognitive-behavioral therapy (CBT)

    Explanation: Cognitive-behavioral therapy (CBT) is a first-line treatment for panic disorder and has been

    shown to be effective in reducing the frequency and severity of panic attacks.

13. Answer 13: A. Panic disorder

    Explanation: Panic disorder is characterized by recurrent unexpected panic attacks, which are abrupt

    surges of intense fear or discomfort that peak within minutes.

14. Answer 14: A. Panic disorder

    Explanation: Panic disorder is characterized by recurrent unexpected panic attacks, which are abrupt

    surges of intense fear or discomfort that peak within minutes.

15. Answer 15: A. Panic disorder

    Explanation: Panic disorder is characterized by recurrent unexpected panic attacks, which are abrupt

    surges of intense fear or discomfort that peak within minutes.

Parkinson's Disease

1. Answer 1: B. Parkinson's disease

   Explanation: Parkinson's disease is characterized by resting tremor, bradykinesia (slowness of movement), rigidity (muscle stiffness), and postural instability. Essential tremor typically occurs with movement and is not associated with other parkinsonian features.

2. Answer 2: A. Degeneration of the basal ganglia

   Explanation: Parkinson's disease is primarily caused by degeneration of dopaminergic neurons in the substantia nigra, a part of the basal ganglia.

3. Answer 3: A. Tremor, rigidity, and bradykinesia

   Explanation: The classic triad of symptoms in Parkinson's disease includes resting tremor, muscle rigidity, and bradykinesia (slowness of movement).

4. Answer 4: B. Essential tremor

   Explanation: Essential tremor is characterized by bilateral action tremor (improves with action) and typically lacks other parkinsonian features seen in Parkinson's disease.

5. Answer 5: A. Freezing of gait

   Explanation: Freezing of gait is a common motor symptom in Parkinson's disease characterized by sudden episodes of being unable to move, often when starting to walk or when turning.

6. Answer 6: A. Levodopa

   Explanation: Levodopa is the most effective medication for treating the motor symptoms of Parkinson's disease by increasing dopamine levels in the brain.

7. Answer 7: A. Dysphagia

   Explanation: Dysphagia (difficulty swallowing) is a common non-motor symptom in Parkinson's disease, which can lead to complications like aspiration pneumonia.

8. Answer 8: A. Dyskinesia

   Explanation: Dyskinesia (involuntary movements) is a potential side effect of long-term levodopa therapy in patients with Parkinson's disease.

9. Answer 9: D. Positron emission tomography (PET)

   Explanation: PET imaging with a dopamine transporter (DaT) scan can help differentiate Parkinson's disease from other parkinsonian syndromes.

10. Answer 10: C. Hyposmia

    Explanation: Hyposmia (reduced sense of smell) is a common non-motor symptom in Parkinson's disease, often occurring years before motor symptoms develop.

11. Answer 11: A. Constipation

    Explanation: Constipation is a common non-motor symptom in Parkinson's disease, attributed to dysregulation of the autonomic nervous system.

12. Answer 12: A. Levodopa

    Explanation: Levodopa is the most effective medication for treating the motor symptoms of Parkinson's disease by increasing dopamine levels in the brain.

13. Answer 13: A. Dysphagia

    Explanation: Dysphagia (difficulty swallowing) is a common non-motor symptom in Parkinson's disease, which can lead to complications like aspiration pneumonia.

14. Answer 14: A. Dyskinesia

    Explanation: Dyskinesia (involuntary movements) is a potential side effect of long-term levodopa therapy in patients with Parkinson's disease.

15. Answer 15: D. Positron emission tomography (PET)

    Explanation: PET imaging with a dopamine transporter (DaT) scan can help differentiate Parkinson's disease from other parkinsonian syndromes.

Peptic Ulcer Disease

1. Answer: B. Peptic ulcer disease (PUD)

   Explanation: The patient's symptoms, including improvement with food and history of NSAID use, are characteristic of PUD.

2. Answer: A. Esophagogastroduodenoscopy (EGD)

   Explanation: EGD is the most appropriate initial test to evaluate for peptic ulcer disease.

3. Answer: B. Duodenal ulcer

   Explanation: Symptoms that improve with food intake are typical of duodenal ulcers.

4. Answer: A. Proton pump inhibitor (PPI)

   Explanation: PPIs are first-line treatment for peptic ulcer disease due to their potent acid suppression.

5. Answer: A. Biopsy of the ulcer

   Explanation: Biopsy of the ulcer is essential to rule out gastric malignancy.

6. Answer: C. Discontinue NSAID use

   Explanation: Discontinuation of NSAID use is crucial in managing NSAID-induced peptic ulcers.

7. Answer: A. Perform endoscopic hemostasis

   Explanation: Endoscopic hemostasis is indicated in cases of bleeding from peptic ulcers.

8. Answer: A. Perform endoscopic hemostasis

   Explanation: Endoscopic hemostasis is indicated in cases of bleeding from peptic ulcers.

9. Answer: A. Immediate surgical consultation

   Explanation: Perforated peptic ulcers require immediate surgical consultation.

10. Answer: A. Perform H. pylori testing

    Explanation: H. pylori testing is indicated to determine the need for eradication therapy.

11. Answer: A. Perform endoscopic hemostasis

    Explanation: Endoscopic hemostasis is indicated in cases of bleeding from peptic ulcers.

12. Answer: A. Start treatment with a PPI

    Explanation: PPIs are first-line treatment for peptic ulcer disease due to their potent acid suppression.

13. Answer: B. Perform endoscopic hemostasis

    Explanation: Endoscopic hemostasis is indicated in cases of bleeding from peptic ulcers.

14. Answer: D. Discontinue NSAID use

    Explanation: Discontinuation of NSAID use is crucial in managing NSAID-induced peptic ulcers.

15. Answer: A. Proton pump inhibitor (PPI)

    Explanation: PPIs are first-line treatment for peptic ulcer disease due to their potent acid suppression.

Peripheral Arterial Disease (PAD)

1. Answer: B) Peripheral Arterial Disease (PAD)

    Explanation: This patient presents with classic symptoms of PAD (intermittent claudication) and diminished pedal pulses, which are indicative of arterial insufficiency.

2. Answer: C) Peripheral Arterial Disease (PAD)

    Explanation: The symptoms of pain at rest, coolness, and pallor suggest severe PAD with ischemic rest pain.

3. Answer: C) Peripheral Arterial Disease (PAD)

    Explanation: Non-healing ulcers in the setting of smoking and diabetes are more likely due to PAD causing chronic ischemia and poor wound healing.

4. Answer: A) Acute arterial thrombosis

    Explanation: Sudden onset of pain, pallor, and paralysis in the absence of trauma is characteristic of acute arterial thrombosis, a complication of PAD.

5. Answer: D) Offloading and wound care

    Explanation: Offloading and wound care are the initial steps in managing ischemic ulcers in patients with PAD. Surgical revascularization may be considered if the ulcer does not heal.

6. Answer: B) Pitting edema

    Explanation: Calf pain worsened by elevation and improved by dependent positioning (dangling) suggests venous insufficiency rather than PAD.

7. Answer: B) Perform angiography with possible intervention

    Explanation: Persistent leg pain at rest and non-healing ulcers are signs of severe PAD requiring evaluation with angiography and possible revascularization.

8. Answer: C) Supervised exercise program (e.g., walking program)

    Explanation: Supervised exercise programs, such as walking programs, are recommended for patients with PAD to improve walking distance and reduce symptoms.

9. Answer: C) Arterial insufficiency

    Explanation: Pain that worsens at night and improves with dependency is characteristic of ischemic rest pain due to PAD.

10. Answer: C) Arterial insufficiency

    Explanation: A decreased ABI indicates arterial insufficiency, which is a hallmark of PAD.

11. Answer: C) Acute arterial thrombosis

    Explanation: Acute onset of numbness and weakness in the leg is concerning for acute arterial thrombosis, a complication of PAD.

12. Answer: B) Perform immediate surgical revascularization

    Explanation: Severe symptoms of pain, pallor, paralysis, and absence of distal pulses indicate acute limb ischemia requiring immediate surgical revascularization.

13. Answer: A) Acute arterial thrombosis

    Explanation: Cyanotic, cold, and pulseless extremity in the absence of trauma suggests acute arterial thrombosis, a critical complication of PAD.

14. Answer: C) Start cilostazol therapy

    Explanation: Cilostazol is a medication used to improve walking distance and symptoms in patients with PAD who have intermittent claudication.

15. Answer: A) Discontinue cilostazol

    Explanation: Palpitations and dizziness are common side effects of cilostazol. Discontinuation is warranted in this case.

Pneumonia

1. Answer:B) Pneumonia

   Explanation: Sudden onset fever, productive cough with purulent sputum, pleuritic chest pain, and coarse crackles on auscultation suggest pneumonia, likely of bacterial origin.

2. Answer:B) Pneumonia

   Explanation: Fever, non-productive cough, pleuritic chest pain, and patchy infiltrates on chest X-ray suggest pneumonia, which can be bacterial in origin and exacerbated by SLE.

3. Answer:B) Pneumonia

   Explanation: Confusion, fever, productive cough with yellowish sputum, decreased breath sounds, and dullness to percussion suggest pneumonia, likely with an associated pleural effusion.

4. Answer:B) Pneumonia

   Explanation: Sudden onset high fever, chills, pleuritic chest pain, and a wedge-shaped infiltrate on chest X-ray suggest pneumonia, possibly due to Streptococcus pneumoniae or other pathogens in the setting of sickle cell disease.

5. Answer:D) Lung abscess

   Explanation: Foul-smelling sputum, a cavitary lesion with an air-fluid level on chest X-ray, and symptoms of cough and shortness of breath suggest a lung abscess.

6. Answer:D) Pneumocystis pneumonia

   Explanation: Fever, cough, shortness of breath, bilateral interstitial infiltrates on chest X-ray, and a history of immunosuppressive therapy (methotrexate) suggest Pneumocystis pneumonia in a patient with rheumatoid arthritis.

7. Answer:B) Pneumonia

   Explanation: Cough, dyspnea, low-grade fever, right middle lobe infiltrate, and a small pleural effusion on chest X-ray suggest pneumonia, possibly bacterial in origin.

8. Answer:B) Pneumonia

   Explanation: Rusty-colored sputum, fever, pleuritic chest pain, and crackles over the right lower lung field suggest pneumonia, likely due to Streptococcus pneumoniae.

9. Answer:C) Pulmonary embolism

   Explanation: Sudden onset sharp chest pain, shortness of breath, recent surgery, and a wedge-shaped infiltrate on chest X-ray are suggestive of pulmonary embolism.

10. Answer:D) Lung abscess

    Explanation: Pleuritic chest pain, cough, fever, and a right lower lobe infiltrate with an air-fluid level on chest X-ray suggest a lung abscess.

11. Answer:D) Lung abscess

    Explanation: Foul-smelling sputum, poor dentition, decreased breath sounds, and dullness to percussion over the right lower lung field suggest a lung abscess.

12. Answer:D) Exacerbation of COPD

    Explanation: Cough, fever, dyspnea, smoking history, and chest X-ray findings of hyperinflation and scattered infiltrates suggest an exacerbation of COPD.

13. Answer:B) Pneumonia

    Explanation: Fever, cough, chest pain, recent travel to Southeast Asia, and patchy infiltrates on chest X-ray suggest pneumonia, which could be due to atypical organisms.

14. Answer:D) Lung abscess

    Explanation: Cough, fever, dyspnea, and a cavitary lesion with an air-fluid level on chest X-ray suggest a lung abscess.

15. Answer:D) Lung cancer

    Explanation: Hemoptysis, fever, cough, and a coin lesion on chest X-ray suggest lung cancer.

Post-Traumatic Stress Disorder (PTSD)

1. Answer: C. Post-Traumatic Stress Disorder (PTSD)

   Explanation: PTSD is characterized by intrusive memories, avoidance of trauma-related stimuli, negative alterations in mood, and hyperarousal.

2. Answer: C. Post-Traumatic Stress Disorder (PTSD)

   Explanation: Symptoms of PTSD typically develop following exposure to a traumatic event and include re-experiencing, avoidance, negative alterations in mood, and hyperarousal.

3. Answer: B. Cognitive-behavioral therapy (CBT)

   Explanation: CBT, particularly trauma-focused CBT, is considered first-line for the treatment of PTSD. It addresses the cognitive and behavioral aspects of the disorder.

4. Answer: A. Depersonalization

   Explanation: Depersonalization refers to feeling detached from oneself or one's body, often seen in PTSD.

5. Answer: B. Alpha-1 adrenergic receptor antagonism

   Explanation: Prazosin, an alpha-1 adrenergic receptor antagonist, is used to treat nightmares and sleep disturbances in PTSD by reducing noradrenergic hyperactivity.

6. Answer: B. Avoidance

   Explanation: Avoidance is a core symptom of PTSD, where individuals actively avoid people, places, activities, or situations that remind them of the traumatic event.

7. Answer: B. Trauma-focused cognitive-behavioral therapy (CBT)

   Explanation: Trauma-focused CBT, including exposure therapy, is recommended as the initial treatment for PTSD to help individuals process and cope with traumatic memories.

8. Answer: A. Hyperarousal

   Explanation: Hyperarousal is one of the symptom clusters of PTSD, characterized by increased startle response, difficulty sleeping, irritability, and hypervigilance.

9. Answer: B. Derealization

   Explanation: Derealization is characterized by a sense of unreality or detachment from one's surroundings, often seen in PTSD.

10. Answer: A. Amnesia

    Explanation: Amnesia refers to difficulty remembering aspects of the traumatic event, a common symptom in PTSD.

11. Answer: B. Avoidance

    Explanation: Avoidance is a core symptom of PTSD, where individuals avoid reminders of the traumatic event, including talking about it or visiting places associated with it.

12. Answer: C. Trauma-focused cognitive-behavioral therapy (CBT)

    Explanation: Trauma-focused CBT, including exposure therapy, is effective in treating intrusive memories and nightmares in PTSD.

13. Answer: B. Selective serotonin reuptake inhibition

    Explanation: SSRIs like sertraline are commonly used to treat PTSD by increasing serotonin levels in the brain, which can improve mood and reduce anxiety.

14. Answer: B. Prazosin

    Explanation: Prazosin, an alpha-1 adrenergic receptor antagonist, is often used to reduce nightmares and improve sleep quality in patients with PTSD.

15. Answer: B. Prolonged exposure therapy (PE)

    Explanation: Prolonged exposure therapy is a type of CBT that helps patients confront and process memories and feelings related to their trauma, reducing avoidance behaviors.

Premenstrual Syndrome (PMS)

1. Answer: A. Premenstrual syndrome (PMS)

   Explanation: PMS is characterized by mood changes, irritability, and physical symptoms such as breast tenderness, which occur cyclically before menstruation.

2. Answer: D. Hot flashes

   Explanation: Hot flashes are not typically associated with PMS. They are more characteristic of menopause.

3. Answer: B. Oral contraceptive pills (OCPs)

   Explanation: OCPs are often used to manage PMS symptoms, as they stabilize hormone levels and can alleviate mood symptoms.

4. Answer: D. Symptom diary

   Explanation: Keeping a symptom diary can help identify patterns and severity of symptoms, which is important for diagnosing and managing PMS.

5. Answer: C. SSRIs

   Explanation: SSRIs can be effective in treating severe emotional symptoms of PMS when other treatments are not sufficient.

6. Answer: B. Calcium supplementation

   Explanation: Calcium supplementation is unlikely to exacerbate weight gain or fluid retention and may help reduce symptoms of PMS.

7. Answer: A. Headaches

   Explanation: Headaches are a common physical symptom of PMS, occurring in a significant number of women.

8. Answer: A. SSRIs

   Explanation: SSRIs are commonly used as first-line pharmacologic treatment for severe emotional symptoms of PMS.

9. Answer: C. Low-salt diet

    Explanation: A low-salt diet may help reduce symptoms of fluid retention associated with PMS.

10. Answer: A. Refer for psychotherapy

    Explanation: Psychotherapy can be beneficial for women with severe PMS symptoms that affect their work and relationships.

11. Answer: C. Symptom diary

    Explanation: A symptom diary is the initial step in diagnosing PMS, as it helps to establish the pattern and severity of symptoms.

12. Answer: A. Exercise

    Explanation: Regular exercise is recommended as a first-line non-pharmacologic treatment for managing symptoms of PMS.

13. Answer: B. Evening primrose oil

    Explanation: Evening primrose oil has been studied for its potential benefit in reducing symptoms of PMS, including breast tenderness and mood changes.

14. Answer: B. By stabilizing hormone levels

    Explanation: OCPs stabilize hormone levels throughout the menstrual cycle, which can help alleviate PMS symptoms.

15. Answer: A. Acupuncture

    Explanation: Acupuncture has some evidence supporting its effectiveness in reducing PMS symptoms such as irritability and mood swings.

Prostate Cancer

1. Answer: C. Perform transrectal ultrasound-guided biopsy

   Explanation: A PSA level of 10 ng/mL and an abnormal DRE warrant further evaluation with a prostate biopsy to rule out prostate cancer.

2. Answer: B. Repeat PSA measurement in 1 year

   Explanation: In asymptomatic patients with a PSA level of 2 ng/mL, repeat measurement in 1 year is recommended as per guidelines.

3. Answer: A. Perform transrectal ultrasound-guided biopsy

   Explanation: The combination of elevated PSA, bone pain, and palpable prostate nodule suggests advanced prostate cancer; thus, a prostate biopsy is indicated.

4. Answer: A. Perform transrectal ultrasound-guided biopsy

   Explanation: Rising PSA levels after radical prostatectomy indicate biochemical recurrence. A prostate biopsy is needed to assess for local recurrence or metastasis.

5. Answer: A. Perform transrectal ultrasound-guided biopsy

   Explanation: Suspicious findings on MRI and abnormal DRE warrant further evaluation with a prostate biopsy to confirm the diagnosis.

6. Answer: B. Start androgen deprivation therapy

   Explanation: Metastatic prostate cancer with a PSA level of 200 ng/mL should be treated with androgen deprivation therapy to control disease progression.

7. Answer: B. Repeat PSA measurement in 1 year

   Explanation: With a PSA level of 3.5 ng/mL and a normal DRE, repeating the PSA measurement in 1 year is appropriate as per guidelines.

8. Answer: A. Perform transrectal ultrasound-guided biopsy

   Explanation: A PSA level of 15 ng/mL and a palpable prostate nodule warrant further evaluation with a prostate biopsy.

9. Answer: C. Repeat PSA measurement in 6 months

    Explanation: In patients with a PSA level of 6 ng/mL and a normal DRE, repeating the PSA

    measurement in 6 months is appropriate before considering biopsy.

10. Answer: A. Perform transrectal ultrasound-guided biopsy

    Explanation: A PSA level of 3 ng/mL and a palpable nodule on DRE warrant further evaluation with a

    prostate biopsy.

11. Answer: C. Monitor PSA every 6 months

    Explanation: In patients with elevated PSA and normal DRE who are not candidates for immediate

    biopsy, monitoring PSA every 6 months is recommended.

12. Answer: A. Perform transrectal ultrasound-guided biopsy

    Explanation: Hematuria, urinary retention, PSA level of 25 ng/mL, and an irregular prostate contour on

    DRE warrant further evaluation with a prostate biopsy.

13. Answer: A. Perform transrectal ultrasound-guided biopsy

    Explanation: In patients with an elevated PSA and normal DRE, a prostate biopsy is indicated to rule out

    prostate cancer.

14. Answer: A. Perform transrectal ultrasound-guided biopsy

    Explanation: In patients with an elevated PSA and normal DRE, a prostate biopsy is indicated to rule out

    prostate cancer.

15. Answer: A. Perform transrectal ultrasound-guided biopsy

    Explanation: In patients with a strong family history of prostate cancer and an elevated PSA, a prostate

    biopsy is indicated to rule out cancer.

Psoriasis

1. Answer: B. Psoriasis

   Explanation: Psoriasis is characterized by well-demarcated, erythematous plaques with silvery scales, commonly affecting extensor surfaces such as elbows and knees.

2. Answer: B. Psoriasis

   Explanation: Psoriasis commonly affects the scalp and intergluteal cleft with scaly, erythematous plaques and can involve the nails, causing nail pitting and onycholysis.

3. Answer: B. Guttate psoriasis

   Explanation: Guttate psoriasis presents with small, droplike papules and plaques with fine scales, commonly seen on the trunk, arms, legs, and scalp.

4. Answer: A. Psoriasis

   Explanation: Psoriasis typically presents with thick, silver-white scales covering sharply demarcated, erythematous plaques, commonly affecting extensor surfaces and the scalp.

5. Answer: B. Psoriasis

   Explanation: Psoriasis can present as palmoplantar psoriasis, characterized by red, scaly plaques on the palms and soles, which can be itchy and painful.

6. Answer: A. Topical corticosteroids

   Explanation: Topical corticosteroids are the first-line treatment for mild to moderate psoriasis, especially in patients with comorbid conditions like hypertension and diabetes mellitus.

7. Answer: D. Biologic therapy

   Explanation: Severe, widespread psoriasis is typically treated with biologic therapies, which are effective in reducing inflammation and improving symptoms.

8. Answer: B. Phototherapy

   Explanation: Phototherapy (UVB or PUVA) is an appropriate initial treatment for psoriasis affecting localized areas, such as knees and elbows, when topical treatments alone are not sufficient.

9. Answer: A. Topical corticosteroids

   Explanation: Topical corticosteroids are generally considered safe during pregnancy and are the preferred initial treatment for localized psoriasis in pregnant patients.

10. Answer: B. Methotrexate

   Explanation: Methotrexate is an appropriate initial treatment for moderate to severe psoriasis in patients with hepatitis B infection, after proper monitoring and screening.

11. Answer: B. Psoriasis

   Explanation: Psoriasis commonly affects the scalp and can extend to involve the external ear canal, presenting with red, scaly plaques and silvery scales.

12. Answer: B. Seborrheic dermatitis

   Explanation: Seborrheic dermatitis commonly affects the face, particularly the nasolabial folds and eyebrows, with red, scaly plaques and thick, adherent scales.

13. Answer: D. Biologic therapy

   Explanation: Biologic therapies are effective and safe in treating psoriasis in patients with HIV infection, as they do not significantly affect the immune system like other systemic treatments.

14. Answer: C. Acitretin

   Explanation: Acitretin is an appropriate initial treatment for moderate to severe psoriasis in patients with chronic alcohol use disorder, as it does not have significant interactions.

15. Answer: A. Psoriasis

   Explanation: Psoriatic arthritis commonly presents with joint involvement (psoriatic arthropathy) along with skin manifestations such as red, scaly plaques.

Pulmonary Embolism

1. Answer 1: B. Pulmonary embolism

    Explanation: This patient presents with classic symptoms of pulmonary embolism (PE) following a recent surgery, which increases the risk of deep vein thrombosis (DVT) and subsequent PE.

2. Answer 2: B. D-dimer assay

    Explanation: D-dimer assay is a sensitive test for excluding PE in patients with a low or moderate pre-test probability. A positive result would necessitate further imaging such as CTPA.

3. Answer 3: B. Pulmonary embolism

    Explanation: This patient presents with symptoms of acute PE, which is a common complication following long periods of immobility, such as during long flights.

4. Answer 4: D. CT pulmonary angiography (CTPA)

    Explanation: Given the high suspicion for PE in a cancer patient with sudden onset dyspnea and syncope, CTPA is the preferred initial imaging modality.

5. Answer 5: B. Pulmonary embolism

    Explanation: This patient presents with symptoms of acute PE and has a risk factor of oral contraceptive use, which increases the risk of thromboembolic events.

6. Answer 6: A. Pulmonary embolism

    Explanation: This patient has symptoms consistent with acute PE following recent surgery, which increases the risk of developing DVT and subsequent PE.

7. Answer 7: A. Administer oxygen and monitor closely

    Explanation: Initial management of suspected PE includes supportive measures such as oxygen therapy and close monitoring, followed by confirmation with imaging and anticoagulation.

8. Answer 8: A. Start heparin therapy

    Explanation: Despite being on warfarin, this patient presents with symptoms concerning for PE. Heparin therapy should be initiated pending further diagnostic evaluation.

9. Answer 9: D. CT pulmonary angiography (CTPA)

   Explanation: Given the high suspicion for PE in a patient with recent major surgery and acute symptoms, CTPA is the preferred initial imaging modality.

10. Answer 10: B. Pulmonary embolism

    Explanation: This patient presents with symptoms of acute PE following a recent surgery, which is a risk factor for developing DVT and subsequent PE.

11. Answer 11: A. Pulmonary embolism

    Explanation: This patient presents with symptoms suggestive of acute PE following immobility, which is a major risk factor for developing DVT and subsequent PE.

12. Answer 12: D. CT pulmonary angiography (CTPA)

    Explanation: Given the high suspicion for PE in a cancer patient with acute symptoms, CTPA is the preferred initial imaging modality.

13. Answer 13: B. Pulmonary embolism

    Explanation: This patient presents with symptoms of acute PE and has a history of lupus, which is a risk factor for developing thromboembolic events.

14. Answer 14: B. Start anticoagulation therapy

    Explanation: Pregnancy is a risk factor for developing venous thromboembolism, including PE. Anticoagulation therapy should be initiated promptly.

15. Answer 15: B. D-dimer assay

    Explanation: D-dimer assay is a sensitive test for excluding PE in patients with low or moderate pre-test probability, such as in this patient with COPD.

Rheumatoid Arthritis

1. Answer 1: B. Rheumatoid arthritis

   Explanation: This patient's symptoms are classic for rheumatoid arthritis, including symmetrical joint involvement, morning stiffness, and rheumatoid nodules.

2. Answer 2: A. Anti-cyclic citrullinated peptide (anti-CCP) antibodies

   Explanation: Anti-CCP antibodies are highly specific for rheumatoid arthritis, while RF can also be positive in other conditions. ESR and ANA are less specific.

3. Answer 3: D. Anti-Ro (SSA) antibodies

   Explanation: Anti-Ro (SSA) antibodies can be found in both rheumatoid arthritis and Sjögren's syndrome, which commonly coexist.

4. Answer 4: D. Fibrinoid necrosis of small vessels

   Explanation: Rheumatoid nodules are caused by fibrinoid necrosis of small vessels in affected tissues, resulting in granulomatous inflammation.

5. Answer 5: C. Pulmonary nodules

   Explanation: Rheumatoid arthritis can present with extra-articular manifestations, including pulmonary nodules, which are more common in patients with severe disease.

6. Answer 6: C. C-reactive protein (CRP)

   Explanation: CRP is an acute phase reactant that reflects systemic inflammation and is used to assess disease activity and response to treatment in rheumatoid arthritis.

7. Answer 7: A. Methotrexate

   Explanation: Methotrexate is contraindicated in patients with significant renal impairment due to its potential nephrotoxicity.

8. Answer 8: A. X-ray

   Explanation: X-ray imaging can show characteristic joint changes such as periarticular osteopenia, joint space narrowing, and erosions, which are typical in rheumatoid arthritis.

9. Answer 9: A. Subchondral cysts

    Explanation: Subchondral cysts, joint space narrowing, and erosions are common radiographic findings in rheumatoid arthritis.

10. Answer 10: C. Anti-Ro (SSA) antibodies

    Explanation: Anti-Ro (SSA) antibodies are commonly found in both rheumatoid arthritis and Sjögren's syndrome, which frequently coexist.

11. Answer 11: B. Smoking

    Explanation: Smoking is a well-established environmental risk factor for developing rheumatoid arthritis, especially in genetically predisposed individuals.

12. Answer 12: A. Proximal interphalangeal (PIP) joints

    Explanation: Rheumatoid arthritis typically involves small joints symmetrically, including the PIP joints, metacarpophalangeal (MCP) joints, and wrists.

13. Answer 13: D. Rheumatoid nodules

    Explanation: Rheumatoid nodules are a common extra-articular manifestation of rheumatoid arthritis, typically located over extensor surfaces.

14. Answer 14: A. Methotrexate

    Explanation: Methotrexate is contraindicated in patients with significant renal impairment due to its potential nephrotoxicity.

15. Answer 15: D. Depression

    Explanation: Depression is a common comorbidity associated with rheumatoid arthritis, likely due to the chronic pain and disability associated with the disease.

Rosacea

1. Answer 1: B. Rosacea

   Explanation: Rosacea presents with facial redness, small red papules or pustules, and flushing, often triggered by factors like sun exposure or spicy foods.

2. Answer 2: C. Phymatous rosacea

   Explanation: Phymatous rosacea is characterized by thickening of the skin and irregular surface nodularities, commonly affecting the nose (rhinophyma).

3. Answer 3: A. Erythematotelangiectatic rosacea

   Explanation: Erythematotelangiectatic rosacea presents with persistent facial redness, flushing, and visible blood vessels (telangiectasias), often triggered by emotional stress.

4. Answer 4: B. Papulopustular rosacea

   Explanation: Papulopustular rosacea is characterized by facial redness, papules, and pustules, with symptoms of burning and stinging.

5. Answer 5: C. Ocular rosacea

   Explanation: Ocular rosacea presents with red, irritated eyes, eyelid swelling, and potential complications like conjunctivitis and blepharitis.

6. Answer 6: D. All of the above

   Explanation: Rosacea symptoms can be triggered by various factors, including sun exposure, cold weather, emotional stress, spicy foods, and certain skin care products.

7. Answer 7: B. Topical metronidazole

   Explanation: Topical metronidazole is a first-line treatment for rosacea, especially for reducing inflammatory lesions and erythema.

8. Answer 8: B. Permanent facial scarring

   Explanation: Untreated or severe phymatous rosacea can lead to permanent facial scarring, such as rhinophyma, due to the thickening and irregular surface nodularities.

9. Answer 9: D. Ocular rosacea

   Explanation: Ocular rosacea presents with red, irritated eyes, eyelid swelling, and potential complications like conjunctivitis and blepharitis.

10. Answer 10: C. Spicy foods

    Explanation: Spicy foods are a common trigger for exacerbating rosacea symptoms, including facial redness and papulopustular lesions.

11. Answer 11: A. Erythematotelangiectatic rosacea

    Explanation: Erythematotelangiectatic rosacea presents with persistent facial redness, flushing, and visible blood vessels (telangiectasias), often triggered by emotional stress.

12. Answer 12: D. Topical metronidazole

    Explanation: Topical metronidazole is a first-line treatment for rosacea, especially for reducing inflammatory lesions and erythema.

13. Answer 13: B. Permanent facial scarring

    Explanation: Untreated or severe phymatous rosacea can lead to permanent facial scarring, such as rhinophyma, due to the thickening and irregular surface nodularities.

14. Answer 14: D. Ocular rosacea

    Explanation: Ocular rosacea presents with red, irritated eyes, eyelid swelling, and potential complications like conjunctivitis and blepharitis.

15. Answer 15: B. Papulopustular rosacea

    Explanation: Papulopustular rosacea is characterized by facial redness, papules, and pustules, with symptoms of burning and stinging.

Schizophrenia

1. Answer: B. Schizophrenia

   Explanation: Auditory hallucinations, disorganized speech, and social withdrawal are characteristic symptoms of schizophrenia.

2. Answer: D. Schizophrenia

   Explanation: Delusions of persecution and disorganized behavior are common symptoms of schizophrenia.

3. Answer: B. Schizotypal personality disorder

   Explanation: Schizotypal personality disorder is characterized by odd beliefs, magical thinking, and social isolation, but lacks the severity and duration required for a diagnosis of schizophrenia.

4. Answer: A. Haloperidol

   Explanation: Haloperidol, an antipsychotic medication, is indicated for the treatment of schizophrenia, especially for symptoms like hallucinations and delusions.

5. Answer: B. Schizophrenia, disorganized type

   Explanation: Disorganized speech, flat affect, and social withdrawal are characteristic of disorganized type schizophrenia.

6. Answer: C. Schizophrenia, catatonic type

   Explanation: Catatonic symptoms, such as mutism and rigid posture, are characteristic of catatonic type schizophrenia.

7. Answer: A. Start antipsychotic medication

   Explanation: Antipsychotic medication is the first-line treatment for acute psychosis, including the first episode of schizophrenia.

8. Answer: A. Increase the dose of the current antipsychotic medication

   Explanation: Worsening of negative symptoms in schizophrenia may warrant an increase in the dose of the current antipsychotic medication.

9. Answer: B. Administer lorazepam

    Explanation: Lorazepam, a benzodiazepine, can be used to manage acute agitation in schizophrenia patients.

10. Answer: B. Switch to a long-acting injectable antipsychotic medication

    Explanation: Long-acting injectable antipsychotic medications can improve adherence in patients with schizophrenia who are non-compliant with oral medications.

11. Answer: A. Increase the dose of the current antipsychotic medication

    Explanation: Visual hallucinations and paranoid delusions indicate an exacerbation of positive symptoms, which may require an increase in the dose of the current antipsychotic medication.

12. Answer: D. Increase the dose of the current antipsychotic medication

    Explanation: Worsening of symptoms in a compliant patient may warrant an increase in the dose of the current antipsychotic medication.

13. Answer: A. Switch to a long-acting injectable antipsychotic medication

    Explanation: Long-acting injectable antipsychotic medications can improve adherence in patients with schizophrenia who are non-compliant with oral medications.

14. Answer: A. Increase the dose of the current antipsychotic medication

    Explanation: Exacerbation of positive symptoms may require an increase in the dose of the current antipsychotic medication.

15. Answer: B. Switch to a different class of antipsychotic medication

    Explanation: Worsening of negative symptoms may warrant a trial of a different class of antipsychotic medication.

Seasonal Affective Disorder (SAD)

1. Answer: C) Seasonal Affective Disorder (SAD)

   Explanation: SAD is characterized by recurrent episodes of major depression that occur during specific seasons, usually fall and winter, and remit in spring and summer.

2. Answer: D) Seasonal Affective Disorder (SAD)

   Explanation: SAD is characterized by recurrent episodes of depression that occur during specific seasons, typically fall and winter.

3. Answer: D) Seasonal Affective Disorder (SAD)

   Explanation: SAD is characterized by recurrent depressive episodes that follow a seasonal pattern, usually starting in fall or winter and remitting in spring or summer.

4. Answer: C) Light therapy

   Explanation: Light therapy is a first-line treatment for Seasonal Affective Disorder (SAD), particularly for those experiencing depressive symptoms during fall and winter.

5. Answer: D) Seasonal Affective Disorder (SAD)

   Explanation: SAD can occur in the spring and summer months, although it is less common than fall and winter onset. Symptoms often include depression, low energy, and changes in sleep and appetite.

6. Answer: C) Seasonal Affective Disorder (SAD)

   Explanation: SAD is characterized by recurrent episodes of depression that follow a seasonal pattern, most commonly in fall and winter.

7. Answer: D) Light therapy

   Explanation: Light therapy is a recommended treatment for Seasonal Affective Disorder (SAD), especially for those experiencing depressive symptoms during fall and winter.

8. Answer: D) Initiate light therapy

   Explanation: For patients with SAD, light therapy is an effective treatment option and can be used as an adjunct to antidepressant medication.

9. Answer: D) Seasonal Affective Disorder (SAD)

    Explanation: SAD is characterized by recurrent depressive episodes that follow a seasonal pattern, typically in fall and winter.

10. Answer: D) Light therapy

    Explanation: Light therapy is a first-line treatment for Seasonal Affective Disorder (SAD), especially for those experiencing depressive symptoms during fall and winter.

11. Answer: D) Seasonal Affective Disorder (SAD)

    Explanation: SAD is characterized by recurrent depressive episodes that follow a seasonal pattern, most commonly in fall and winter.

12. Answer: D) Light therapy

    Explanation: Light therapy is a recommended treatment for Seasonal Affective Disorder (SAD), especially for those experiencing depressive symptoms during fall and winter.

13. Answer: D) Seasonal Affective Disorder (SAD)

    Explanation: SAD is characterized by recurrent episodes of depression that follow a seasonal pattern, most commonly in fall and winter.

14. Answer: D) Seasonal Affective Disorder (SAD)

    Explanation: SAD is characterized by recurrent episodes of depression that follow a seasonal pattern, most commonly in fall and winter.

15. Answer: D) Light therapy

    Explanation: Light therapy is a first-line treatment for Seasonal Affective Disorder (SAD), especially for those experiencing depressive symptoms during fall and winter.

Sickle Cell Disease

1. Answer:A)Vaso-occlusive crisis

   Explanation: Severe pain in the arms and legs, fever, and tenderness over long bones are characteristic of vaso-occlusive crisis in sickle cell disease.

2. Answer:B) Acute chest syndrome

   Explanation: Sudden onset chest pain, cough, dyspnea, tachypnea, and hypoxia are characteristic of acute chest syndrome in sickle cell disease.

3. Answer:D) Cervical lymphadenitis

   Explanation: Fever, sore throat, difficulty swallowing, neck swelling, and tenderness are suggestive of cervical lymphadenitis in sickle cell disease.

4. Answer:C) Aplastic crisis

   Explanation: Pallor, fatigue, weakness, dizziness, tachycardia, and evidence of transient aplastic crisis (decreased reticulocyte count) are characteristic findings.

5. Answer:D) Splenic sequestration crisis

   Explanation: Sudden onset severe abdominal pain and distension, hypotension, and a palpable spleen are characteristic of splenic sequestration crisis.

6. Answer:A)Deep vein thrombosis

   Explanation: Pain, swelling, calf tenderness, and erythema in the leg are suggestive of deep vein thrombosis in a patient with sickle cell disease.

7. Answer:D) Ocular infarction

   Explanation: Pain in the eye, decreased vision, conjunctival injection, and a cherry-red spot on the retina suggest ocular infarction in sickle cell disease.

8. Answer:B) Acute hepatic sequestration crisis

   Explanation: Sudden onset severe abdominal pain, tenderness over the liver, and jaundice suggest acute hepatic sequestration crisis in sickle cell disease.

9. Answer:B) Acute chest syndrome

    Explanation: Fever, cough, pleuritic chest pain, decreased breath sounds, and dullness to percussion suggest acute chest syndrome in sickle cell disease.

10. Answer:B) Vaso-occlusive crisis

    Explanation: Bone pain, tenderness, swelling, and warmth over the right humerus are characteristic of vaso-occlusive crisis in sickle cell disease.

11. Answer:B) DVT

    Explanation: Pain, swelling, erythema, warmth over the calf, and confirmation of DVT on Doppler ultrasound suggest deep vein thrombosis.

12. Answer:C) Aplastic crisis

    Explanation: Fever, oliguria, hypotension, pallor, and severe anemia (hemoglobin 6 g/dL) suggest aplastic crisis in sickle cell disease.

13. Answer:B) Acute hepatic sequestration crisis

    Explanation: Sudden onset severe abdominal pain, tenderness over the liver, and increased bilirubin levels suggest acute hepatic sequestration crisis in sickle cell disease.

14. Answer:D) Cellulitis

    Explanation: Acute onset severe pain, swelling, erythema, and warmth in the right leg are characteristic of cellulitis in sickle cell disease.

15. Answer:A)Meningitis

    Explanation: Fever, headache, altered mental status, and nuchal rigidity are characteristic of meningitis in sickle cell disease.

Sinusitis

1. Answer: B. Acute bacterial sinusitis

    Explanation: Acute bacterial sinusitis presents with facial pain and pressure, purulent nasal discharge, and fever, typically following a viral upper respiratory infection.

2. Answer: C. Chronic sinusitis

    Explanation: Chronic sinusitis is diagnosed when symptoms persist for more than 12 weeks, often accompanied by nasal congestion, facial pain, and postnasal drip.

3. Answer: C. Antibiotics

    Explanation: Acute bacterial sinusitis is treated with antibiotics if symptoms persist for more than 10 days or worsen after an initial period of improvement.

4. Answer: A. Acute bacterial sinusitis

    Explanation: Acute bacterial sinusitis commonly follows a viral upper respiratory infection and presents with fever, facial pain, and purulent nasal discharge.

5. Answer: C. Chronic sinusitis

    Explanation: Chronic sinusitis is characterized by symptoms persisting for more than 12 weeks, including nasal congestion, facial pain, and thick nasal discharge.

6. Answer: B. Maxillary sinus

    Explanation: The maxillary sinus is the most commonly affected sinus in acute bacterial sinusitis, causing pain and pressure over the cheeks and teeth.

7. Answer: B. Chronic sinusitis

    Explanation: Chronic sinusitis is characterized by symptoms lasting more than 12 weeks, which may be associated with nasal polyps and recurrent infections.

8. Answer: B. Allergic rhinitis

    Explanation: Allergic rhinitis commonly presents with nasal congestion, sneezing, and postnasal drip, often associated with allergies to dust, pollen, or other allergens.

9. Answer: C. Chronic sinusitis with nasal polyps

   Explanation: Chronic sinusitis with nasal polyps presents with symptoms such as nasal congestion, facial pain, and headaches, often accompanied by polyps visible on nasal exam.

10. Answer: C. Orbital cellulitis

    Explanation: Orbital cellulitis is a serious complication of sinusitis characterized by periorbital swelling, proptosis, fever, and difficulty with eye movements.

11. Answer: B. Topical nasal corticosteroid spray

    Explanation: Topical nasal corticosteroids are often used as initial therapy in chronic sinusitis to reduce inflammation and improve symptoms.

12. Answer: D. Aspirin-exacerbated respiratory disease (AERD)

    Explanation: Aspirin-exacerbated respiratory disease (AERD) is characterized by chronic rhinosinusitis, nasal polyps, asthma, and aspirin sensitivity.

13. Answer: A. CT scan of the sinuses

    Explanation: CT scan of the sinuses is the imaging modality of choice for evaluating sinusitis, providing detailed images of the paranasal sinuses.

14. Answer: A. Change to a different class of antibiotics

    Explanation: If symptoms of acute bacterial sinusitis do not improve after 10-14 days of initial antibiotic therapy, changing to a different class of antibiotics is recommended.

15. Answer: A. By reducing inflammation and shrinking polyps

    Explanation: Intranasal corticosteroids reduce inflammation and help shrink nasal polyps, improving symptoms of chronic sinusitis.

Stroke

1. Answer: B. Ischemic stroke

   Explanation: Ischemic stroke is characterized by sudden onset neurological deficits due to a blockage of blood flow to the brain.

2. Answer: C. Hemorrhagic stroke

   Explanation: Hemorrhagic stroke occurs due to bleeding in the brain, leading to sudden onset of symptoms like severe headache, nausea, and vomiting.

3. Answer: C. Transient ischemic attack (TIA)

   Explanation: TIAs are transient episodes of neurological dysfunction caused by temporary focal ischemia without acute infarction.

4. Answer: A. IV thrombolysis with alteplase

   Explanation: IV thrombolysis with alteplase is the standard of care for eligible patients presenting within 4.5 hours of symptom onset with acute ischemic stroke.

5. Answer: B. Hemorrhagic stroke

   Explanation: Hemorrhagic stroke typically presents with sudden severe headache, altered mental status, and focal neurological deficits due to bleeding in the brain.

6. Answer: B. Cardiogenic embolism

   Explanation: Cardiogenic embolism, often from atrial fibrillation, is a common cause of ischemic stroke due to emboli from the heart.

7. Answer: C. Non-contrast CT scan of the brain

   Explanation: A non-contrast CT scan of the brain is the initial imaging study to evaluate for hemorrhagic stroke and to assess for early signs of ischemic stroke.

8. Answer: A. Time of symptom onset

   Explanation: Time of symptom onset is crucial for determining eligibility for thrombolytic therapy, with the window typically being within 4.5 hours from symptom onset.

9. Answer: A. Left middle cerebral artery

   Explanation: Left middle cerebral artery territory stroke typically presents with right hemiparesis and right gaze preference due to cortical and subcortical involvement.

10. Answer: D. Non-contrast CT scan of the brain

    Explanation: A non-contrast CT scan of the brain is the initial imaging study to evaluate for hemorrhagic stroke and guide management.

11. Answer: A. Atherosclerosis

    Explanation: Atherosclerosis causing carotid artery stenosis is a common cause of ischemic stroke, particularly in patients with risk factors such as hypertension and smoking.

12. Answer: C. Non-contrast CT scan of the brain

    Explanation: A non-contrast CT scan of the brain is the initial imaging study to evaluate for hemorrhagic stroke and early signs of ischemic stroke.

13. Answer: A. Large artery atherosclerosis

    Explanation: Large artery atherosclerosis is a common cause of ischemic stroke, especially in patients with risk factors such as smoking and hyperlipidemia.

14. Answer: C. Anticoagulation therapy

    Explanation: Anticoagulation therapy is indicated for patients with atrial fibrillation to prevent cardiogenic embolism and recurrent ischemic stroke.

15. Answer: D. Non-contrast CT scan of the brain

    Explanation: A non-contrast CT scan of the brain is the initial imaging study to evaluate for hemorrhagic stroke and assess for early signs of ischemic stroke.

Systemic Lupus Erythematosus (SLE)

1. Answer: B. Systemic Lupus Erythematosus (SLE)

    Explanation: SLE commonly presents with a butterfly-shaped rash (malar rash), fatigue, joint pain, and positive ANA and anti-dsDNA antibodies.

2. Answer: B. Systemic Lupus Erythematosus (SLE)

    Explanation: Oral ulcers, photosensitivity, arthritis, positive ANA, and anti-Sm antibodies are characteristic of SLE.

3. Answer: B. Systemic Lupus Erythematosus (SLE)

    Explanation: Rash worsened by sun exposure (photosensitivity), joint pain, hair loss, positive ANA, and anti-Ro (SSA) antibodies are characteristic of SLE.

4. Answer: B. Systemic Lupus Erythematosus (SLE)

    Explanation: Fever, weight loss, malar rash, low complement levels, positive ANA, and anti-dsDNA antibodies are characteristic of SLE.

5. Answer: B. Systemic Lupus Erythematosus (SLE)

    Explanation: Fatigue, hair loss, malar rash worsened by sun exposure, oral ulcers, arthritis, positive ANA, and anti-dsDNA antibodies are characteristic of SLE.

6. Answer: C. Sjögren's syndrome

    Explanation: Dry eyes, dry mouth, fatigue, positive ANA, and anti-Ro (SSA) antibodies are characteristic of Sjögren's syndrome.

7. Answer: B. Systemic Lupus Erythematosus (SLE)

    Explanation: Fatigue, joint pain, malar rash, mouth ulcers, alopecia, low complement levels, positive ANA, and anti-dsDNA antibodies are characteristic of SLE.

8. Answer: B. Systemic Lupus Erythematosus (SLE)

    Explanation: Joint pain, fatigue, malar rash, photosensitivity, hair loss, positive ANA, and anti-Smith (anti-Sm) antibodies are characteristic of SLE.

9. Answer: B. Systemic Lupus Erythematosus (SLE)

    Explanation: Chest pain, shortness of breath, malar rash, oral ulcers, joint pain, positive ANA, anti-dsDNA antibodies, and pericarditis are characteristic of SLE.

10. Answer: B. Systemic Lupus Erythematosus (SLE)

    Explanation: Fatigue, joint pain, malar rash, oral ulcers, alopecia, low complement levels, positive ANA, and anti-dsDNA antibodies are characteristic of SLE.

11. Answer: B. Systemic Lupus Erythematosus (SLE)

    Explanation: Fever, joint pain, malar rash, oral ulcers, fatigue, positive ANA, and anti-dsDNA antibodies are characteristic of SLE.

12. Answer: D. Antiphospholipid syndrome

    Explanation: Headache, visual disturbances, joint pain, fatigue, malar rash, positive ANA, and anti-dsDNA antibodies can be seen in SLE, but the presence of antiphospholipid antibodies would suggest coexisting antiphospholipid syndrome.

13. Answer: B. Systemic Lupus Erythematosus (SLE)

    Explanation: Fever, joint pain, malar rash, oral ulcers, hair loss, low complement levels, positive ANA, and anti-dsDNA antibodies are characteristic of SLE.

14. Answer: B. Systemic Lupus Erythematosus (SLE)

    Explanation: Fatigue, joint pain, malar rash, oral ulcers, photosensitivity, positive ANA, and anti-Ro (SSA) antibodies are characteristic of SLE.

15. Answer: B. Systemic Lupus Erythematosus (SLE)

    Explanation: Fever, joint pain, malar rash, oral ulcers, hair loss, low complement levels, positive ANA, and anti-dsDNA antibodies are characteristic of SLE.

Testicular Cancer

1. Answer: C. Testicular cancer

   Explanation: Testicular cancer typically presents as a painless, firm mass within the testicle. It is important to differentiate from other causes of scrotal mass.

2. Answer: A. Ultrasound of the scrotum

   Explanation: Ultrasound of the scrotum is the initial investigation of choice to evaluate testicular masses and is highly sensitive for detecting testicular tumors.

3. Answer: A. Seminoma

   Explanation: Seminomas are a type of germ cell tumor that commonly present with elevated β-hCG and LDH levels, but normal AFP levels.

4. Answer: B. Embryonal carcinoma

   Explanation: Embryonal carcinoma is a non-seminomatous germ cell tumor that commonly presents with elevated AFP and β-hCG levels.

5. Answer: A. Seminoma

   Explanation: Seminomas typically present with normal serum markers (AFP, β-hCG, LDH), distinguishing them from non-seminomatous germ cell tumors.

6. Answer: A. Yolk sac tumor

   Explanation: Yolk sac tumors (endodermal sinus tumors) are a type of non-seminomatous germ cell tumor that commonly presents with elevated AFP levels.

7. Answer: B. Embryonal carcinoma

   Explanation: Embryonal carcinoma is a non-seminomatous germ cell tumor that commonly presents with elevated β-hCG and LDH levels.

8. Answer: C. Choriocarcinoma

   Explanation: Choriocarcinoma is a rare type of germ cell tumor that can present with elevated β-hCG levels, distinguishing it from other testicular tumors.

9. Answer: A. Seminoma

   Explanation: Seminomas typically present with normal serum markers (AFP, β-hCG, LDH), distinguishing them from non-seminomatous germ cell tumors.

10. Answer: A. Yolk sac tumor

    Explanation: Yolk sac tumors (endodermal sinus tumors) are a type of non-seminomatous germ cell tumor that commonly presents with elevated AFP levels.

11. Answer: B. Embryonal carcinoma

    Explanation: Embryonal carcinoma is a non-seminomatous germ cell tumor that commonly presents with elevated β-hCG and LDH levels.

12. Answer: C. Choriocarcinoma

    Explanation: Choriocarcinoma is a rare type of germ cell tumor that can present with elevated β-hCG levels, distinguishing it from other testicular tumors.

13. Answer: A. Seminoma

    Explanation: Seminomas typically present with normal serum markers (AFP, β-hCG, LDH), distinguishing them from non-seminomatous germ cell tumors.

14. Answer: A. Yolk sac tumor

    Explanation: Yolk sac tumors (endodermal sinus tumors) are a type of non-seminomatous germ cell tumor that commonly presents with elevated AFP levels.

15. Answer: B. Embryonal carcinoma

    Explanation: Embryonal carcinoma is a non-seminomatous germ cell tumor that commonly presents with elevated β-hCG and LDH levels.

Thyroid Cancer

1. Answer: A. Total thyroidectomy

   Explanation: Total thyroidectomy is the recommended initial treatment for papillary thyroid carcinoma to remove the primary tumor.

2. Answer: C. Repeat FNAB with molecular testing

   Explanation: Follicular neoplasms on FNAB require molecular testing (e.g., BRAF, RAS mutations) to help determine if surgical resection (total thyroidectomy) is necessary.

3. Answer: B. Chemotherapy and radiation therapy

   Explanation: Anaplastic thyroid carcinoma is aggressive, and initial management involves chemotherapy and radiation therapy due to the poor prognosis and lack of benefit from surgery.

4. Answer: A. Total thyroidectomy with central neck dissection

   Explanation: Medullary thyroid carcinoma requires total thyroidectomy with central neck dissection due to the risk of lymph node involvement.

5. Answer: B. Chemotherapy and radiation therapy

   Explanation: Lymphoma involving the thyroid gland is managed with chemotherapy and radiation therapy, not surgery.

6. Answer: A. Total thyroidectomy

   Explanation: Total thyroidectomy is recommended for follicular variant of papillary thyroid carcinoma due to the increased risk of recurrence and metastasis.

7. Answer: B. Graves' disease

   Explanation: Graves' disease is the most common cause of hyperthyroidism and diffuse goiter in young patients.

8. Answer: C. Trial of radioactive iodine (RAI) therapy

   Explanation: Radioactive iodine therapy can be used for management of thyroid nodules in patients who are not surgical candidates, especially if the nodule is hyperfunctioning or has suspicious cytology.

9. Answer: A. Total thyroidectomy

   Explanation: Hurthle cell neoplasms are indeterminate on FNAB and require surgical resection (total thyroidectomy) for definitive diagnosis and treatment.

10. Answer: A. Total thyroidectomy

    Explanation: BRAF V600E mutation is associated with aggressive behavior in papillary thyroid carcinoma, and total thyroidectomy is recommended.

11. Answer: A. Total thyroidectomy

    Explanation: Follicular neoplasms with RAS mutations are associated with a higher risk of malignancy, and total thyroidectomy is recommended.

12. Answer: C. Observation with repeat FNAB in 6 months

    Explanation: Follicular adenomas are benign, and observation with repeat FNAB is appropriate to monitor for any changes.

13. Answer: C. Observation with periodic follow-up

    Explanation: Benign cytology on FNAB does not require immediate intervention. Observation with periodic follow-up is appropriate.

14. Answer: A. Total thyroidectomy with central neck dissection

    Explanation: Medullary thyroid carcinoma requires surgical resection (total thyroidectomy with central neck dissection) due to the high risk of lymph node involvement.

15. Answer: B. Chemotherapy and radiation therapy

    Explanation: Lymphoma involving the thyroid gland is managed with chemotherapy and radiation therapy, not surgery.

Ulcerative Colitis

1. Answer: B. Ulcerative colitis

   Explanation: Ulcerative colitis typically presents with bloody diarrhea, abdominal cramps, and weight loss, often in young adults without a family history of gastrointestinal diseases.

2. Answer: C. Continuous colonic involvement with friable mucosa and pseudopolyps

   Explanation: Ulcerative colitis typically presents with continuous colonic involvement starting from the rectum, with a characteristic appearance of friable mucosa and pseudopolyps.

3. Answer: A. Toxic megacolon

   Explanation: Fever, abdominal pain, leukocytosis, and abdominal tenderness in a patient with ulcerative colitis suggest toxic megacolon, a serious complication that requires urgent management.

4. Answer: A. Reactive arthritis (Reiter's syndrome)

   Explanation: Reactive arthritis is associated with ulcerative colitis and presents with asymmetric oligoarthritis, often involving the lower extremities, along with extra-articular manifestations like uveitis.

5. Answer: C. Systemic corticosteroids

   Explanation: Pyoderma gangrenosum-like lesions in patients with ulcerative colitis are managed with systemic corticosteroids.

6. Answer: C. Azathioprine-induced myelosuppression

   Explanation: Azathioprine can cause myelosuppression, leading to symptoms such as diarrhea and abdominal pain.

7. Answer: A. Perianal fistula

   Explanation: In ulcerative colitis, perianal fistulas can develop and present with symptoms of pain, fever, and pus collection adjacent to the colon.

8. Answer: D. Start infliximab

   Explanation: In patients with refractory ulcerative colitis, biologic therapies such as infliximab (anti-TNF therapy) may be indicated.

9. Answer: C. Start mesalamine suppositories

   Explanation: Mesalamine is often used as first-line treatment for mild to moderate ulcerative colitis in pregnancy.

10. Answer: C. Continuous involvement with pseudopolyps

    Explanation: Pseudopolyps are a characteristic endoscopic finding in ulcerative colitis, representing areas of mucosal regeneration.

11. Answer: C. Ankylosing spondylitis

    Explanation: Ankylosing spondylitis is an extraintestinal manifestation associated with ulcerative colitis.

12. Answer: A. Toxic megacolon

    Explanation: Toxic megacolon is a serious complication of ulcerative colitis characterized by colonic dilatation, fever, and abdominal pain.

13. Answer: A. Intravenous fluids and antibiotics

    Explanation: This patient presents with symptoms suggestive of severe colitis and should initially receive intravenous fluids and antibiotics.

14. Answer: A. Surgical drainage

    Explanation: Perianal abscesses in patients with ulcerative colitis often require surgical drainage.

15. Answer: B. Pleuritis

    Explanation: Pleuritis can occur as an extraintestinal manifestation in patients with ulcerative colitis.

Urinary Tract Infection (UTI)

1. Answer: C. Nitrofurantoin

   Explanation: Nitrofurantoin is a first-line agent for uncomplicated lower urinary tract infections (UTIs) in non-pregnant women.

2. Answer: B. Obtain a urine culture and start antibiotics

   Explanation: This patient likely has acute uncomplicated pyelonephritis. Empirical antibiotics should cover both gram-negative rods and enterococci until culture results are available.

3. Answer: A. Empirical treatment with TMP/SMX

   Explanation: This patient likely has catheter-associated UTI. Empirical treatment should cover common pathogens including Escherichia coli and Enterococcus species.

4. Answer: B. Amoxicillin-clavulanate

   Explanation: Nitrofurantoin and TMP/SMX are contraindicated in pregnancy due to potential fetal harm. Amoxicillin-clavulanate is safe and effective for treating UTIs in pregnancy.

5. Answer: B. Obtain a urine culture and start antibiotics

   Explanation: Diabetic patients with UTI are at higher risk for complicated UTI. Empirical antibiotics should cover gram-negative rods and enterococci until culture results are available.

6. Answer: A. Empirical treatment with TMP/SMX

   Explanation: This patient likely has a UTI with risk factors for complicated infection (benign prostatic hyperplasia). Empirical treatment should cover common pathogens including Escherichia coli and enterococci.

7. Answer: B. Obtain a urine culture and start antibiotics

   Explanation: This patient likely has uncomplicated cystitis. Empirical treatment should cover common pathogens including Escherichia coli and enterococci until culture results are available.

AI PLUS EXAM REVIEW

8. Answer: D. Start intravenous vancomycin

   Explanation: This patient likely has catheter-associated UTI with signs of systemic infection. Initial broad-spectrum antibiotics should cover gram-negative rods and enterococci until culture results are available.

9. Answer: B. Obtain a urine culture and start antibiotics

   Explanation: This patient likely has uncomplicated recurrent UTIs. Empirical antibiotics should cover common pathogens until culture results are available.

10. Answer: D. Start intravenous piperacillin-tazobactam

    Explanation: Renal transplant recipients with UTI are at risk for severe infections. Initial broad-spectrum antibiotics should cover gram-negative rods and enterococci until culture results are available.

11. Answer: B. Obtain a urine culture and start antibiotics

    Explanation: This patient likely has acute uncomplicated pyelonephritis. Empirical antibiotics should cover both gram-negative rods and enterococci until culture results are available.

12. Answer: D. Remove urinary catheter and start ciprofloxacin

    Explanation: This patient likely has catheter-associated UTI. Immediate removal of the urinary catheter and initiation of broad-spectrum antibiotics are indicated.

13. Answer: B. Amoxicillin-clavulanate

    Explanation: Nitrofurantoin and TMP/SMX are contraindicated in pregnancy due to potential fetal harm. Amoxicillin-clavulanate is safe and effective for treating UTIs in pregnancy.

14. Answer: B. Obtain a urine culture and start antibiotics

    Explanation: Diabetic patients with UTI are at higher risk for complicated UTI. Empirical antibiotics should cover gram-negative rods and enterococci until culture results are available.

15. Answer: A. Empirical treatment with TMP/SMX

    Explanation: This patient likely has a UTI with risk factors for complicated infection (benign prostatic hyperplasia). Empirical treatment should cover common pathogens including Escherichia coli and enterococci.

Venous Thromboembolism (VTE)

1. Answer: A. Deep vein thrombosis (DVT)

   Explanation: The classic presentation of DVT includes unilateral leg swelling, pain, warmth, and tenderness. Risk factors such as recent surgery increase suspicion for DVT.

2. Answer: D. Perform a CT pulmonary angiography (CTPA)

   Explanation: A Wells score of 5 indicates high clinical probability of pulmonary embolism (PE), warranting immediate imaging with CTPA.

3. Answer: B. Compression ultrasonography of the right leg

   Explanation: Compression ultrasonography is the preferred initial test for diagnosing DVT in patients with suspected lower extremity symptoms.

4. Answer: B. Pulmonary embolism (PE)

   Explanation: The combination of sudden dyspnea, chest pain, and risk factors such as recent surgery raises suspicion for PE.

5. Answer: C. CTPA

   Explanation: In patients with suspected PE and high clinical suspicion, CTPA is the imaging modality of choice to confirm the diagnosis.

6. Answer: D. Perform a CTPA

   Explanation: Pleuritic chest pain and hemoptysis in a high-risk patient suggest PE, requiring immediate CTPA to confirm the diagnosis.

7. Answer: B. Compression ultrasonography of the left leg

   Explanation: Compression ultrasonography is the preferred initial test for diagnosing DVT in patients with suspected lower extremity symptoms.

8. Answer: D. Perform a CTPA

   Explanation: A Wells score of 4 indicates moderate clinical probability of PE, necessitating immediate imaging with CTPA.

9. Answer: D. Perform a compression ultrasonography of the right leg

    Explanation: Compression ultrasonography is the initial test of choice for diagnosing DVT in patients with suspected lower extremity symptoms.

10. Answer: C. CTPA

    Explanation: In patients with suspected PE and high clinical suspicion, CTPA is the imaging modality of choice to confirm the diagnosis.

11. Answer: C. CTPA

    Explanation: In patients with suspected PE and high clinical suspicion, CTPA is the imaging modality of choice to confirm the diagnosis.

12. Answer: D. Perform a CTPA

    Explanation: Pleuritic chest pain and hemoptysis in a high-risk patient suggest PE, requiring immediate CTPA to confirm the diagnosis.

13. Answer: B. Compression ultrasonography of the left leg

    Explanation: Compression ultrasonography is the preferred initial test for diagnosing DVT in patients with suspected lower extremity symptoms.

14. Answer: D. Perform a CTPA

    Explanation: A Wells score of 4 indicates moderate clinical probability of PE, necessitating immediate imaging with CTPA.

15. Answer: D. Perform a compression ultrasonography of the right leg

    Explanation: Compression ultrasonography is the initial test of choice for diagnosing DVT in patients with suspected lower extremity symptoms.

Vitiligo

1. Answer: C) Vitiligo

   Explanation: Vitiligo presents with depigmented patches that progressively increase in size. It is an autoimmune condition where melanocytes are destroyed, leading to loss of skin pigmentation.

2. Answer: A) Autoimmune destruction of melanocytes

   Explanation: Vitiligo is an autoimmune disorder where the immune system mistakenly attacks melanocytes, leading to depigmentation of the skin.

3. Answer: B) Hypopigmented macules with irregular borders

   Explanation: Vitiligo lesions are typically hypopigmented macules with irregular borders. They may occur on sun-exposed areas like the face, hands, elbows, and knees.

4. Answer: B) Autoimmune inflammation affecting nerves

   Explanation: Vitiligo can be associated with autoimmune inflammation affecting nerves (vitiligo-associated neural symptoms), leading to tingling sensation and pain in affected areas.

5. Answer: A) Wood's lamp examination

   Explanation: Wood's lamp examination is useful in confirming the diagnosis of vitiligo, as depigmented patches appear vividly under the ultraviolet light.

6. Answer: A) Initiate topical corticosteroid therapy

   Explanation: Topical corticosteroids are a first-line treatment for vitiligo, especially in patients with new patches or active disease.

7. Answer: B) Immune-mediated destruction of melanocytes

   Explanation: Vitiligo is often associated with autoimmune diseases such as Hashimoto's thyroiditis and type 1 diabetes mellitus, suggesting a common autoimmune pathogenesis.

8. Answer: D) Monitor without intervention

   Explanation: Stable vitiligo patches may not require active treatment. Observation and reassurance are often appropriate in these cases.

9. Answer: B) Refer for phototherapy

   Explanation: Phototherapy with narrow-band UVB is effective in treating vitiligo that is resistant to topical treatments like corticosteroids.

10. Answer: B) Psychological stress

    Explanation: Psychological stress is a known trigger for the development or exacerbation of vitiligo lesions due to its effects on immune function.

11. Answer: B) Phototherapy with narrow-band UVB

    Explanation: Phototherapy with narrow-band UVB is an effective treatment for vitiligo, especially in patients with widespread disease.

12. Answer: C) Segmental or localized

    Explanation: Vitiligo can have different patterns of distribution. Segmental or localized vitiligo often occurs unilaterally and follows a dermatomal or segmental distribution.

13. Answer: B) Recommend camouflage makeup

    Explanation: Camouflage makeup can help improve the cosmetic appearance of vitiligo patches, providing a non-invasive option for managing patient concerns.

14. Answer: B) Autoimmune inflammation affecting nerves

    Explanation: Vitiligo can be associated with autoimmune inflammation affecting nerves (vitiligo-associated neural symptoms), leading to tingling sensation and pain in affected areas.

15. Answer: D) Monitor without intervention

    Explanation: Stable vitiligo patches may not require active treatment. Observation and reassurance are often appropriate in these cases.

www.ingramcontent.com/pod-product-compliance
Lightning Source LLC
Chambersburg PA
CBHW062346220526
45472CB00008B/1720